Improving Patient Treatment Adherence

T0234364

Hayden Bosworth
Editor

Improving Patient Treatment Adherence

A Clinician's Guide

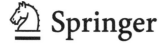 Springer

Editor
Hayden Bosworth
Duke University Medical Center
Erwin Road 2424
Suite 1105
27705 Durham, NC
USA
hayden.bosworth@duke.edu

ISBN 978-1-4419-5865-5   e-ISBN 978-1-4419-5866-2
DOI 10.1007/978-1-4419-5866-2
Springer New York Dordrecht Heidelberg London

Library of Congress Control Number: 2010926922

Printed on acid-free paper

Springer is part of Springer Science+Business Media (www.springer.com)

Contents

Contributors

Kelli Allen, PhD Associate Research Professor, General Internal Medicine; Research Health Scientist, Durham Veterans Affairs Medical Center, Duke University, Durham, NC, USA, domin004@mc.duke.edu

Lori A. Bastian, MD, MPH Center for Health Services Research in Primary Care, Durham Veterans Affairs Medical Center; Cancer Prevention, Detection and Control Research Program, Duke Comprehensive Cancer Center, Duke University Medical Center; Department of Medicine, Duke University Medical Center, Durham, NC, USA, basti001@mc.duke.edu

Hayden B. Bosworth, PhD Associate Director, Center for Health Services Research in Primary Care, Durham Veterans Affairs Medical Center; Research Professor, Departments of Medicine, Psychiatry and Behavioral Sciences, School of Nursing, Duke University Medical Center, Durham, NC, USA, hayden.bosworth@duke.edu

Patrick S. Calhoun, PhD Assistant Professor, Medical Psychology, Duke University Medical Center, Durham, NC, USA, patrick.calhoun2@va.gov

Jeanette R. Chin, MD Center for Health Services Research in Primary Care, Durham Veterans Affairs Medical Center, Duke University, Durham, NC, USA, jeanette.chin@duke.edu

A. Meade Eggleston, PhD Psychology Fellow, Veterans Affairs Mid-Atlantic Mental Illness, Research, and Clinical Center; Durham Veterans Affairs Medical Center, Durham, NC, USA, a.meade.eggleston@gmail.com

Laura J. Fish, PhD Cancer Prevention, Detection and Control
Research Program, Duke Comprehensive Cancer Center; Department
of Community and Family Medicine, Duke University Medical
Center, Durham, NC, USA, laura.fish@duke.edu

Serina E. Floyd, MD, MPH Assistant Professor, Department of
Obstetrics and Gynecology, Duke University Medical Center,
Durham, NC, USA, floyd013@mc.duke.edu

Jennifer M. Gierisch, PhD, MPH Postdoctoral Scholar, General
Internal Medicine, Duke University Medical Center, Durham, NC,
USA, j.gierisch@duke.edu

Karen Moore Goldstein, MD, MSPH Staff Physician, The
Jonathan Lax Treatment Center; Clinical Assistant Professor,
Department of General Internal Medicine, University of
Pennsylvania, Philadelphia, PA, USA,
karen.goldstein@uphs.upenn.edu

Vito S. Guerra Postdoctoral Scholar, Psychology, Durham Veterans
Affairs Medical Center, Durham, NC, USA, vito.guerra@va.gov

S. Nicole Hastings, MD, MHS Assistant Professor, Geriatrics, Duke
University Medical Center, Durham, NC, USA,
hasti003@mc.duke.edu

Mike Hill, MSW Center for Health Services Research in Primary
Care, Durham Veterans Affairs Medical Center, Durham, NC, USA,
michael.hill1b9a@va.gov

Francis J. Keefe, PhD Professor, Medical Psychology, Duke
University Medical Center, Durham, NC, USA,
keefe003@mc.duke.edu

Alex R. Kemper, MD, MPH, MS Division of Children's Primary
Care, Department of Pediatrics, Duke University Medical Center,
Durham, NC, USA, kempe006@mc.duke.edu

Janine C. Kosmoski, Pharm.D Christiana Health Care System,
Newark, DE, USA, janine.kosmoski@va.gov

Elizabeth Landolfo, MD Assistant Professor, Division of Primary
Care, Department of Pediatrics, Duke University Medical Center,
Durham, NC, USA, lando002@mc.duke.edu

Brigid Lynn, MPH Center for Health Services Research in Primary Care, Durham Veterans Affairs Medical Center, Durham, NC, USA, brigid.lynn@va.gov

Christine E. Marx Associate Professor, Biological Psychiatry, Duke University Medical Center, Durham, NC, USA, christine.marx@va.gov

Miriam Morey, PhD Associate Professor, Division of Geriatrics, Duke University Medical Center, Durham, NC, USA, morey002@mc.duke.edu

Jason M. Moss, PharmD Geriatric Pharmacy Fellow, Department of Clinical Research, Campbell University College of Pharmacy and Health Sciences; Durham Veterans Affairs Geriatrics Research Education and Clinical Center, Durham, NC, USA, jason.moss@va.gov

Lesley Rohrer, MPH Center for Health Services Research in Primary Care, Durham Veterans Affairs Medical Center, Durham, NC, USA, lesley.rohrer@va.gov

Carol D. Saur Clinical Nurse Specialist, Department of Medicine, Duke University Medical Center, Durham, NC, USA, carol.saur@duke.edu

Rebecca A. Shelby Assistant Professor, Medical Psychology, Duke University Medical Center, Durham, NC, USA, shelb003@mc.duke.edu

David C. Steffens Head, Geriatric Psychiatry; Professor, Departments of Psychiatry and Medicine, Duke University Medical Center, Durham, NC, USA, david.steffens@duke.edu

Jennifer L. Strauss Assistant Professor, Department of Psychiatry and Behavioral Sciences, Duke University Medical Center; Investigator, Mid-Atlantic Research Educational and Clinical Center Health Scientist, Durham VAMC Center for Health Services Research in Primary Care, Durham, NC, USA, jennifer.strauss@duke.edu

Geeta K. Swamy, MD Assistant Professor, Department of Obstetrics and Gynecology, Duke University Medical Center, Durham, NC, USA, swamy002@mc.duke.edu

Corrine I. Voils, PhD Associate Professor, General Internal Medicine, Duke University Medical Center, Durham, NC, USA, corrine.voils@duke.edu

Emmanuel B. Walter, MD, MPH Professor, Division of Children's Primary Care, Department of Pediatrics, Duke University Medical Center, Durham, NC, USA, walte002@mc.duke.edu

William S. Yancy, Jr., MD, MHS Associate Professor, General Internal Medicine, Duke University Medical Center, Durham, NC, USA, yancy006@mc.duke.edu

Chapter 1
Introduction

Hayden B. Bosworth

While the United States national debate on health care is getting a lot of publicity, there has been limited focus on treatment adherence and prevention. In fact, less than 3% of the United States massive health budget goes toward population-based prevention and more than 90% is spent on treating diseases and their complications – many of which are easily preventable [1, 2]. The remaining health-care resources are directed toward financing and delivery of medical care, with substantially less emphasis on other determinants of health, such as behavioral choices, social circumstances, and environmental conditions [3].

The lack of focus on treatment adherence is a shame given the clear relationships between health behaviors and outcomes. Despite advances in health care, all too often the benefits of these treatments are not fully realized because of patient nonadherence. Almost all medical and behavioral health treatments require at least some degree of adherence to treatment (e.g., coming to appointments, picking up medications, agreeing to have procedures performed, use of contraception, obtaining immunizations, attending follow-up appointments), and many treatments require significant behavior change (e.g., following long-term demanding and complex medication regimens, improving

---

H.B. Bosworth (✉)
Center for Health Services Research in Primary Care, Durham Veterans Affairs Medical Center; Departments of Medicine, Psychiatry and Behavioral Sciences, School of Nursing, Duke University Medical Center, Durham, NC, USA
e-mail: hayden.bosworth@duke.edu

H. Bosworth (ed.), *Improving Patient Treatment Adherence*,
DOI 10.1007/978-1-4419-5866-2_1,
© Springer Science+Business Media, LLC 2010

1

diet and physical activity, reducing alcohol consumption, and cigarette smoking). Adherence has been defined as the extent to which a person's behavior – taking medication, following a diet, and/or executing lifestyle changes – corresponds with agreed recommendations from a health-care provider.

Unfortunately as reviewed in this book, few patients fail to make these behavior changes. When the major multiple health-protective behaviors are studied, few individuals meet the criteria for a healthy lifestyle. About one-third of adults adhere with most – six or more out of nine recommendations which include two to four servings of fruit per day, three to five servings of vegetables per day, less than 2,400 mg of sodium per day, less than 10% of kilocalories from saturated fat per day, at least 150 min of physical activity per week, not smoke, moderate alcohol use, blood cholesterol checked in the last 5 years, and blood pressure checked in past 2 years [4]. In the United States, only 3% of adults meet all four health behavior goals of being a nonsmoker, having a healthy weight, being physically active, and eating five or more fruits and vegetables a day [5].

Despite the low levels of adherence to recommended health behaviors, there is growing evidence of the impact of adherence to health behaviors. The major causes of morbidity and premature mortality in the United States – heart disease, cancer, and stroke – are influenced by multiple health risk behaviors, including smoking, alcohol abuse, physical inactivity, and poor diet. The 52-nation INTERHEART study identified tobacco use, obesity, lipids, and psychosocial factors as accounting for about 90% of the population-attributable risks for myocardial infarction [6, 7]. In a recent study of 77,782 middle-aged United States women, never smoking, engaging in regular physical activity, eating a healthy diet, and avoiding becoming overweight were each associated with a markedly lower mortality during 24 years of follow-up. It was estimated that 55% of all cause mortality, 44% cancer mortality, and 72% of cardiovascular mortality during the follow-up could have been avoided by adherence to these four lifestyle guidelines [8]. Mental illness, as well as stress and distress more broadly, also places a significant burden on health and productivity in the United States and globally [9].

Rates of nonadherence to treatment generally range from 20 to 40% for acute illness regimens, 20 to 60% for chronic illness regimens, and 50 to 80% preventive regimens [10]. Nonadherence to treatment has been found to be high in psychotherapy and behavior therapy, with premature treatment dropout rates ranging from 30 to 60% [11]. Adherence to treatment by children and adolescents ranges from 43 to 100%, with an average of 58% in developed countries [12]. Several studies have suggested that adolescents are less adherent than younger children [13].

While there is increasing evidence documenting the problems and impact of nonadherence to treatment, other factors to consider and make the focus of treatment adherence all that more important are that improving treatment adherence also enhances patients' safety. Because most of the care needed for chronic conditions is based on patient self-management (usually requiring complex multi-therapies), use of medical technology for monitoring, and changes in the patient's lifestyle, patients face several potentially life-threatening risks if not appropriately supported by the health system.

Increasing the effectiveness of adherence interventions may have a far greater impact on the health of the population than any improvement in specific medical treatments. Increasingly studies find significant cost savings and increases in the effectiveness of health interventions that are attributable to low-cost intervention for improving treatment adherence. Without a system that addresses the determinants of treatment adherence, advances in biomedical technology will fail to realize their potential to reduce the burden of chronic illness.

Given that patient nonadherence is such a significant barrier to effective and efficient health-care delivery, better recognition, understanding, and methods for reducing the impact of this problem are crucial steps toward promoting patient care, outcomes, and treatment costs.

Defining Treatment Adherence

To define treatment adherence, multiple terms have been used including compliance, co-operation, concordance, mutuality, and therapeutic alliance, and operational definitions of these terms vary widely across studies [14]. Most definitions contain elements relating to patients' self-care responsibilities, their role in the treatment process, and their collaboration with health-care providers. In recent years, patients have been encouraged to participate more actively in decision making regarding their health care. The terms "adherence" and "concordance" have been more preferred lately [15]. The term adherence will be used throughout this book and connotes the patient's participation and engagement in maintaining a regimen she/he believes will be beneficial, strongly implying a therapeutic partnership with providers that is essential to the individuals' success in following the prescribed treatment regimen. Similar to the World Health Organization recommendation, it is also recognized that adherence to a regimen may reflect behaviors ranging from seeking medical attention, filling prescriptions, obtaining immunizations, and executing behavioral modifications that address self-management of disease, smoking, contraception, unhealthy diet, and insufficient levels of physical activity.

Clinical Measurement of Medical Regimen Adherence

Accurate assessment of adherence behavior is necessary for effective and efficient treatment planning. However, the challenge lies in that there is often no "gold standard" for measuring adherence behavior [16, 17] and often the use of a variety of strategies has been recommended in the literature. Relying on providers' rating of the degree to which their patients follow their recommendations often results in overestimated adherence [18, 19]. Similarly, relying on patients' subjective reports may be problematic as well. Patients who reveal that they have not followed treatment advice tend to describe their behavior accurately, whereas patients who deny their failure or are not aware of that they are not following recommendations report their behavior inaccurately [17].

In summary, measurement of treatment adherence provides useful information that outcome monitoring alone cannot provide, but it remains only an estimate of a patient's actual behavior. The goals of the provider, the accuracy requirements associated with the regimen, the available resources, the response burden on the patient, and how the results will be used should all be taken. No single measurement strategy has been deemed optimal. A multi-method approach that combines feasible self-reporting and reasonable objective measures supported by effective patient–provider communication is likely to be the best method for identifying problems with treatment adherence.

Take Home Messages of the Book

There continues to be a tendency to focus on patient-related factors as the causes of problems with adherence with limited consideration of provider and health system-related contributing factors. Oftentimes, treatment adherence for a particular behavior is influenced by several factors – whether these factors are social and economic factors, the health-care team/system, the characteristics of the disease or health issue, therapies, and patient-related factors. In addition, individuals need to contend with adherence to multiple health recommendations and each behavior/health condition is likely to have a separate source of barriers to adherence. Similarly, whether the problem is acute/chronic or the behavior involves initiating or maintaining, there are likely to be different factors that influence treatment adherence. Additional recommendations readers will find in the book include

1. Patient-centered tailored interventions are likely required to improve treatment adherence given that there is no single intervention strategy that has been shown to be effective across all patients, conditions, and settings. Although teaching patients about their treatment regimen and disease/condition is important, additional focus on behavioral strategies to increase treatment adherence is needed. Patient education should involve less verbal instruction, and individuals should be provided clear succinct written instructions that they can refer to at home.
2. Adherence is a dynamic process that needs to be followed up. For many behaviors there are typically at least four phases to treatment adherence, contemplating, initiating, maintaining, and sustaining long-term behavior – phases that all have potentially different barriers and facilitators. For example, in Chapter 3, Drs. Yancy and Voils discuss differences in initiating diet interventions and maintaining them. The lack of a match between patient's stage and the practitioner's attempts at intervention means that treatments are frequently prescribed to patients who are not ready to follow them.
3. Incorporating family, community, and organizations is a likely key factor for success in improving adherence. Social support consisting of informal or formal support received by patients from other members of their community has been consistently reported as an

important factor affecting treatment adherence. There is growing evidence that support among patients can improve adherence to therapy while reducing the amount of time devoted by the health professionals to the care of chronic conditions.

4. There is a need for health professionals to be trained in identifying and alleviating treatment adherence. As recognized by the World Health Organization, health providers can have a significant impact on treatment adherence by assessing risk of nonadherence and delivering interventions to optimize adherence. Beyond training practitioners, the systems in which they work must design and support delivery systems that support this objective. Training will likely need to address three topics: knowledge (information on adherence) including the factors that have been reported to influence adherence and effective interventions available; clinically useful ways of using this information which includes ways to assess adherence and how priorities should be ranked and best available intervention chosen, when and how should patient progress be followed up and assessed; and behavioral tools for health professionals for creating and maintaining habits – this component should be taught using "role-play" and other educational strategies to ensure that health professionals incorporate behavioral tools for enhancing adherence into their daily practice (WHO).

Conclusions

Clinicians are all challenged by identifying and addressing treatment nonadherence among their patients. Poor treatment adherence accounts for substantial worsening of disease, death, and increased health-care costs in the United States. Adherence to treatments with proven efficacy is a primary determinant of the effectiveness of treatment. Adherence clearly and directly optimizes clinical benefit and health-related quality of life of patients with disease (secondary and tertiary prevention), as well as prevents onset of disease (primary prevention). In addition, higher rates of adherence confer direct economic benefits by, for example, reducing costs associated with acute exacerbations of disease (e.g., hospitalizations, emergency department visits, expensive treatments). Indirect savings may result by enhancing patients' quality of life and decreasing work days lost to illness. When adherence programs are combined with regular treatment and disease-specific education, significant improvements in health-promoting behaviors, symptom management, communication, and disability management have been observed. Despite these benefits, adherence is often far from optimal; this is especially true for lifestyle behaviors where, for example, poor diet and lack of exercise contribute to the growing obesity epidemic.

While increasing work has focused on examining treatment adherence, there remains a lack of a summary of proven methods for identifying and addressing patient nonadherence. Thus, this book provides (a) a summary of the impact of treatment nonadherence (e.g., costs, clinical outcomes, health-related quality of life); (b) a review of patient factors related to treatment adherence for specific behaviors (i.e., diet, exercise, medication use), as well as across diseases and special populations (e.g., children); and (c) proven methods for improving treatment adherence.

References

1. Satcher D, Higginbotham EJ. The public health approach to eliminating disparities in health. *Am J Public Health*. 2008;98(9 Suppl):S8–S11.
2. Woolf SH. A closer look at the economic argument for disease prevention. *JAMA*. 20094;301(5):536–538.
3. Schroeder SA. Shattuck lecture. We can do better – improving the health of the American people. *N Engl J Med*. 2007;357(12):1221–1228.
4. Wright JD, Hirsch R, Wang C-Y. *One-third of U.S. adults embraced heart health behaviors in 1999–2002*. NCHS data brief, no. 17. Hyattsville, MD: National Center for Health Statistics; 2009.
5. Reeves MJ, Rafferty AP. Healthy lifestyle characteristics among adults in the United States, 2000. *Arch Intern Med*. 2005;165(8):854–857.
6. Lanas F, Avezum A, Bautista LE, Diaz R, Luna M, Islam S, et al. Risk factors for acute myocardial infarction in Latin America: the INTERHEART Latin American study. *Circulation*. 2007;115(9):1067–1074.
7. Yusuf S, Hawken S, Ounpuu S, Dans T, Avezum A, Lanas F, et al. Effect of potentially modifiable risk factors associated with myocardial infarction in 52 countries (the INTERHEART study): case-control study. *Lancet*. 2004;364(9438):937–952.
8. van Dam RM, Li T, Spiegelman D, Franco OH, Hu FB. Combined impact of lifestyle factors on mortality: prospective cohort study in US women. *BMJ*. 2008;337:a1440.

9. United States Department of Health and Human Services (USDHHS). *1999 USDHHS, mental health: A report of the surgeon general*. Washington, DC: Department of Health and Human Services; 1999.

10. Christensen AJ. *Patience adherence to medical treatment regimens: Bridging the gap between behavioral science and biomedicine*. New Haven, CT: Yale University Press; 2004.

11. Wierzbicki M, Pekarik, G. A meta-analysis of psychotherapy dropout. Prof *Psychol Res Pract*. 1993;24:190–195.

12. Burkhart P, Dunbar-Jacob J. Adherence research in the pediatric and adolescent populations: a decade in review. In: Hayman LMM, Turner R, ed. *Chronic illness in children: An evidence-based approach*. New York, NY: Springer; 2002:199–229.

13. Fotheringham MJ, Sawyer MG. Adherence to recommended medical regimens in childhood and adolescence. *J Paediatr Child Health*. 1995;31(2): 72–78.

14. Farmer KC. Methods for measuring and monitoring medication regimen adherence in clinical trials and clinical practice. *Clin Ther*. 1999;21(6):1074–1090; discussion 3.

15. Mullen PD. Compliance becomes concordance. BMJ. 1997;314(7082): 691–692.

16. Farmer K. Methods for measuring and monitoring medication regimens adherence in clinical trials and clinical practice. *Clin Ther*. 1999;21:1074–1090.

17. Bosworth H. Medication adherence. In: Bosworth HB, Oddone EZ, Weinberger M, eds. *Patient treatment adherence: Concepts, interventions, and measurement*. Mahwah, NJ: Lawrence Erlbaum Associates; 2006.

18. DiMatteo M, DiNicola, DD. *Achieving patient compliance*. Elmsford, NY: Pergamon Press; 1982.

19. Norell SE. Accuracy of patient interviews and estimates by clinical staff in determining medication compliance. *Soc Sci Med E*. 1981;15(1):57–61.

Chapter 2
Physical Activity and Adherence

Kelli Allen and Miriam C. Morey

Adherence to Physical Activity

There is abundant evidence supporting the health benefits of physical activity, including reduced risk for cardiovascular disease, stroke, some cancers, type 2 diabetes, osteoporosis, hypertension, high cholesterol, obesity, osteoarthritis, and all-cause mortality [1]. Physical activity is also associated with improved psychological health and functional status, as well as reduced health-care expenditures [2]. It has been estimated that the direct costs of physical inactivity account for approximately $24 billion, or 2.4% of US health-care expenditures [1, 2]. Furthermore, about 12% of all deaths in the USA can be attributed to physical inactivity [3].

This chapter provides a synopsis of research related to physical activity adherence, with a primary focus on adults. We discuss recommendations for physical activity, the problem of non-adherence to physical activity recommendations and factors associated with non-adherence, screening for non-adherence, and interventions to increase

K. Allen (✉)
General Internal Medicine; Durham Veterans Affairs Medical Center, Duke University, Durham, NC, USA
e-mail: domin004@mc.duke.edu

H. Bosworth (ed.), *Improving Patient Treatment Adherence*,
DOI 10.1007/978-1-4419-5866-2_2,
© Springer Science+Business Media, LLC 2010

physical activity. Finally, we will discuss clinical and policy implications of physical activity adherence research.

Physical Activity Guidelines and Recommendations

There has been substantial debate and study regarding the amount of physical activity required for achieving health and fitness benefits. Guidelines from Healthy People 2010 (HP2010), the American College of Sports Medicine (ACSM), the American Heart Association (AHA), and the US Department of Health and Human Services (DHHS) advise the following [4–6] (Boxes 2.1 and 2.2):

Box 2.1 Physical Activity Recommendations for Adults Under Age 65

* Do at least 30 or up to 60 (for greater benefit) min per day of moderate intensity aerobic activity, in bouts of at least 10 min each, to total 150–300 min per week

OR

* Do at least 20–30 min per day or more of vigorous intensity aerobic activity to total 75–150 min per week

OR

* Do an equivalent combination of moderate and vigorous activity

AND

* Do 8–10 strength training exercises, 8–12 repetitions of each, twice a week

Box 2.2 Physical Activity Recommendations for Adults Age 65 and Older

* Follow the same guidelines for aerobic activity as those for adults under age 65

AND

* 8–10 strength training exercises, 10–15 repetitions each, 2–3 times per week

AND

* Do balance exercises, if at risk for falling

* When older adults cannot do these recommended amounts of physical activity because of chronic conditions they should be as physically active as their abilities and conditions allow.

The guidelines emphasize that all adults should avoid inactivity. Some activity is better than none. The guidelines also emphasize that additional health benefits can be gained by performing physical activity in amounts greater than the minimum recommendations. It should also be noted that physical activity performed in the context of regular occupational, household, and leisure activities can produce benefits similar to those of structured exercise, as long as the frequency, intensity, and duration are sufficient [7].

The Problem of Non-adherence to Physical Activity Recommendations

Estimates of the proportion of adults who do not meet physical activity recommendations vary slightly according to the specific set of guidelines being considered (HP2010, ACSM/AHA, and DHHS). The Centers for Disease Control and Prevention (CDC) analyzed physical activity data from the 2007 Behavioral Risk Factor Surveillance System, which is a nationally representative sample of adults ≥ 18 years. These data showed that when considering the HP2010 guidelines, 48.8% of adults met physical activity recommendations compared with 64.5% who met recommendations according to the 2008 DHHS guidelines. Nevertheless, these and other data show that a large proportion of adults do not meet physical activity recommendations, and this is a significant public health problem [8]. These data also likely underestimate the problem of non-adherence, as adults tend to overreport physical activity levels in comparison to objective measures [9, 10].

Long-term adherence to physical activity is essential for the maintenance of health benefits. For example, Morey et al. reported that among older adults enrolled in a physical activity program for over 10 years, participants classified as adherent had a long-term survival benefit by time compared to a non-adherent group [11]. Other research showed that individuals who are more adherent to regular exercise programs, compared to those who are less adherent, experience greater improvements in fitness, physical function, quality of life, and disease-specific outcomes [12]. However, studies suggest that about 50% of adults who start a physical activity program will drop out within a few months [13].

Risk Factors for Non-adherence to Physical Activity Recommendations

There have been several comprehensive reviews of the correlates and predictors of physical activity, covering over 380 studies [14–17]. This section describes prior research on key correlates of physical activity, focusing on seven categories of factors: demographic, health-related and biological, cognitive and psychological, behavioral, social, program-related, and environmental. Table 2.1 also provides a comprehensive summary of factors associated with physical inactivity.

Table 2.1 Factors associated with physical inactivity

Demographic factors
  Older age
  Female gender
  Non-white race/ethnicity
  Low socioeconomic status

Health-related and clinical factors
  Chronic illnesses
  Poor general health and physical function
  Overweight/obesity

Cognitive and psychological factors
  Greater perceived barriers to physical activity
  Lack of enjoyment of physical activity
  Low expectations of benefits from physical activity
  Poor psychological health
  Low self-efficacy for physical activity
  Low self-motivation for physical activity
  Lack of readiness to change physical activity behaviors
  Poor fitness level

Behavioral factors
  Prior physical activity
  Smoking
  Type A behavior[a]

Social factors
  Lack of cohesion in exercise group
  Lack of physician influence/advice for physical activity
  Lack of social support for physical activity

Program-related factors
  High physical activity intensity
  Long physical activity duration

Environmental factors
  Lack of access to facilities/parks/trails
  Lack of neighborhood safety

---

[a]Type A behavior associated with poorer adherence in supervised exercise programs but greater overall physical activity levels

Demographic Factors

The demographic factors most strongly associated with physical activity levels in prior research include the following:

Age

While the benefits and safety of physical activity for older adults have been well established, increasing age is still one of the most consistent predictors of decreased physical activity [8, 9, 14, 18, 19]. About 60% of older adults in the USA do not meet physical activity recommendations [18, 20]. Some data suggest that physical activity levels increase slightly around the typical age of retirement (60–65), but then decline shortly afterward [21]. Studies have also shown that there is a greater age-related decline in physical activity among older women in comparison to older men [22].

Not surprisingly, poor health status is one of the most important and consistent correlates of physical inactivity among older adults [23]. Some specific health-related variables associated with reduced activity among older adults include poor perceptions of overall health, presence of chronic diseases, depressive symptoms, injuries, activity and mobility limitations, pain, and fear of pain [16, 24]. There are several other factors that seem to be particularly salient with respect to older adults' physical activity levels. First, some research suggests that social support for physical activity decreases substantially with age [25], and this may negatively affect activity among older adults. Second, older adults may be more likely than younger individuals to report lack of skill as a barrier to physical activity [26]. Third, misconceptions about physically activity are problematic among older adults. Specifically, older adults may be deterred from physical activity because of beliefs that activity must be vigorous or uncomfortable to produce benefits [27]. Fourth, physicians are less likely to ask older adults about physical activity and less likely to counsel their patients to become more physically active [28]. The US Preventive Task Force's conclusion that there was insufficient evidence that physical activity counseling by primary care providers was effective may have hindered incorporation of physical activity counseling into primary care [29]. However, more recent studies in primary care settings have reported significant improvements in physical activity among elders, and physician advice appears to play a key role in older adults' physical activity [30, 31].

Gender

Gender has also been a consistent predictor of physical activity, with men showing greater levels of activity than women [9, 14, 15, 18, 19]. While many barriers to physical activity are similarly influential among both women and men, there are some factors that are particularly relevant to women. First, previous physical activity guidelines emphasized fairly vigorous activity, which may have discouraged participation among women. Research has shown that only about 5% of women adopt vigorous activities (such as running) annually, but about 34% adopt moderate activities (such as walking) [32]. Newer physical activity guidelines focus more on moderate level activities, and this change may have a positive influence on women's activity levels as these recommendations continue to be conveyed. Second, women may experience a social environment that is not as supportive or conducive to activity as men. Women's frequent multiple roles, involving both work and family responsibilities, may be a particularly significant barrier to regular physical activity. For example, data show that women with young children at home are less active than women without young children [33].

Race and Ethnicity

Racial and ethnic minorities suffer disproportionately from chronic illnesses that are associated with physical inactivity, and elimination of these health disparities is a national health priority [34]. Yet there are still considerable racial and ethnic differences in physical activity levels [35]. Blacks, Hispanics, Asian and Pacific Islanders, and American Indians/Alaska Natives all report lower levels of physical activity compared to non-Hispanic Whites [19, 34]. Data from the CDC's Behavioral Risk Factor Surveillance System show that when considering the 2008 DHHS guidelines, 68% of non-Hispanic Whites meet physical activity recommendations compared with only 57% of non-Hispanic Black and Hispanic participants [18].

While racial/ethnic differences in physical activity may partly be mediated by socioeconomic status (SES) [15], some studies have controlled for income, work status, or education in statistical models and still observed racial differences in physical activity level [36, 37]. Barriers and facilitators of physical activity have not been as well examined among racial and ethnic minority groups as among non-Hispanic Whites. However, these data are emerging, and in particular, there is a growing literature on physical activity among racial and ethnic minority women [38–43]. These studies indicate that among racial and ethnic minority women, family disapproval, family needs, and child care are particularly important barriers to physical activity [42, 43]. Research also shows that among racial and ethnic minorities in general, two key strategies for increasing physical activity may be enhancing social support for physical activity and augmenting access to places for physical activities [44].

Socioeconomic Status

Overall, SES has been a fairly consistent correlate of physical activity [14, 19]. "Blue collar" occupational status (typically manual and industrial labor), low income, and lower education level have all been associated with less physical activity (especially leisure time physical activity) in some studies [14]. Women with low SES and low-skilled occupations are at particular risk for being physically inactive [45].

There are several likely reasons that physical activity levels are lower among individuals with low SES. First, these individuals are more likely to live in communities that have fewer parks or recreational facilities, are more likely to lack financial resources to purchase home exercise equipment, may lack social support or encouragement to lead a physically active lifestyle, and may also lack understanding about the health benefits of activity [46]. Second, some research suggests that individuals with lower income levels receive less advice from their physicians about preventive health behaviors such as physical activity [47]. Third, low SES is associated with poor adherence during and following clinical exercise programs such as cardiac rehabilitation [48], and this may be related to financial constraints, health-care coverage, and lack of work flexibility.

Health-Related and Clinical Factors

Individuals with chronic diseases and overall poorer levels of health and physical function are less likely to be physically active [49]. For individuals with some chronic health conditions, involvement in a formal, structured exercise program can facilitate physical activity adherence. Alternatively, the use of group-mediated cognitive-behavioral therapy has been successful at integrating physical activity into daily life rather than delivered as an independent center-based activity among adults with chronic conditions [50].

Overweight/obesity is also strongly associated with lower activity levels [14, 18]. For example, Brownson et al. found that among a national sample of women in the USA, those who were overweight were significantly less likely to report being regularly active and more likely to report having no leisure time physical activity compared to women who were not overweight [51].

Cognitive and Psychological Factors

A wide array of cognitive and psychological variables have been examined as potential correlates of physical activity adherence (see Table 2.1) [14, 15, 17]. Among these variables, studies have shown that the following are most consistently associated with greater physical activity levels: fewer perceived barriers, greater enjoyment of physical activity, greater expected benefits, better psychological health, greater self-efficacy for physical activity, greater self-motivation for physical activity, greater readiness to change, and better perceived health or fitness [14, 17].

Self-efficacy for physical activity, defined as an individual's confidence in his or her ability to be physically active on a regular basis, has been one of the strongest and most consistent cognitive correlates of activity level [14, 15, 17]. Self-efficacy is related to both adoption and maintenance of physical activity [32]. It has been correlated with physical activity in a variety of settings, including large population-based community samples, exercise groups for healthy individuals, and clinical exercise programs [14]. Self-efficacy has also been shown to predict future physical activity levels in longitudinal studies [17]. Furthermore, self-efficacy may be enhanced through training and feedback [52] and therefore could be a particularly important target for interventions.

Perceived barriers also correlate strongly with physical activity [14, 15, 17]. The most commonly reported barrier to physical activity among US samples is lack of time [15]. Some other common barriers include lack of facilities, bad weather, safety, lack of exercise partner, fatigue or lack of energy, poor health, and self-consciousness about appearance [14]. Perceived barriers may incorporate both subjective and objective components. Objective barriers, such as lack of exercise facilities, may be modified by policy interventions, and subjective barriers may be modified through cognitive interventions that refute beliefs that hinder activity.

Behavioral Factors

Behavioral factors that have been associated with current physical activity level include prior physical activity history, smoking, and Type A behavior. Of these, prior activity history has shown the most consistent association with current activity level [14, 17]. While not all studies have shown a significant association between smoking and physical activity, most have found an inverse relationship [14]. Type A behavior has been defined as a behavioral syndrome or style of living characterized by competitiveness, feelings of being under the pressures of time, striving for achievement, and aggressiveness [53]. Studies have indicated that Type A behavior is associated with greater overall levels of physical activity but lower adherence within supervised exercise programs [15, 17]. These results have implications for interventions, suggesting that individuals with greater Type A behavior may be better suited to individual or home-based physical activity programs.

Social Factors

Social factors that have been studied as correlates of physical activity include exercise group cohesion, physician influence, and social support. Group cohesion has shown a modest positive correlation with adherence in some studies [17]. However, physician influence and social support have been stronger and more consistent correlates of physical activity level and adherence [14, 17]. Physician advice to exercise has been reported as a correlate of physical activity among the general adult population [54]. Social support has been significantly associated with physical activity in cross-sectional and prospective studies, both in community samples and within organized exercise groups [14, 55]. While both family and friend support for physical activity appear to be influential [14, 17], the role of the spouse seems to be particularly important [55].

Program-Related Factors

In addition to person-level characteristics, specific aspects of the physical activity regimen or program can influence adherence. Adherence may be poorer for high-intensity physical activity versus lower intensity levels [56]. With respect to exercise duration, some evidence indicates that completing several shorter bouts of activity may result in greater adherence than one longer bout, while retaining some health benefits [57]. Shorter, intermittent exercise periods may be particularly beneficial for reducing rates of attrition at the beginning of an exercise program [58].

Studies have also compared group- or center-based programs versus home-based programs. Some studies have found that home-based exercise is associated with greater adherence and higher levels of activity [59, 60]. However, some research has shown an advantage of center-based programs [61], and this may vary according to individual needs and preferences. Within the context of group- or center-based programs, there are several factors that have been shown to enhance adherence, including convenient time and location, reasonable cost, variety of exercise modalities, flexibility in exercise goals, and quality of the exercise leader [62].

Environmental Factors

There is growing recognition that environmental factors have a tremendous influence on individuals' physical activity behavior [14]. Perhaps the most prominent theme to emerge in recent research involving environmental factors is that of convenient access. Studies show that simply having convenient access to parks, walking or biking trails, or other physical activity facilities is strongly associated with greater activity levels [63, 64]. Neighborhood safety is also another key factor, particularly among older adults, women, and individuals with lower education levels [64].

Screening for Non-adherence to Physical Activity Recommendations

There are numerous options for assessing physical activity. Most commonly, physical activity is measured via subjective self-report, using one of many available validated questionnaires [65]. While there is no single best questionnaire for assessing physical activity, some have been developed for specific patient groups (i.e., older adults), and this should be considered when selecting a measure. There are also objective measures of physical activity, including pedometers and accelerometers. While these objective measures may provide a more accurate assessment of activity level, use of this equipment may not be feasible in clinical settings and in some large-scale studies.

In clinical settings, a brief screening assessment for physical activity level is typically most appropriate. Many validated physical activity questionnaires, though useful in research settings, may be too time consuming to administer as part of a clinical screening process. However, brief assessments can be used to identify patients who are physically inactive [66, 67]. For example, Smith et al. found that the two-item assessment shown in Box 2.3 was feasible to use in a clinical setting and enabled physicians to ascertain the overall activity levels of patients [66]. These questions can be used to assess whether patients are meeting the guidelines for aerobic activity described in Boxes 2.1 and 2.2.

Box 2.3 Physical Activity Screening Assessment

1. How many times a week do you usually do 20 min or more of vigorous intensity activity that makes you sweat or puff and pant (e.g., heavy lifting, digging, jogging, aerobics, or fast bicycling)?

   ☐ 3 or more times a week   ☐ 1–2 times a week   ☐ None

2. How many times a week do you usually do 30 min or more of moderate intensity physical activity or walking that increases your heart rate or makes you breathe harder than normal (e.g., carrying light loads, bicycling, at a regular pace, or doubles tennis)?

□ 5 or more times per week   □ 3–4 times a week   □ 1–2 times a week   □ None

Source: Ref. [66]

Physical Activity Adherence Intervention Studies

There have been numerous studies designed to identify successful physical activity interventions. These studies have varied widely with respect to participant samples, settings, theoretical models, and intervention strategies. Physical activity interventions can be grouped into two main categories: public health/environmental/policy interventions and individual-based interventions (which also encompass small group classes). While this chapter focuses primarily on individual interventions that can be implemented in clinical settings, we first provide a brief overview of broad public health interventions.

Public Health, Environmental, and Policy Interventions

Because the problem of physical inactivity is pervasive, large-scale, population-based strategies to this problem are an important counterpart to intensive individualized and small group interventions. Public health, environmental, and policy strategies to enhance physical activity adherence can range from very simple, low-cost interventions to complex policies involving budget allocation and transportation restructuring [68]. In general, broad mass media educational approaches seem to have little influence on physical activity levels within communities [69]. However, other types of environmental and policy interventions have shown promising results [70, 71]. These interventions have included posting signs in public areas to encourage the use of stairways, adding bicycle trails, organizing activity clubs, and providing additional exercise facilities in the community. While community- and population-based strategies are clearly important for facilitating physical activity, the costs of implementation are often a significant barrier [72].

Individual Interventions

Systematic reviews have concluded that there is good evidence to support the overall efficacy of individual interventions to increase physical activity and improve fitness [73, 74]. The following are brief descriptions of specific intervention components that have been shown to enhance physical activity levels and/or adherence:

1. *Health Education* [52, 75] While health education alone is not sufficient to promote long-term changes in exercise adherence, this can be a foundational component of broader interventions. It is important to provide individuals with information about the benefits of exercise, proper exercise techniques, and normal physiological responses that can be expected during exercise.
2. *Health Risk Appraisal* [76] Health risk appraisals provide participants with information about various aspects of their current health, risk factors, and/or fitness level. Health risk appraisals are also not typically sufficient to engender long-term behavior change, but they can help to enhance motivation and be used to monitor changes over time.
3. *Goal Setting* [52, 75] This strategy has been used widely in behavior change studies and involves asking participants to identify and document personal goals related to their physical activity behavior. Individuals should be encouraged to set goals that are realistic, specific, and relatively short term. Individuals should also be asked to identify specific steps toward meeting their physical activity goals.
4. *Contracts* [77] This strategy involves asking participants to write out specific physical activity behaviors they agree to do. Participants also identify individuals who will be responsible for verifying they have fulfilled their contract.

5. *Self-Monitoring* [78, 79] Self-monitoring is a commonly used strategy that involves asking participants to document their physical activity behavior. Participants can be asked to turn in their self-monitoring records to group leaders or other participants, which helps to facilitate adherence.

6. *Reinforcement and Incentives* [78, 80] These strategies are often combined with self-monitoring and/or goal setting and involve provision of some type of reward when participants attain an activity-related goal.

7. *Problem Solving* [52, 75, 79, 80] Problem-solving interventions teach individuals to identify obstacles or barriers that hinder their physical activity, generate and implement solutions, evaluate the outcome, and choose other solutions if needed.

8. *Relapse Prevention* [52, 75, 76] Similar to problem solving, this intervention involves instructing participants to identify future situations that may lead to lapses in adherence. Participants are then taught to develop specific strategies to deal with these potential situations.

9. *Stimulus Control* [52, 77] This strategy is built on the principle that environmental cues exert an important influence on behavior. Stimulus control interventions involve teaching participants to structure their environment in ways that encourage physical activity.

10. *Cognitive Restructuring* [77] Maladaptive thoughts and beliefs can contribute to non-adherence. For example, individuals may believe that exercise must be vigorous or painful to produce any health benefit. Cognitive restructuring is a process of teaching individuals to recognize these thoughts and replace them with more positive self-statements that can help to promote regular physical activity.

11. *Enhancing Social Support* [52, 75, 77, 80] Social support for physical activity can be enhanced through a group program, friend or family involvement, or interactions with personal trainers or health professionals.

12. *Modeling* [77] Modeling involves providing examples of peers who are successfully engaging in physical activity. This can occur in a group program context or through videos or other media that include examples of peers engaging in physical activity.

13. *Motivational Interviewing* [81] Motivational interviewing is a technique for negotiating behavior changes with people who are reluctant or ambivalent about changing [82]. The goal of this method is to increase individuals' intrinsic motivation for physical activity, as well as self-efficacy for physical activity.

There is no clear "best" strategy for increasing individuals' physical activity levels. Because many interventions have incorporated more than one of the components described above, it is difficult to disentangle the effectiveness of specific elements. Rather, these intervention components can be considered a "toolbox" of strategies to incorporate into physical activity interventions. In addition, the following general principles are important for effective physical activity interventions:

- *Incorporate Multiple Components* Interventions involving multiple components (of those described above) are generally more successful than those employing a single strategy [52, 77].
- *Include Cognitive-Behavioral Strategies* Studies that include some type of cognitive-behavioral component, such as goal setting or self-monitoring, seem to be the most effective [74, 83, 84].
- *Sufficient Intensity* Brief interventions (such as a one-time advice or health risk appraisals) are generally not a sufficient stimulus to promote behavior change [85]. However, provision of professional guidance about starting an exercise program, supplemented by some type of ongoing support, can be an effective strategy for increasing physical activity [74].
- *Use a Tailored Approach* Tailoring interventions to individual needs and preferences may result in better outcomes and improved adherence [86, 87].
- *Lifestyle Approach* Several studies have now shown that interventions designed to enhance lifestyle physical activity (including all leisure, occupational, or household activities) produce health and fitness benefits similar to those of structured exercise [7, 88, 89]. Furthermore, research suggests that lifestyle physical activity interventions are associated with greater adherence and activity levels than structured programs [90].

Settings for Delivery of Individual Interventions

There are many possible settings for delivering physical activity interventions, including community settings, worksites, and health-care settings. While there have been successful models of physical activity programs in each of these settings, and all are important, we focus here on interventions delivered in the health-care context. This is an attractive and important venue for delivering physical activity interventions for two main reasons. First, the majority of adults have contact with physicians on at least a yearly basis and average over three office visits per year [91]. Therefore, this method has the potential to reach a larger number of individuals than other in-person strategies. Second, clinicians' recommendations regarding health behaviors are generally valued and trusted by patients, and research shows that patients want to receive information about physical activity from their physicians [92]. However, studies show that physicians provide physical activity counseling infrequently and typically do not spend more then 3–5 min providing this type of counseling [93–95]. Lack of time, counseling training, organizational support, materials, and standardized protocols are barriers to provision of physical activity counseling by health-care providers [94].

Despite the challenges of delivering physical activity counseling in a health-care setting, reviews of prior research indicate that supplemental interventions in this context can be effective [29, 83, 85, 96]. Three examples of large trials that have shown the efficacy of health-care provider-based physical activity interventions include the Activity Counseling Trial [97], the Physical Activity for Life program [98], and the Patient-Centered Assessment and Counseling for Exercise (PACE) program [99]. The PACE program was designed to be incorporated into health-care settings with minimal involvement from medical staff. Briefly, PACE involves completion of a short questionnaire to assess readiness to begin a physical activity program, a 3–5 min physician-delivered physical counseling session based on the patient's stage of readiness to engage in physical activity, and a brief booster telephone call by a health educator approximately 2 weeks after the visit. PACE materials, including a Provider Manual, assessment forms, and three counseling protocols (for patients in different stages of readiness), are available for use (Project PACE, Centers for Disease Control and Prevention, Cardiovascular Health

Branch). These materials have also been modified for older adults (http://www.research.va.gov/resources/pubs/LIFE-modules.cfm).

Physical activity programs in the health-care settings should incorporate the general principles described above for effective interventions. Also, the US Preventive Services Task Force has adopted the following general approach to clinically based behavior programs (including physical activity) [100]:

- *Assess*: Ask about or assess behavioral health risk(s) and factors affecting a patient's choice of behavior change goals and methods. Physical activity behaviors should be assessed *routinely at each visit.*
- *Advise*: Give clear, specific, and personalized behavior change advice, including information about personal health harms and benefits.
- *Agree*: Collaboratively select appropriate treatment goals and methods based on the patient's interest in and willingness to change the behavior.
- *Assist*: Using behavior change techniques (self-help and/or counseling), aid the patient in achieving agreed-on goals by acquiring the skills, confidence, and social/environmental supports for behavior change, supplemented with adjunctive medical treatments when appropriate.
- *Arrange*: Schedule follow-up contacts (in person or by telephone) to provide ongoing assistance/support and to adjust the treatment plan as needed, including referral to more intensive or specialized treatment.

Historically, physical activity programs have been delivered face to face. However, there has been movement toward developing alternative modes of delivery, particularly telephone and Internet-based programs. Studies have shown that overall these approaches are effective in increasing physical activity levels [69, 101]. Some research has even suggested that adherence rates may even be higher in telephone or Internet-assisted, home-based interventions compared to programs involving face-to-face contact [59, 60]. Telephone or Internet-based follow-up should be considered as an approach to follow-up of brief in-person physical activity counseling in primary case settings, as well as other contexts.

Physical Activity Adherence Interventions in Special Populations

There are several demographic groups known to have lower levels of physical activity, including older adults, women, ethnic and racial minorities, and individuals with low SES. When considering physical activity interventions for these groups, the same general principles described above should be followed. In addition, the following key points should be considered:

Older Adults

- All older adults should avoid inactivity. Some physical activity is better than none, and older adults who participate in any amount of physical activity gain some health benefits.
- Older adults with chronic conditions should understand whether and how their conditions affect their ability to do regular physical activity safely.
- Older adults should begin with low-intensity exercise and gradually increase to moderate levels [102].
- Cognitive mediators, particularly self-efficacy, seem to be of particular importance in this group [103, 104]. Therefore strategies to enhance self-efficacy for physical activity (i.e., goal setting, modeling) should be included in interventions.
- Individually tailored interventions should be stressed to allow incorporation of strategies that address unique barriers such as intermittent illness and the burden of caregiving [24].

Ethnic and Racial Minorities

- Physical activity programs should be tailored to meet specific cultural concerns, perspectives, and values [105]. For example, interventions may need to address cultural norms, perspectives, and beliefs regarding physical activity.
- Communities should be directly involved in planning and implementation of physical activity programs [106].
- Among some African American communities, church-based programs may be an appropriate setting for delivery of physical activity interventions [107].

Individuals with Low Socioeconomic Status

- Individuals with low SES are underrepresented in physical activity intervention research, therefore optimal strategies to promote exercise adherence in this demographic group are not well understood [106].
- Access to exercise facilities and safe areas for outdoor recreation may be limitations. Interventions that assist with providing these resources may be particularly effective.
- Interventions combining telephone and mailed counseling have been effective in promoting increased physical activity among low-income women [108] and may be suitable in general for this demographic group.

Women

- Research suggests that women may be particularly responsive to intensive behavioral counseling [75].
- Physical activity interventions should consider and incorporate family and caregiving responsibilities [109, 110].
- Interventions should also incorporate social support from peers of family members [33].

Clinical and Policy Implications

Research has confirmed the importance of health-care provider influence on patients' physical activity. Studies have not yet identified an optimal strategy for enhancing physical activity within the health-care settings. However, research does suggest that clinicians can improve patients' adherence simply by assessing and encouraging physical activity on a *regular and repeated* basis. Current rates of physical activity recommendation by physicians are low and must be increased. There are several specific steps that may improve current practice in this area:

- First, more attention should be given to training medical students regarding physical activity (and other health behavior) recommendations and counseling. Since physical activity guidelines change over time, continuing education for clinicians at all stages of their career would also be valuable.

- Second, physical activity assessment and recommendations could be included as a quality indicator within medical systems. This would provide both a reminder system and accountability for physicians to speak with patients about their physical activity.
- Third, physicians should be informed about local resources related to physical activity, including both clinical and community facilities. This would allow easy referral for patients who are interested in group activities, specific types of facilities, or more intensive exercise counseling.
- Fourth, physicians' time with patients is clearly limited, and there is a need to develop and implement programs that enhance physician recommendations with more detailed behavioral counseling, delivered by a nurse or health educator.

Research has also highlighted the significant influence of the environment on physical activity behavior. Public health initiatives and policies that enhance opportunities for physical activity within communities may have a tremendous impact on nationwide activity levels. There is a need to increase the number, safety, and accessibility of parks and recreational facilities within communities. In addition to community-based efforts, worksites can play an important role in encouraging physical activity. Some practical strategies for worksites include onsite exercise groups, provision of onsite shower facilities for employees, and financial incentives that encourage physical activity (such as reduced costs for health club memberships).

Summary

Physical activity is associated with many physical and psychological health benefits. Yet despite decades of effort to improve physical activity levels, many Americans do not meet physical activity recommendations, and this remains an important public health problem. Health-care visits are an important but underutilized venue for encouraging individuals to adopt and maintain physically active lifestyles. While there are demographic groups who are at greater risk for physical inactivity (older adults, women, racial and ethnic minorities, individuals with low SES), the problem of inactivity is pervasive, and this health behavior should be addressed for all adults as part of routine health care.

While time limitations and competing demands during health-care visits are barriers to physical activity counseling, it should be considered that outcomes for many chronic health conditions can be substantially improved by increasing physical activity levels. Therefore discussion of physical activity should be treated as a priority. The following are recommendations for incorporating physical activity screening and counseling into health-care visits:

- Ask patients about physical activity behaviors *routinely* during visits. (Use questions such as those listed in Box 2.3 to assess whether patients are meeting physical activity recommendations described in Boxes 2.1 and 2.2.)
- Clearly advise that patients become and remain physically active and stress that physical activity is a key component to maintaining health and managing disease.
- Provide written information on physical activity recommendations and advise that patients set a goal to achieve that amount of physical activity weekly.
- Assist patients with specific plans for incorporating physical activity into their daily life.
- For physically inactive patients, ask about main barriers to physical activity and provide recommendations for dealing with these. Physical inactivity should not be an acceptable lifestyle.
- Become familiar with community resources for physical activity (i.e., organized exercise classes, parks and trails, recreation facilities) and recommend these to patients. Consider maintaining a written list of these resources to give to patients.
- Consider possibilities for incorporating more intensive physical activity interventions into a clinical practice, such as

  - Regular follow-up calls from a nurse or health educator to discuss progress toward physical activity goals
  - Internet-based programs for recording physical activity that can be accessed by the health-care provider prior to visits

- Facilitate creation of physical activity groups among patients and their family members (i.e., walking club)
- Become familiar with insurance companies that provide incentives or benefits aimed at promoting physical activity
- Access national organizations that provide materials aimed at promoting physical activity, such as the American College of Sports Medicine and the Centers for Disease Control and Prevention

References

1. U.S. Department of Health and Human Services. *Physical activity fundamental to preventing disease.* Washington, DC; 2002.
2. Colditz GA. Economic costs of obesity and inactivity. *Med Sci Sports Exerc.* 1999;31(11):S663–S667.
3. McGinnis JM, Foege WH. Actual causes of death in the United States. *JAMA.* 1993;270:2207–2212.
4. U.S. Department of Health and Human Services. *Healthy people 2010: Understanding and improving health. 2nd Ed.* Washington, DC: US Government Printing Office; 2000.
5. U.S. Department of Health and Human Services. *2008 Physical activity guidelines for Americans*; 2008.
6. Haskell WL, Lee I-M, Pate RR, et al. Physical activity and public health: updated recommendation for adults from the American College of Sports Medicine and the American Heart Association. *Med Sci Sports Exerc.* 2007;39(8):1423–1434.
7. Dunn AL, Marcus BH, Kampert JB, Garcia ME, Kohl HW, Blair SN. Comparison of lifestyle and structured interventions to increase physical activity and cardiorespiratory fitness: a randomized trial. *JAMA.* 1999;281:327–334.
8. Matthews CE, Chen KY, Freedson PS, et al. Amount of time spent in sedentary behaviors in the United States, 2003–2004. *Am J Epidemiol.* 2008;167(7):875–881.
9. Troiano RP, Berrigan D, Dodd KW, Masse LC, Tilert T, McDowell M. Physical activity in the United States measured by accelerometer. *Med Sci Sports Exerc.* 2008;40:181–188.
10. Sallis JF, Swelens BE. Assessment of physical activity by self-report: status, limitations, and future directions. *Res Q Exerc Sport.* 2000;71:S1–S14.
11. Morey MC, Pieper CF, Crowley GM, Sullivan RJ, Puglisi CM. Exercise adherence and 10-year mortality in chronically ill older adults [comment]. *J Am Geriatr Soc.* 2002;50(12):1929–1933.
12. Belza B, Topolski T, Kinne S, Patrick DL, Ramsey SD. Does adherence make a difference? Results from a community-based aquatic exercise program. *Nurs Res.* 2002;51(5):285–291.

13. Dishman RK. Overview. In: Dishman RK, ed. *Exercise adherence: It's impact on public health.* Champaign, IL: Human Kinetics; 1988.
14. Trost SG, Owen N, Bauman AE, Sallis JF, Brown W. Correlates of adults' participation in physical activity: review and update. *Med Sci Sports Exerc.* 2002;34(12):1996–2001.
15. Dishman RK, Sallis JF. Determinants and interventions for physical activity and exercise. In: Bouchard C, Shephard RJ, Stephens T, eds. *Physical activity, fitness and health: International proceedings and consensus statement.* Champaign, IL: Human Kinetics; 1994:214–238.
16. Rhodes RE, Martin AD, Taunton JE, Rhodes EC, Donnelly M, Elliot J. Factors associated with exercise adherence among older adults. An individual perspective. *Sports Med.* 1999;28(6):397–411.
17. Sallis JF, Owen N. Determinants of physical activity. *Physical activity and behavioral medicine.* Thousand Oaks, CA: Sage; 1999:110–134.
18. Centers for Disease Control and Prevention. Prevalence of self-reported physically active adults, United States, 2007. *MMWR.* 2008;57(48):1297–1300.
19. Barnes PM, Schoenborn CA. *Physical activity among adults: United States 2000. Advance data from vital and health statistics; no. 333.* Hyattsville, MD: National Center for Health Statistics; 2003.
20. U.S. Department of Health and Human Services. *Physical activity and health: A report to the surgeon general.* Atlanta, GA: U.S. Department of Health and Human Services; 1996.
21. Stephens T, Caspersen CJ. The demography of physical activity. In: Bouchard C, Shephard RJ, Stephens T, eds. *Physical activity, fitness, and health.* Champaign, IL: Human Kinetics; 1995:204–213.
22. Caspersen CJ, Merritt RK, Stephens T. International physical activity patterns: a methodological perspective. In: Dishman RK, ed. *Advances in exercise adherence.* Champaign, IL: Human Kinetics; 1994:73–110.
23. Schutzer KA, Graves BS. Barriers and motivations to exercise in older adults. *Prev Med.* 2004;39:1056–1061.
24. Brawley LR, Rejeski WJ, King AC. Promoting physical activity for older adults: the challenges for changing behavior. *Am J Prev Med.* 2003;25(3Sii):172–183.
25. Stephens T, Craig CL. *The well-being of Canadians: highlights from the 1988 Campbell's soup survey.* Ottawa, ON: Canadian Fitness and Lifestyle Research Institute; 1990.
26. Craig CL, Russell SJ, Cameron C, Beaulieu A. *1997 Physical activity benchmarks report.* Ottawa, ON: Canadian Fitness and Lifestyle Research Institute; 1998.
27. Burton LC, Shapiro S, German PS. Determinants of physical activity and maintenance among community-dwelling older persons. *Prev Med.* 1999;29:422–430.
28. Morey MC, Sullivan RJ. Medical assessment for health advocacy and practical strategies for exercise initiation. *Am J Prev Med.* 2003;25(3Sii):204–208.

29. Eden KB, Orleans CT, Mulrow CD, Pender NJ, Teutsch SM. Does counseling by clinicians improve physical activity? A summary of the evidence for the U.S. Preventive Services Task Force. *Ann Intern Med.* 2002;137: 208–215.

30. Kerse NM, Elley CR, Robinson E, Arroll B. Is physical activity counseling effective for older people? A cluster randomized, controlled trial in primary care. *J Am Geriatr Soc.* 2005;53(11):1951–1956.

31. Kolt GS, Schofield GM, Kerse N, Garrett N, Oliver M. Effect of telephone counseling on physical activity for low-active older people in primary care: a randomized, controlled trial. *J Am Geriatr Soc.* 2007;55(7):986–992.

32. Sallis JF, Haskell WL, Fortmann SP, Vranizan KM, Taylor CB, Solomon DS. Predictors of adoption and maintenance of physical activity in a community sample. *Prev Med.* 1986;15:331–341.

33. Vrazel J, Saunders RP, Wilcox S. An overview and proposed framework of social-environmental influences on the physical-activity behavior of women. *Am J Health Promot.* 2008;23(1):2–12.

34. Crespo CJ. Encouraging physical activity in minorities: eliminating disparities by 2010. *Physician Sports Med.* 2000;28(10):36–51.

35. Crespo CJ, Smit E, Andersen RE, Carter-Pokras O, Ainsworth BE. Race/ethnicity, social class and their relation to physical activity during leisure time: results from the Third National Health and Nutrition Examination Survey, 1988–1994. *Am J Prev Med.* 2000;18(1):46–53.

36. Washburn RA, Kline G, Lackland DT, Wheeler FC. Leisure time physical activity: are there black/white differences? *Prev Med.* 1992;21:127–135.

37. Wilcox S, Castro C, King AC, Housemann R, Brownson RC. Determinants of leisure time physical activity in rural compared to urban older and ethnically diverse women in the United States. *J Epidemiol Community Health.* 2000;54:667–672.

38. Henderson KA, Ainsworth BE. Sociocultural perspectives on physical activity in the lives of older African American and American Indian women: a cross cultural activity participation study. *Women Health.* 2000;31(1): 1–20.

39. Whitt MC, Kumanyika SK. Tailoring counseling on physical activity and inactivity for African-American women. *Ethn Dis.* 2002;12(4):62–71.

40. Dergance JM, Calmbach WL, Dhanda R, Miles TP, Hazuda HP, Mouton CP. Barriers and benefits of leisure time physical activity in the elderly: differences across cultures. *J Am Geriatr Soc.* 2003;51(6):863–868.

41. Henderson KA, Ainsworth BE. A synthesis of perceptions about physical activity among older African American and American Indian women. *Am J Public Health.* 2003;93(2):313–317.

42. Richter DL, Wilcox S, Greaney ML, Henderson KA, Ainsworth BE. Environmental, policy, and cultural factors related to physical activity in African American women. *Women Health.* 2002;36(2):91–109.

43. Wilcox S, Richter DL, Henderson KA, Greaney ML, Ainsworth BE. Perceptions of physical activity and personal barriers and enablers in African American women. *Ethn Dis.* 2002;12(3):353–362.

44. Van Duyn MAS, McCrae T, Wingrove BK, et al. Adapting evidence-based strategies to increase physical activity among African Americas, Hispanics, Hmong, and Native Hawaiians: a social marketing approach. *Prev Chronic Dis.* 2007;4(4):1–11.

45. Salmon JW, Owen N, Bauman A, Schmitz MKH, Booth M. Leisure-time, occupational, and household activity among professional, skilled, and less-skilled workers and homemakers. *Prev Med.* 2000;30:191–199.

46. Rimmer JH, Nicola T, Riley B, Creviston T. Exercise training for African Americans with disabilities residing in difficult social environments. *Am J Prev Med.* 2002;23(4):290–295.

47. Billings J, Zeitel L, Lukomnik J, Carey T, Blank A, Newman L. Impact of socioeconomic status on hospital use in New York City. *Health Aff (Millwood).* 1993;12:162–173.

48. Daly J, Sindone AP, Thompson DR, Hancock K, Chang E, Davidson P. Barriers to participation in and adherence to cardiac rehabilitation programs: a critical literature review. *Prog Cardiovasc Nurs.* 2002;17(1):8–17.

49. King AC, Blair SN, Bild DE, et al. Determinants of physical activity and interventions in adults. *Med Sci Sports Exerc.* 1992;24(6): S221–S236.

50. Brawley LR, Rejeski WJ, Lutes L. A group-mediated cognitive behavioral intervention for increasing adherence to physical activity in older adults. *J Appl Biobehav Res.* 2000;5:47–65.

51. Brownson RC, Eyler AA, King AC, Brown DR, Shyu YL, Sallis JF. Patterns and correlates of physical activity among US women 40 years and older. *Am J Public Health.* 2000;90:267–270.

52. Rejeski WJ, Brawley LR, Ambrosius WT, et al. Older adults with chronic disease: benefits of group-mediated counseling in the promotion of physically active lifestyles. *Health Psychol.* 2003;22(4):414–423.

53. Pargman D, Green L. The Type A behavior pattern and adherence to a regular running program by adult males ages 25–39 years. *Percept Mot Skills.* 1990;70(3 Pt 1):1040–1042.

54. Kreuter MW, Chheda SG, Bull FC. How does physician advice influence patient behavior? Evidence for a priming effect. *Arch Fam Med.* 2000;9(5):426–433.

55. Wallace JP, Raglin JS, Jastremski CA. Twelve month adherence of adults who joined a fitness program with a spouse vs without a spouse. *J Sports Med Phys Fit.* 1995;35(3):206–213.

56. Perri MG, Anton SD, Durning PE, et al. Adherence to exercise prescriptions: effects of prescribing moderate versus higher levels of intensity and frequency. *Health Psychol.* 2002;21(5):452–458.

57. Murphy MH, Hardman AE. Training effects of short and long bouts of brisk walking in sedentary women. *Med Sci Sports Exerc.* 1998;30(1): 152–157.

58. Jacobsen DJ, Donnelly JE, Snyder-Heelan K, Livingston K. Adherence and attrition with intermittent and continuous exercise in overweight women. *Int J Sports Med.* 2003;24(6):459–464.

59. King AC, Haskell WL, Taylor CB, Kraemer HC, DeBusk RF. Group-vs home-based exercise training in healthy older men and women. A community-based clinical trial. *JAMA.* 1991;266(11):1535–1542.

60. Carlson JJ, Johnson JA, Franklin BA, VanderLaan RL. Program participation, exercise adherence, cardiovascular outcomes, and program cost of traditional versus modified cardiac rehabilitation. *Am J Cardiol.* 2000;86(1): 17–23.

61. Cox KL, Burke V, Gorely TJ, Beilin LJ, Puddey IB. Controlled comparison of retention and adherence in home- vs center-initiated exercise interventions in women ages 40–65 years: the S.W.E.A.T. Study (Sedentary Women Exercise Adherence Trial). *Prev Med.* 2003;36(1):17–29.

62. Franklin BA. Program factors that influence exercise adherence: Practical adherence for the clinical staff. In: Dishman RK, ed. *Exercise adherence: Its impact on public health.* Champaign, IL: Human Kinetics; 1988:237–258.

63. Huston SJ, Evenson KR, Bors P, Gizlice Z. Neighborhood environment, access to places for activity, and leisure time physical activity in a diverse North Carolina population. *Am J Health Promot.* 2003;18(1):58–69.

64. Powell KE, Martin LM, Chowdhury PP. Places to walk: convenience and regular physical activity. *Am J Public Health.* 2003;93(9):1519–1521.

65. Kriska A, Caspersen C. Introduction to a collection of physical activity questionnaires. *Med Sci Sports Exerc.* 1997;29(6):5–9.

66. Smith BJ, Marshall AL, Huang N. Screening for physical activity in family practice: evaluation of two brief assessment tools. *Am J Prev Med.* 2005;29(4):256–264.

67. Taylor-Piliae RE, Norton LC, Haskell WL, et al. Validation of a new brief activity survey among men and women aged 60–69 years. *Am J Epidemiol.* 2006;164(6):598–606.

68. Sallis JF, Bauman A, Pratt M. Environmental and policy interventions to promote physical activity. *Am J Prev Med.* 1998;15(4):379–397.

69. Marcus BH, Owen N, Forsyth LH, Cavill NA, Fridinger F. Physical activity interventions using mass media, print media, and information technology. *Am J Prev Med.* 1998;15(4):362–378.

70. Blamey A, Mutrie N, Aitchison T. Health promotion by encouraged use of stairs. *Br Med J.* 1995;311:289–290.

71. Brownell KD, Stunkard AJ, Albaum JM. Evaluation and modification of exercise patterns in the natural environment. *Am J Psychiatry.* 1980;137:1540–1545.

72. Brownson RC, Ballew P, Dieffenderfer B, et al. Evidence-based interventions to promote physical activity: what contributes to dissemination by state health departments. *Am J Prev Med.* 2007;33(1S):S66–S78.

73. Kahn EB, Ramsey LT, Brownson RC, et al. The effectiveness of interventions to increase physical activity: a systematic review. *Am J Prev Med.* 2002;22(4S):73–107.

74. Foster C, Hillsdon M, Thorogood M. Interventions for promoting physical activity. *Cochrane Database Syst Rev.* 2005;1. Art No.: CD003180. DOI: 003110.001002/14651858.CD14003180.pub14651852.

75. The Writing Group for the Activity Counseling Trial Research Group. Effects of physical activity counseling in primary care: the activity counseling trial: a randomized controlled trial. *JAMA.* 2001;286: 677–687.

76. Friedman RH. Automated telephone conversations to assess health behavior and deliver behavioral interventions. *J Med Syst.* 1998;22(2):95–102.

77. Sullivan T, Allegrante JP, Peterson MG, Kovar PA, MacKenzie CR. One-year followup of patients with osteoarthritis of the knee who participated in a program of supervised fitness walking and supportive patient education. *Arthritis Care Res.* 1998;11(4):228–233.

78. Noland MP. The effects of self-monitoring and reinforcement on exercise adherence. *Res Q Exerc Sport.* 1989;60(3):216–224.

79. King AC, Pruitt LA, Phillips W, Oka R, Rodenburg A, Haskell WL. Comparative effects of two physical activity programs on measured and perceived physical functioning and other health-related quality of life outcomes in older adults. *J Gerontol Ser A-Biol Sci Med Sci.* 2000;55(2): M74–83.

80. Heesch KC, Masse LC, Dunn AL, Frankowski RF, Mullen D. Does adherence to a lifestyle physical activity intervention predict changes in physical activity. *J Behav Med.* 2003;26(4):333–348.

81. Wilson DK, Friend R, Teasley N, Green S, Reaves IL, Sica D. Motivational versus social cognitive interventions for promoting fruit and vegetable intake and physical activity in African American adolescents. *Ann Behav Med.* 2002;24(4):310–319.

82. Miller WC, Pollock S. *Motivational interviewing: Preparing people to change addictive behaviour.* London: Gilford Press; 1991.

83. Marcus BH, Williams DM, Dubbert PM, et al. Physical activity intervention studies: what we know and what we need to know: a scientific statement from the American Heart Association Council on Nutrition, Physical Activity, and Metabolism (Subcommittee on Physical Activity); Council on Cardiovascular Disease in the Young; and the Interdisciplinary Working Group on Quality of Care and Outcomes Research. *Circulation.* 2006;114:2739–2752.

84. Conn VS, Hafdahl AR, Brown SA, Brown LM. Meta-analysis of patient interventions to increase physical activity among chronically ill adults. *Patient Educ Couns.* 2008;70:157–172.

85. Simons-Morton DG, Calfas KJ, Oldenburg B, Burton NW. Effects of interventions in health care settings on physical activity or cardiorespiratory fitness. *Am J Prev Med.* 1998;15(4):413–430.

86. Blissmer B, McAuley E. Testing the requirements of stages of physical activity among adults: the comparative effectiveness of stage-matched, mismatched, standard care, and control interventions. *Ann Behav Med.* 2002;24(3):181–189.

87. Peterson TR, Aldana SG. Improving exercise behavior: an application of the stages of change model in a worksite setting. *Am J Health Promot.* 1999;13:229–232.

88. Dunn AL, Gracia ME, Marcus BH, Kampert JB, Kohl HW, Blair SN. Six-month physical activity and fitness changes in Project Active, a randomized trial. *Med Sci Sports Exerc.* 1998;30(7):1076–1083.

89. Andersen RE, Bartlett SJ, Moser CD, Evangelisti MI, Verde TJ. Lifestyle or aerobic exercise to treat obesity in dieting women. *Med Sci Sports Exerc.* 1997;29(Suppl 5):S46.

90. Cardinal BJ, Sachs ML. Effects of a mail-mediated, stage-matched exercise behavior change strategies on female adults' leisure-time exercise behavior. *J Sports Med Phys Fit.* 1996;36(2):100–107.

91. Schappert SM. *National ambulatory medical care survey: 1991. 230th Ed.* Hyattsville, MD: National Center for Health Statistics; 1993.

92. Godin G, Shephard R. An evaluation of the potential role of the physician in influencing community exercise behavior. *Am J Health Promot.* 1990;4: 225–229.

93. Wee CC, McCarthy EP, Davis RB, Phillips RS. Physician counseling about exercise. *JAMA.* 1999;282(16):1583–1588.

94. Lewis CE, Clancy C, Leake B, Schwartz JS. The counseling practices of internists. *Ann Intern Med.* 1991;114:54–58.

95. Centers for Disease Control and Prevention. Missed opportunities in preventive counseling for cardiovascular disease – United States, 1995. *MMWR.* 1998;47:91–95.

96. Eakin EG, Glasgow RE, Riley KM. Review of primary care-based physical activity intervention studies: effectiveness and implications for practice and future research. *J Fam Pract.* 2000;49:158–168.

97. The ACT Writing Group. Effects of physical activity counseling in primary care. The activity counseling trial: a randomized controlled trial. *JAMA.* 2001;286:677–687.

98. Pinto BM, Goldstein MG, Marcus BH. Activity counseling by primary care physicians. *Prev Med.* 1998;27:506–513.

99. Calfas KJ, Long BJ, Sallis JF, Wooten WJ, Pratt M, Patrick K. A controlled trial of physician counseling to promote the adoption of physical activity. *Prev Med.* 1996;25(3):225–233.

100. US Preventive Services Task Force. *Guide to clinical preventive services. 2nd Ed.* Baltimore, MD: Williams & Wilkins; 1996.

101. Castro CM, King AC. Telephone-assisted counseling for physical activity. *Exerc Sport Sci Rev.* 2002;30(2):64–68.

102. Cress ME, Buchner DM, Prohaska T, et al. Best practices for physical activity programs and behavior counseling in older adult populations. *J Aging Phys Act.* 2004;13(1):61–74.

103. Brassington GS, Atienza AA, Perczek RE, DiLorenzo TM, King AC. Intervention-related cognitive versus social mediators of exercise adherence in the elderly. *Am J Prev Med.* 2002;23(2 Suppl):80–86.

104. Conn VS, Minor MA, Burks KJ, Rantz MJ, Pomeroy SH. Integrative review of physical activity intervention research with aging adults. *J Am Geriatr Soc.* 2003;51:1159–1168.

105. Pasick RJ, D'Onofrio CN, Otero-Sabogal R. Similarities and differences across cultures: questions to inform a third generation for health promotion research. *Health Educ Q*. 1996;23:S142–S161.
106. Taylor WC, Baranowski T, Young DR. Physical activity interventions in low-income, ethnic minority, and populations with disability. *Am J Prev Med*. 1998;15(4):334–313.
107. Kumanyika SK, Charleston JB. Lose weight and win: a church-based weight loss program for blood pressure control among black women. *Patient Educ Couns*. 1992;19:19–32.
108. Albright CL, Pruitt L, Castro C, Gonzales A, Woo S, King AC. Modifying physical activity in a multiethnic sample of low-income women: one-year results from the IMPACT (Increasing Motivation for Physical Activity) project. *Ann Behav Med*. 2005;50(3):191–200.
109. Miller YD, Trost SG, Brown WJ. Mediators of physical activity behavior changes among women with young children. *Am J Prev Med*. 2002;23(2S):98–103.
110. King AC, Baumann K, O'Sullivan P, Wilcox S, Castro C. Effects of moderate-intensity exercise on physiological, behavioral, and emotional responses to family caregiving: a randomized controlled trial. *J Gerontol Ser A-Biol Sci Med Sci*. 2002;57(1):M26–M36.

Chapter 3
Improving Dietary Adherence

William S. Yancy Jr. and Corrine I. Voils

Introduction

Of the many challenges clinicians face, those associated with unhealthy diet practices may be the most widespread and the most difficult to address and overcome. This is because everyone has performed the ritual of eating (and drinking) more frequently and for longer than any other health habit. Food and drink are associated with a number of factors that can make adherence to a new diet regimen quite challenging, including a person's sense of comfort and pleasure, underlying physiology, social interactions, ethnic and family traditions, and cravings.

The difficulty of adhering to healthy dietary practices is evidenced by the high prevalence of obesity. From 1980 to 2004, the prevalence of obesity (defined as body mass index [BMI] ≥ 30 kg/m^2) increased from 14.5 to 32.2% [1, 2]. When overweight individuals (BMI 25–29.9 kg/m^2) are considered, then the proportion of Americans who are above the recommended weight rises to 66% [2]. Obesity is associated with a host of acute and chronic diseases, including diabetes mellitus (DM), hypertension, coronary heart disease (CHD), congestive heart failure, hyperlipidemia, cancer, gall bladder disease,

W.S. Yancy Jr. (✉)
General Internal Medicine, Duke University Medical Center, Durham, NC, USA
e-mail: yancy006@mc.duke.edu

H. Bosworth (ed.), *Improving Patient Treatment Adherence*,
DOI 10.1007/978-1-4419-5866-2_3,
© Springer Science+Business Media, LLC 2010

osteoarthritis, gastroesophageal reflux disease (GERD), and obstructive sleep apnea [3–5]. The prevalence of these diseases has increased as the rates of obesity have increased [6]. As a result, obesity is the second most prominent contributor to mortality in the United States, superseded only by tobacco use [7, 8]. Due to the high prevalence of obesity and overweight, and their associated health problems, dietary adherence for the purpose of weight management will be a major focus of this chapter.

The detrimental health effects of obesity are generally well known by the public. It is perhaps for this reason that so many American adults have, at one time or another, attempted to lose weight. In two separate nationwide surveys of adults, at least 28% of men and 44% of women who were overweight or obese were attempting to lose weight [9, 10]. Those percentages climb to nearly 65% for men and 80% for women when taking into account people actively trying to maintain their current weight (i.e., avoiding weight gain) [10]. In one study, although diet was the most commonly reported strategy for weight loss, only about 50% of those trying to lose weight reported actually consuming fewer calories, which is the best proven method for weight loss.

Initiating weight loss (i.e., weight loss over a short period of time) can be difficult for an individual but various diet interventions have been proven successful for this purpose. Once initial weight loss is achieved, however, maintaining the weight loss is much more difficult [11]. On average, patients who lose weight will regain 1/3–2/3 of that weight after 1 year and nearly all of it by 5 years [12]. Because adherence to dietary interventions tends to decrease over time, clinicians and patients often discount lifestyle modification in favor of second-line therapies such as medication and even surgery. Such interventions may be useful in some situations, but before they are tried, more effort could be devoted to enhancing the success of first-line therapies (i.e., lifestyle changes). To develop successful strategies for long-term weight loss, an understanding of the mechanisms underlying weight loss initiation and maintenance is necessary.

Weight Loss Initiation Versus Maintenance

Initiation refers to early attempts to make a behavior change, whereas maintenance refers to continuing the new behaviors after some period of time. A popular model of behavior change, the transtheoretical model (TTM), specifically distinguishes these behaviors according to the length of time they have been enacted [13]. In TTM, *action* refers to a behavior change lasting from 1 day to 6 months, whereas *maintenance* is achieved if patients have sustained the behavior for 6 months or longer. Consequently, many researchers consider 6 months the minimum amount of time that a newly initiated behavior (e.g., diet, exercise) should be performed before it is considered to be maintained [14–16]. Over the past decade, efforts have been made to understand the psychological processes and contextual factors involved in behavior maintenance [14, 17–19]. This research, the bulk of which has focused on smoking cessation, weight loss, and physical activity, has identified important differences between initiation and maintenance, which we summarize in Table 3.1.

Table 3.1 Cognitive and behavioral strategies involved in weight loss initiation versus maintenance

Initiation	Maintenance
Self-regulatory goal: *approach* of a favorable end state (i.e., normal weight)	Self-regulatory goal: *avoidance* of a less favorable end state (i.e., overweight)
Motivational self-efficacy	Recovery self-efficacy
Favorable expectations	Satisfaction with outcomes derived from weight loss
Guided goal setting	Self-directed goal setting
Monitoring by clinician or interventionist	Self-monitoring
Primary source of social support is interventionist or similar others	Primary source of support is social network

One primary difference between behavior initiation and maintenance lies in the self-regulatory goal [17]. Self-regulation refers to efforts to minimize the discrepancy between the current state and an alternative state. In weight loss initiation, the objective is to *approach* a favorable end state (i.e., goal weight) by minimizing the discrepancy between that state and the current state. In contrast, in weight loss maintenance, in which patients are already at their goal weight, the objective is to *avoid* an alternative, less favorable end state (reverting back to being overweight) by sustaining the discrepancy between that state and the current state.

Another difference between initiation and maintenance is the source of self-efficacy (i.e., confidence to perform a behavior) that drives behavior [20]. *Motivational self-efficacy* refers to the confidence one has in enacting a new behavior. *Recovery self-efficacy* refers to the confidence one has in being able to "get back on track after being derailed" [20].

Yet another difference between weight loss initiation and maintenance is consideration of the benefits that may result [18]. When deciding whether to adopt a new dietary pattern, one typically considers the benefits of the new diet (e.g., improved mobility resulting from weight loss) relative to those of the current behavior (e.g., impaired mobility due to excess weight). If the perceived benefits of the new diet outweigh the benefits of the current diet, weight loss should occur. However, expectations about the benefits of weight loss may be detrimental to weight loss maintenance if the expectations are too high to be achieved. Weight loss maintenance is better determined by the satisfaction with the outcomes resulting from the weight loss. Thus, very high expectations are more likely to promote weight loss initiation, whereas modest expectations linked to realistic, achievable outcomes are more likely to promote weight loss maintenance.

Weight loss initiation and weight maintenance also differ in how goal setting is enacted. Weight loss initiation in the context of an intervention is typically guided by an interventionist, who helps patients set weight loss goals and specific plans to achieve those goals. Likewise, monitoring of progress toward the weight loss goal is often done by the interventionist, although self-monitoring may be incorporated as well. In contrast, during weight loss maintenance, the individual takes over primary responsibility for goal setting and monitoring.

Finally, a key difference between weight loss initiation and maintenance is the primary source of social support. In the context of a weight loss intervention, the primary source of support for achieving a weight loss goal is the interventionist and/or similar others (e.g., participants in a group dietary intervention). When the intervention ceases, the primary source of support for weight loss maintenance necessarily shifts from the interventionist to an individual's social network members such as family members, friends, or coworkers.

The ultimate public health goal is to have individuals maintain weight loss so as to sustain a new, healthy state over the long term. From our review of the processes required for weight loss maintenance, it is no surprise that the beneficial effects of weight loss interventions are short lived and that people often regain weight. This is likely because weight loss interventions typically focus on the processes of weight loss initiation and do not consider the processes of weight loss maintenance, which can actually be at odds with weight loss initiation [17]. Therefore, to maintain a new dietary pattern over the long term, a brief transition period may be needed in which patients are taught, and gain confidence in, weight maintenance strategies. During this period, the focus, if not the intensity, of the weight management intervention will need to change.

How can clinicians better promote weight loss initiation and maintenance? Strategies for weight loss initiation and maintenance following from the previously described behavioral principles are listed in Table 3.2.

Barriers to and Facilitators of Diet Adherence

Prior to initiating a weight loss intervention, and periodically during the process, it is important for both clinicians and patients to consider the barriers to and facilitators of diet adherence. These factors may differ depending on the individual patient, so a thorough knowledge of them will help a clinician to address a wide variety of patient situations.

Barriers to Diet Adherence

The prominent impact that barriers can have on dietary adherence can be exemplified by the recent rise in obesity prevalence. To combat obesity, the US Department of Agriculture (Dietary Guidelines) [21] and the National Heart, Lung, and Blood Institute (NHLBI) of the NIH (Clinical Guidelines) [22] have recommended a decrease in total caloric intake, including reducing portion sizes, for patients to achieve weight loss. Neilsen and Popkin examined adherence to these recommendations using consumer surveys from 1977 to 1996, when the prevalence of obesity in the United States was increasing rapidly. They found that food portion sizes increased both inside and outside the home for almost all food categories [23]. These data have given rise

Table 3.2 Weight loss initiation and maintenance strategies and intervention implications

Weight loss initiation		Weight loss maintenance	
Strategy	Intervention implication	Strategy	Intervention implication
Self-regulatory goal: *approach* of a favorable end state	• Clinician frames behavioral goals as helping patients to achieve weight loss • Patients develop lists of healthy eating habits they would like to initiate	Self-regulatory goal: *avoidance* of a less favorable end state	• Clinician frames goals as helping patients to avoid weight regain • Patients identify high-risk situations to avoid • Patients develop lists of healthy eating habits they have already initiated and wish to continue
Motivational self-efficacy	• Patients develop a specific dietary plan • Patients anticipate and plan for barriers (e.g., eating at work, in a restaurant) • Patients maximize facilitators (e.g., eat with friends who are also losing weight, take lunch to work)	Recovery self-efficacy	• Patients prepare contingency plans for high-risk situations • Patients imagine and role-play responses for potential situations (e.g., eating in restaurant or at a party)
Favorable expectations	• Patients list the perceived benefits of eating healthier and losing weight • Patients emphasize the benefits of eating healthier and being normal weight over the benefits of their current eating patterns and being overweight	Satisfaction with outcomes of the behavior change	• Patients list the perceived costs and benefits of new dietary habits and weight loss achieved • Patients reflect on satisfaction with past weight loss

Table 3.2 (Continued)

Weight loss initiation		Weight loss maintenance	
Strategy	Intervention implication	Strategy	Intervention implication
Guided goal setting	• Clinician helps patients establish weight loss goals • Clinician helps patients develop specific dietary plan to achieve weight loss goals	Self-directed goal setting	• Clinician emphasizes the need to set own goals • Patients practice goal setting, receiving feedback from clinician or interventionist
Monitoring by clinician or interventionist	• Clinician monitors patients frequently to track their progress • Clinician develops standards for determining when a lapse occurs (e.g., gain >5 lbs, plateau) and intervenes (e.g., new goal setting) when appropriate	Self-monitoring	• Patients identify relevant behaviors that will allow them to monitor their health status (e.g., daily weighing) • Patients develop standards for determining when a lapse occurs (e.g., gain >5 lbs) • Patients keep a diary
Primary source of support is interventionist or similar others	• Clinician provides positive reinforcement for success • Clinician provides emotional support	Primary source of support is social network	• Patients identify supportive members of their social networks • Patients share goals with spouses, friends, coworkers • Patients suggest specific supportive behaviors (e.g., exchange of healthy eating tips)

to the concept of a toxic environment that "...pervasively surrounds [Americans] with inexpensive, convenient foods high in both fat and calories" [24]. This toxic environment is essentially a multitude of barriers making weight management challenging for every individual (see Table 3.3). Identifying and addressing these barriers may be the first step to improving diet adherence.

Table 3.3 Barriers to diet adherence

Educational barriers
Inadequate dietary knowledge
Inability to understand food labels
Inability to estimate portion sizes
Conflicting public recommendations
Internal barriers
Lack of self-regulatory resources to overcome internal (e.g., attitudes toward food, hunger) and external (time of day, place, social situations) cues
Competing motivations
Low self-esteem
Psychological comorbidities
Eating disorders
External barriers
Cost
Low availability of healthy food choices
High availability of unhealthy food choices
Cultural and ethnic factors
Social situations
Lack of empathy from health-care provider
Medication side effects (e.g., increased appetite)

Educational Barriers

Lack of patient knowledge is a barrier common to the successful implementation of many healthy behaviors. Educating the patient is the main goal of diet counseling, and knowledge is a necessary albeit insufficient condition for dietary adherence. Yet learning the right thing to do is perhaps more difficult for dietary change than other behavior changes because of the complexities of nutrition information and of food choices available. The information needed for successful diet adherence includes not only appropriate and inappropriate food choices but also portion sizes, recommended daily intakes of nutrients (e.g., maximum recommended sodium intake, minimum recommended calcium intake), and how to read food labels.

Learning the healthiest food selections is more difficult today than ever because of the lack of consensus over what types of foods should be eaten for optimal health [25–27]. Further complicating this issue is that different diets may be effective for different health problems, e.g., elevated serum LDL cholesterol versus metabolic syndrome versus hypertension. Regarding the problem of obesity, lack of consensus is quite prominent. Clinical guidelines and public recommendations for weight management support lowering dietary fat, yet evidence from a systematic review suggests that low-fat diets are actually less effective than calorie restriction for achieving and maintaining weight loss over a 12- to 18-month period [28]. Further, the largest randomized diet trial to date, the Women's Health Initiative (WHI), found that a low-fat diet was ineffective for reducing risk for cardiovascular disease or cancer [29–31]. Recently, greater weight loss and improvement in certain serum lipids has been reported with a low-carbohydrate/high-fat diet, suggesting that the role of dietary fat in weight gain and cardiovascular disease risk requires re-evaluation [32–37]. Of course, the low-carbohydrate dietary pattern has not been tested in a long-term trial with meaningful clinical outcomes (e.g., mortality or myocardial infarction rates), as with the WHI trial. With these data in mind, and the controversy they have created, it is not surprising that patients receive streams of conflicting diet information from health professionals, friends, and media. In fact, the recent interest in these diets by researchers and consumers has resulted in sudden shifts in the food industry, which have alternately promoted low-fat products and low-carbohydrate products.

Internal Barriers

Several individual-level factors may be barriers to diet adherence or to weight loss. For example, diet adherence will be difficult for individuals who are too distracted or have too many competing demands to overcome internal and external cues. Internal cues include attitudes toward certain foods and hunger. External cues are situations that stimulate food cravings such as time of day or location. Individuals who are too distracted or have too many competing demands may be less likely to resist eating in certain situations when they are not actually hungry. Further, because of being in a particular situation, individuals may have less capacity to resist *over*eating even though they are eating at an appropriate time (i.e., when hungry). Competing motivations frequently interfere with diet adherence, especially as daily schedules become more and more hectic. It can be difficult to adhere to one's diet when work, family, social, and physical activity interests/demands conflict with one's diet goals.

Other individual-level factors that interfere with diet adherence include low self-esteem and psychological disorders. When present, these issues may be some of the most potent barriers to modifying diet. Obese people are particularly vulnerable to symptoms of low self-esteem with possible contributors including repeated unsuccessful weight loss attempts, failure to measure up to the thin ideal promoted by the media, weight-related discrimination, increased physical pain, and decreased physical ability [38–40]. Obese individuals have a higher than average prevalence of depression, and depression has been linked strongly with non-adherence [41–44]. Intuitively, this means that diet modification and weight loss will be extremely challenging in a depressed patient until the depression is treated. Clinicians should assess obese patients for depressive symptoms and treat accordingly, being mindful of the weight gain that has been associated with several antidepressants (see below for examples of weight neutral antidepressants).

Obese people are also at increased risk for having two distinct psychological disorders associated with eating: binge-eating syndrome and night-eating syndrome. A person's eating habits become ingrained over time with certain foods or eating times used to relax, relieve stress, or adapt to difficult situations. These habits can become maladaptive, leading to eating disorders. Binge eating is a loss of control that results in a person eating an amount of food that is considerably more than usual. Binge eating disorder is twice as prevalent in obese patients than in non-obese patients [45]. For example, among bariatric surgery patients, the prevalence of binge eating (prior to surgery) ranges from 13 to 49% [46]. Night-eating syndrome was recognized by Stunkard in 1955 and is defined by the following: (1) consumption of half of the daily caloric intake after the evening meal, (2) awakening at least once a night for three nights a week to eat, and (3) morning anorexia. In obese patients, the prevalence of night-eating syndrome may be as high as 26%, and is higher in men than women [47]. Restrained eating (i.e., dieting) may be an important precursor for these disorders, which are often unrecognized by family members, friends, and clinicians due to the surreptitious manner in which patients binge. These complex psychological illnesses can thwart even comprehensive weight loss interventions; recognition and focused treatment may be necessary before dietary adherence can be addressed.

External Barriers

Other barriers to diet modification may be more external to the individual, including economic, environmental, and cultural/social factors. Following a healthy diet is felt to be more costly and time-consuming than less healthy diets [48]. Therefore, resource constraints are frequently identified as a significant barrier to healthy eating. Disparities in access to healthy foods may contribute to this obstacle because many low socioeconomic communities have few restaurants and food stores with healthy food options but ample access to unhealthy food options [49]. Even people in wealthy communities, however, may find that unhealthy food options are easier to find than healthy options. Further complicating weight management in our society are cultural, ethnic, and social factors, which can interfere with the best efforts by patients and health practitioners during a lifestyle modification intervention [50]. Culture's influence on diet is so powerful that eating habits are one of the last of the aspects a person incorporates from a new culture after relocating from another culture [51]. Social situations can also have a profound impact on eating behaviors. For example, research shows that the number of people present at a meal is correlated with the size of the meal [52]. Furthermore, data from the Framingham cohort demonstrated that a person's likelihood of becoming obese increased 57% by having a friend who also became obese and increased 37–40% by having a sibling or spouse who became obese [53].

Yet another barrier to weight loss involves side effects from chronically used medications. For example, many tricyclic antidepressant and antipsychotic medications can lead to weight gain. On the other hand, bupropion and fluoxetine (for depression) may induce mild weight loss, and quetiapine (for psychotic or bipolar disorders) does not affect weight. Other medications associated with weight gain include beta-antagonists (particularly propranolol), alpha-antagonists (particularly terazosin), most diabetes medications, several anti-seizure medications, and corticosteroids (e.g., pred-nisone). A recently published clinical practice guideline has a table listing culprit medications and their weight neutral alternatives (http://www.healthquality.va.gov/obesity/obe06_final1.pdf) [54].

Lack of empathy from health-care providers can also impede dietary adherence and weight loss attempts. Discrimination against obese people can be profound and is present in a multitude of settings, including the workplace, educational institutions, and the health-care environment. Biases against patients with obesity have been noted in physicians and nurses as well as dietitians, fitness experts, and obe-sity specialists [55–57]. In these studies, health professionals often consider obese patients to be unmotivated, non-adherent, and lacking self-control. In a survey of 400 physicians, one-third of the sample listed obesity as one of the diagnostic categories or social character-istics of patients to which they responded most negatively, ranking it behind only drug addiction, alcoholism, and mental illness [58]. From the patient's perspective, one study surveyed approximately 2,500 women and found that over 50% had received inappropriate comments about their weight from a health professional. Given that building rap-port with patients can be critical to adherence to therapy, health-care providers must maintain an empathetic attitude when working with obese patients, and avoid accusatory or derogatory remarks. Providers will experience more success treating obesity if they work with their patients to identify barriers such as those listed above and then help the patient to overcome these barriers.

Facilitators of Diet Adherence

Intervention-Related Factors

The design of the intervention (i.e., its components, mode of delivery, frequency, and duration) can meaningfully impact how successfully patients adhere to the diet changes that are prescribed. For example, interventions that combine more than one component, such as diet *and* behavioral counseling, are more likely to be successful than those focusing on one component [59]. Further, interventions, whether in person, by telephone, or by the Internet, can be characterized accord-ing to dose. Dosing can refer to the duration of each individual session, the frequency of the sessions, and the period of time over which sessions occur; these latter two aspects (frequency and period of time) of dosing have been shown to impact weight loss. For instance, longer duration interventions have been shown to result in better weight loss than shorter ones, and many interventions have shown that adherence wanes after the delivery of diet counseling ends [59, 60]. Similarly, higher frequency of counseling sessions results in greater weight loss than lower frequency [61]. These findings have led the US Preventive Services Task Force (USPSTF) to recommend only multi-component, high-intensity (more than one counseling session per month for at least the first 3 months), person-to-person (individual or group counseling) interventions as effective for obesity treatment [62] (Table 3.4).

Table 3.4 Facilitators of adherence to diet recommendations

Intervention-related factors
Frequency of sessions [61, 62]
Duration of intervention [60]
Behavioral factors
Patient prepares own meals [66]
Attendance of counseling sessions [63–67]
Self-monitoring [63, 68, 69]
Social factors
Spousal support [77, 120]
Marital satisfaction [77]
Satisfactory home/work environment [121]
Perceived social support [67]
Autonomy [88–90]

Behavioral Factors

Behavioral approaches have been a mainstay of dietary modification interventions and weight management through the years. Several components of behavioral programs have been independently associated with successful weight loss. One important facilitator of diet adherence and weight loss is self-monitoring [63–69]. Self-monitoring might refer to body weight or dietary intake. Simply weighing oneself regularly improves weight management [70–72]. Similarly, self-monitoring of dietary intake has been shown to enhance weight loss but is also useful for several other reasons (see section "Assessing Dietary Intake" for more information on food records) [68]. The act of recording what and how much one eats can favorably alter intake at that moment. It also teaches the patient about portion sizes, composition of prepared foods, and food label reading. The resulting dietary log can then be used to inform both the patient and the clinician of dietary successes and pitfalls.

Social Support

Eating behavior can be profoundly influenced by the interpersonal context; support from family members, friends, and coworkers can be effective for assisting patients to change eating habits [52]. Social support is a common component of clinical interventions and commercial programs to improve adherence to diet recommendations. Social support can be educational, emotional (e.g., verbal reinforcement), or instrumental (e.g., preparing healthier foods) in nature. Spousal involvement can increase patient adherence to weight loss regimens, particularly when spouses are actively involved in purchasing and preparing foods for the patient [73].

Despite the potential benefit of including spouses in dietary interventions, studies of the effect of spousal involvement on dietary adherence have demonstrated mixed results. In a systematic review of four studies with a minimum of 1-year follow-up, spousal support was associated with greater long-term weight loss among intervention than control group patients in only one trial [74–78]. One explanation for the non-significant association between spousal support and weight loss is that some trials had many treatment arms, each with a relatively small sample size, resulting in inadequate power to detect significant effects. Another explanation is that spouses did not play an active role in the intervention and were not taught how to engage in supportive rather than detrimental (e.g., nagging) behaviors; rather, spouses only observed during educational sessions and/or provided emotional support [73]. Interventions might be more effective if (1) spouses became actively involved in food choices and preparation, (2) spouses were informed of patients' goals, and (3) spouses received suggestions for enhancing emotional and instrumental support.

Other members of patients' social networks are commonly recruited into weight loss interventions. For example, one study found that weight loss and maintenance were greater in subjects who entered an intervention with three friends or family members compared with subjects who were recruited alone [79]. In another study, standard behavioral therapy plus social support was more effective for avoiding weight gain than standard behavioral therapy alone.

, Commercial weight loss programs (e.g., Weight Watchers) harness this salutary effect of social support on weight loss, combining it with several other established behavioral approaches. Participants in these programs attend frequent group counseling sessions, which can be more effective at inducing weight loss than individual therapy [80]. These group sessions are not only interactive, allowing exchange of diet tips, recipes, and behavioral techniques but also foster social relationships among people with a common goal of weight management. Participants have a "weigh-in" at each session, creating not only a sort of accountability among facilitators (and peers) but also the opportunity for peers to celebrate with a participant after successes or console and encourage a participant after setbacks. In the scientific literature, these programs have been shown to help participants achieve moderate long-term weight loss on average and have proven more effective than self-help in a randomized controlled trial [81–83]. Despite growing worldwide interest in social networking Internet sites, Internet-based weight loss programs that incorporate social support have been only mildly successful when tested [84–86].

Autonomy

Autonomy refers to the experience of freedom to determine one's behavior and outcomes; level of autonomy contributes significantly to a person's level of intrinsic motivation. When patients are instructed to follow a physician's recommendations without opportunity for collaborative decision making, motivation becomes less intrinsic and more extrinsic. When this happens, patients may become motivated to reestablish freedom, possibly resulting in decreased adherence [87]. Even if this does not occur, and patients instead agree to follow the recommendations, their behavior is less likely to persist because it is partially or fully motivated by sources external to the self, such as rewards, deadlines, approval from others, or social norms. Autonomy can be enhanced by allowing patients to choose several aspects of a dietary intervention, including the following: different diet regimens, preferred food types within a particular diet regimen, magnitude of caloric restriction, specific dietary goals, and format of the diet counseling (e.g., group versus individual; meeting frequency; in person, by telephone, or via the Internet).

For example, one study prescribed a very low-calorie diet for 6 months followed by 23 months of follow-up and examined the relationship between levels of autonomy, intrinsic motivation, and weight loss [88]. Greater autonomy level was associated with greater intrinsic motivation, which in turn was associated with more regular attendance of the weight loss program, greater weight loss at 6 months, and greater maintenance of the weight loss at 23 months. Interestingly, actually having choice is not as important as having the perception of having choice. In a small study in overweight children, all children received the same diet but half were led to believe that they had chosen the diet they received, whereas the other half did not perceive that they had a choice. Children who perceived having a choice lost more weight than children who did not [89]. In another study, 24 obese women were randomly assigned to behavioral choice treatment (whereby participants were taught to cognitively restructure health behaviors as choices) or traditional behavioral treatment [90]. The traditional group experienced greater weight loss at 3 months but then regained weight, whereas the behavioral choice group experienced more gradual weight loss resulting in greater net weight loss at 12 months. These studies demonstrate how enhancing autonomy can be an important part of a weight loss program and improve the long-term adherence to healthy behavior change.

Diet Composition

Whether individuals can lose more weight following a diet of one macronutrient composition versus another (low-fat versus low-carbohydrate diets, in particular) has been examined in a number of recent trials [32–35, 37]. Given our current understanding of caloric balance and assuming that energy expenditure does not change, greater weight loss with one diet approach implies that adherence is better to that diet approach. In a meta-analysis of low-carbohydrate, calorie-unrestricted versus low-fat, calorie-restricted diets, weight loss at 6 months was greater in participants following a low-carbohydrate diet, but comparable at 12 months [91]. In three long-term studies published since the meta-analysis, weight loss was comparable at 1 year in one study [92] and was greater in the low-carbohydrate participants at 1 year in one study [93] and at 2 years in another study [36]. Some insight into how well participants adhere to an assigned diet can also be inferred from completion rates in each of the intervention arms. In one study, retention was greater in the carbohydrate-restricted diet group than in the low-fat diet group [35]. Other studies (with two exceptions [92, 94]) had greater retention in the carbohydrate-restricted diet group but the comparisons were not statistically significant or not examined statistically [32–34, 37, 93, 95].

These results indicate that adherence to the carbohydrate-restricted diet may be easier than a low-fat, energy-restricted diet in the context of a clinical trial. There are several potential reasons for why adherence may be easier with a low-carbohydrate diet. First, the carbohydrate-restricted diet might be simpler to understand – it restricts only carbohydrates, as compared with the low-fat diet, which restricts fat, saturated fat, cholesterol, and calories. In addition, it is fairly easy to restrict carbohydrates to the recommended level simply by focusing on certain foods (i.e., meat, eggs, non-starchy vegetables, and cheese) and avoiding starchy and sugary foods, negating the need to count even carbohydrate grams. Second, compared with a low-fat diet, a carbohydrate-restricted diet may result in less hunger. This satiating effect was demonstrated in many of the studies, in which subjects substantially reduced energy intake despite the instruction to eat low-carbohydrate foods until satiated and to disregard calories [32, 35, 37, 93]. A possible explanation may be the diet's high content of protein, the most satiating of the macronutrients [96]. Finally, subjects might adhere to the diet better because of positive reinforcement from initial weight loss. On the other hand, the fact that carbohydrate restriction has yet to garner widespread acceptance as a healthy option may be an impediment to adherence that other diets do not face and may partially explain why adherence to a low-carbohydrate diet can be low outside of the clinical research setting.

Assessing Dietary Intake

In order to determine what diet modifications are needed, and then whether and to what extent the diet modifications were actually made, an assessment of dietary intake is necessary. In this section, we review various methods which include food records, diet recall, food frequency questionnaires, and biomarkers [97]. Although these methods can be remarkably revealing, clinicians should recognize their limitations, particularly when it comes to accurately portraying calorie intake. When compared against doubly labeled water, an elaborate method used to estimate total energy expenditure, researchers have found that patients typically underestimate energy intake when using diet assessment instruments [98–103]. Moreover, obese patients and patients trying to lose weight may underestimate food intake by a greater amount than do others, and the foods they most often underreport are high-caloric desserts and snack-type foods eaten between meals [98, 99, 101, 104–107].

Food Records

Food records (or a dietary log) are similar to other logs (e.g., blood pressure, blood glucose, sleep habits) recorded by patients to help clinicians monitor clinically important factors as they occur *outside of clinic*. For food records, patients typically write down all food and liquid that they consume over a certain period of time, usually 3–5 days. To be most accurate, patients should document as specific information as possible regarding the type, amount, brand, preparation method, etc., of the food. Data can then be analyzed using computer software aimed toward professionals (e.g., Nutritionist Pro, NutriBase, Food Processor) or toward individual dieters (e.g., DietMaster, Nutrinote, DietPower) to produce estimates of nutrient intake. The USDA also has a Web site where individuals can analyze their diets at no cost via the Internet (www.mypyramidtracker.gov). To increase the accuracy of food records, patients should be advised to include both week and weekend days in their log and trained on what details to record and how to estimate (or measure) portion sizes. Food record forms, instructions, and examples can be found on the Web (e.g., http://www.nhlbi.nih.gov/health/public/heart/obesity/lose_wt/diary.htm; http://www.k-state.edu/lafene/foodrecords.htm); some sites have printouts that patients can refer to when estimating portion sizes, making the task much easier.

An advantage to food records is that multiple days can be recorded so the impact of day-to-day variation is minimized. Another advantage is that it is less cognitively taxing than other methods (e.g., involving recall) and so may produce more accurate estimates. Furthermore, the process of recording what is eaten can increase awareness of food choices and serving sizes, resulting in the accumulation of knowledge that might lead to long-term diet modifications. Conversely, patients may instead adhere to the diet recommendations only during the period they are recording the food intake (i.e., the Hawthorne effect); therefore, food records might not accurately reflect their adherence over longer durations. Other drawbacks include the time required to complete the food records and the necessity of the patient being literate [108].

Twenty-Four-Hour Diet Recall

A typically less burdensome method of diet assessment is the 24-h diet recall, in which patients recall all food and drink consumed over the past 24 h. This can be performed in a few minutes in person during a clinical encounter or over the phone, thereby increasing the convenience to the patient. This method may be the most useful to the clinician because the results are immediately available and can inform treatment plans. Further, if done unannounced, it might be more likely than other methods to identify diet indiscretions. Some disadvantages, which are also common to food records, are that the data may not be representative of dietary patterns over time [108, 109] and that trained personnel may be necessary to obtain the most accurate recording of diet intake. Inaccuracy may occur if patients are not able to recall all foods or portion sizes consumed. Accuracy can be improved by certain techniques that are typically available to dietitians only. A multiple-pass method, which uses five separate approaches to probe the patient about food intake, may help the patient remember foods that might otherwise have been forgotten. Dietitians can also provide pictures or models of foods to demonstrate portion sizes. These methods increase the complexity and duration of the assessment, however, and may still underestimate energy intake by up to 13% [110].

Food Frequency Questionnaire

Food frequency questionnaires (FFQ) ask patients detailed questions about what types and amounts of foods they have eaten, and at what frequencies, over longer, investigator-specified (e.g., 3 months, 1 year) time periods. These instruments can be self-administered by the patient and scored by personnel who do not have a nutrition background or mailed to a company for scoring. They are typically used to determine eating patterns in research subjects who are part of a large population-based sample, rather than to determine adherence to a focused dietary intervention. FFQs should be culturally appropriate for the targeted patients in order to increase accuracy. Advantages to FFQs are that they escape the need for a nutritionally knowledgeable facilitator, which can reduce cost. Moreover, they can help identify eating patterns over a longer period of time than food records or food recall and thus provide a potentially more representative picture of patients' eating habits. Disadvantages are that more comprehensive FFQs can be quite long (100–180 questions) and take more than an hour to complete. Additionally, fairly high levels of health literacy and numeracy are required.

Other Methods

Certain biochemical markers, such as serum or urine measurements, can be used to examine diet adherence. For example, the urinary sodium level can be used to monitor adherence in patients following a low-salt diet [66, 111]. Other examples include urine ketones for ketogenic diets [35, 112], urinary nitrogen for protein intake [111, 113, 114], and various serum vitamin and mineral levels [111, 114–116]. These methods have their own limitations. For instance, urine ketone levels appear to decline over time even in study participants who are strictly following a low-carbohydrate diet [117]. Assessing the fat content of the diet is more difficult and less available clinically; some research studies have examined the fatty acid composition of serum cholesterol esters or fat tissue [118, 119]. Most importantly, no biomarker exists for calorie intake; self-report remains the only assessment method available to the clinician.

Conclusion

Although dietary adherence can be a daily struggle for many people, a number of practical points and strategies can assist clinicians when counseling patients on dietary modifications, including the following:

- recognize that obesity is a chronic disease and that successful treatment often requires lifelong monitoring, therapy, and support, as with any chronic disease;
- help patients to detect and overcome barriers to adherence;
- validate the difficulties patients confront;
- recognize eating disorders and refer patients to the appropriate specialist when needed;
- help patients to incorporate facilitators of dietary adherence into their therapeutic plans;
- develop strategies to help motivate patients into making beneficial changes to their diet;
- have patients design specific goals that describe exactly what they plan to do;
- help patients to choose goals that are not only meaningful but also achievable;
- recognize and congratulate patients for any success at dietary change or weight loss (i.e., positive reinforcement);
- avoid judging or disparaging patients when they are unsuccessful at changing their habits or losing weight.

Recognition of these issues can go a long way toward building a therapeutic alliance with patients and increasing their motivation to initiate and maintain changes. Use of these simple strategies can make the difference between a patient following a diet temporarily with transient health improvement and a patient making a successful lifestyle change leading to sustained improvements in satisfaction and quality of life, decreased morbidity, and increased longevity. Although work still needs to be done to help patients improve dietary adherence, many patients will benefit substantially from an empathic clinician who is informed about existing strategies and is supportive of their efforts.

References

1. Flegal KM, Carroll MD, Kuczmarski RJ, Johnson CL. Overweight and obesity in the United States: prevalence and trends, 1960–1994. *Int J Obes Relat Metab Disord.* 1998;22(1):39–47.
2. Ogden CL, Carroll MD, Curtin LR, McDowell MA, Tabak CJ, Flegal KM. Prevalence of overweight and obesity in the United States, 1999–2004. *JAMA.* 2006;295(13):1549–1555.

3. Nilsson M, Johnsen R, Ye W, Hveem K, Lagergren J. Obesity and estrogen as risk factors for gastroesophageal reflux symptoms. *JAMA*. 2003;290(1): 66–72.

4. Pi-Sunyer FX. Medical hazards of obesity. *Ann Intern Med*. 1993;119(7 Pt 2):655–660.

5. Kenchaiah S, Evans JC, Levy D, et al. Obesity and the risk of heart failure. *N Engl J Med*. 2002;347(5):305–313.

6. National Institutes of Health, National Heart Lung and Blood Institute, North American Association for the Study of Obesity. *The practical guide: Identification, evaluation and treatment of overweight and obesity in adults*. Washington, DC: U.S. Department of Health and Human Services, Public Health Service; 2000. NIH Publication No. 00-4084.

7. McGinnis JM, Foege WH. Actual causes of death in the United States. *JAMA*. 1993;270(18):2207–2212.

8. Mokdad AH, Marks JS, Stroup DF, Gerberding JL. Actual causes of death in the United States, 2000. *JAMA*. 2004;291(10):1238–1245.

9. Kruger J, Galuska DA, Serdula MK, Jones DA. Attempting to lose weight: specific practices among U.S. adults. *Am J Prev Med*. 2004;26(5):402–406.

10. Serdula MK, Mokdad AH, Williamson DF, Galuska DA, Mendlein JM, Heath GW. Prevalence of attempting weight loss and strategies for controlling weight. *JAMA*. 1999;282(14):1353–1358.

11. McCann BS, Retzlaff BM, Dowdy AA, Walden CE, Knopp RH. Promoting adherence to low-fat, low-cholesterol diets: review and recommendations. *J Am Diet Assoc*. 1990;90(10):1408–1414.

12. Methods for voluntary weight loss and control. NIH technology assessment conference panel. Consensus Development Conference, 30 March to 1 April 1992. *Ann Intern Med*. 1993;119(7 Pt 2):764–770.

13. Prochaska JO. *Systems of psychotherapy: A transtheoretical analysis. 2nd Ed*. Pacific Grove, CA: Brooks-Cole; 1984.

14. Jeffery RW, Drewnowski A, Epstein LH, et al. Long-term maintenance of weight loss: current status. *Health Psychol*. 2000;19(1 Suppl):5–16.

15. Kumanyika SK, Van Horn L, Bowen D, et al. Maintenance of dietary behavior change. *Health Psychol*. 2000;19(1 Suppl):42–56.

16. Marcus BH, Dubbert PM, Forsyth LH, et al. Physical activity behavior change: issues in adoption and maintenance. *Health Psychol*. 2000;19(1 Suppl):32–41.

17. Rothman AJ. Toward a theory-based analysis of behavioral maintenance. *Health Psychol*. 2000;19(1 Suppl):64–69.

18. Hertel AW, Finch EA, Kelly KM, et al. The impact of expectations and satisfaction on the initiation and maintenance of smoking cessation: an experimental test. *Health Psychol*. 2008;27(3 Suppl):S197–S206.

19. Fuglestad PT, Rothman AJ, Jeffery RW. Getting there and hanging on: the effect of regulatory focus on performance in smoking and weight loss interventions. *Health Psychol*. 2008;27(3 Suppl):S260–S270.

20. Schwarzer R, Schuz B, Ziegelmann JP, Lippke S, Luszczynska A, Scholz U. Adoption and maintenance of four health behaviors: theory-guided longitudinal studies on dental flossing, seat belt use, dietary behavior, and physical activity. *Ann Behav Med.* 2007;33(2):156–166.

21. Dietary Guidelines Advisory Committee. *Report of the dietary guidelines advisory committee on the dietary guidelines for Americans, 1995.* Washington, DC: US Department of Agriculture, Agricultural Research Services; 1995.

22. NHLBI Obesity Education Initiative. *Clinical guidelines on the identification, evaluation, and treatment of overweight and obesity in adults: The evidence report.* Bethesda, MD: U.S. Department of Health and Human Services, Public Health Service, National Institutes of Health, National Heart, Lung, and Blood Institute; 1998. NIH Publication No. 98-4083.

23. Nielsen SJ, Popkin BM. Patterns and trends in food portion sizes, 1977–1998. *JAMA.* 2003;289(4):450–453.

24. Wadden TA, Brownell KD, Foster GD. Obesity: responding to the global epidemic. *J Consult Clin Psychol.* 2002;70(3):510–525.

25. Willett WC. Low-carbohydrate diets: a place in health promotion? *J Intern Med.* 2007;261(4):363–365.

26. Bloch AS. Low carbohydrate diets, pro: time to rethink our current strategies. *Nutr Clin Pract.* 2005;20(1):3–12.

27. Kushner RF. Low-carbohydrate diets, con: the mythical phoenix or credible science? *Nutr Clin Pract.* 2005;20(1):13–16.

28. Pirozzo S, Summerbell C, Cameron C, Glasziou P. Advice on low-fat diets for obesity. *Cochrane Database Syst Rev.* 2008;3:CD003640.

29. Howard BV, Van Horn L, Hsia J, et al. Low-fat dietary pattern and risk of cardiovascular disease: the Women's Health Initiative Randomized Controlled Dietary Modification Trial. *JAMA.* 2006;295(6):655–666.

30. Prentice RL, Caan B, Chlebowski RT, et al. Low-fat dietary pattern and risk of invasive breast cancer: the Women's Health Initiative Randomized Controlled Dietary Modification Trial. *JAMA.* 2006;295(6):629–642.

31. Beresford SA, Johnson KC, Ritenbaugh C, et al. Low-fat dietary pattern and risk of colorectal cancer: the Women's Health Initiative Randomized Controlled Dietary Modification Trial. *JAMA.* 2006;295(6):643–654.

32. Brehm BJ, Seeley RJ, Daniels SR, D'Alessio DA. A randomized trial comparing a very low carbohydrate diet and a calorie- restricted low fat diet on body weight and cardiovascular risk factors in healthy women. *J Clin Endocrinol Metab.* 2003;88(4):1617–1623.

33. Sondike SB, Copperman N, Jacobson MS. Effects of a low-carbohydrate diet on weight loss and cardiovascular risk factor in overweight adolescents. *J Pediatr.* 2003;142(3):253–258.

34. Foster GD, Wyatt HR, Hill JO, et al. A randomized trial of a low-carbohydrate diet for obesity. *N Engl J Med.* 2003;348(21):2082–2090.

35. Yancy WS, Jr., Olsen MK, Guyton JR, Bakst RP, Westman EC. A low-carbohydrate, ketogenic diet versus a low-fat diet to treat obesity and hyperlipidemia: a randomized, controlled trial. *Ann Intern Med.* 2004;140(10): 769–777.

36. Shai I, Schwarzfuchs D, Henkin Y, et al. Weight loss with a low-carbohydrate, Mediterranean, or low-fat diet. *N Engl J Med.* 2008;359(3): 229–241.

37. Samaha FF, Iqbal N, Seshadri P, et al. A low-carbohydrate as compared with a low-fat diet in severe obesity. *N Engl J Med.* 2003;348(21):2074–2081.

38. Rand CS, Macgregor AM. Morbidly obese patients' perceptions of social discrimination before and after surgery for obesity. *South Med J.* 1990;83(12):1390–1395.

39. Yancy WS, Jr., Olsen MK, Westman EC, Bosworth HB, Edelman D. Relationship between obesity and health-related quality of life in men. *Obes Res.* 2002;10(10):1057–1064.

40. Wooley SC, Garner DM. Obesity treatment: the high cost of false hope. *J Am Diet Assoc.* 1991;91(10):1248–1251.

41. Sheslow D, Hassink S, Wallace W, DeLancey E. The relationship between self-esteem and depression in obese children. *Ann NY Acad Sci.* 1993;699:289–291.

42. Goldstein LT, Goldsmith SJ, Anger K, Leon AC. Psychiatric symptoms in clients presenting for commercial weight reduction treatment. *Int J Eat Disord.* 1996;20(2):191–197.

43. Carpenter KM, Hasin DS, Allison DB, Faith MS. Relationships between obesity and DSM-IV major depressive disorder, suicide ideation, and suicide attempts: results from a general population study. *Am J Public Health.* 2000;90(2):251–257.

44. DiMatteo MR, Lepper HS, Croghan TW. Depression is a risk factor for noncompliance with medical treatment: meta-analysis of the effects of anxiety and depression on patient adherence. *Arch Intern Med.* 2000;160(14): 2101–2107.

45. Smith DE, Marcus MD, Lewis CE, Fitzgibbon M, Schreiner P. Prevalence of binge eating disorder, obesity, and depression in a biracial cohort of young adults. *Ann Behav Med.* 1998;20(3):227–232.

46. Powers PS, Perez A, Boyd F, Rosemurgy A. Eating pathology before and after bariatric surgery: a prospective study. *Int J Eat Disord.* 1999;25(3): 293–300.

47. Rand CS, Macgregor AM, Stunkard AJ. The night eating syndrome in the general population and among postoperative obesity surgery patients. *Int J Eat Disord.* 1997;22(1):65–69.

48. Sherman AM, Bowen DJ, Vitolins M, et al. Dietary adherence: characteristics and interventions. *Control Clin Trials.* 2000;21(5 Suppl): 206S–211S.

49. Morland K, Wing S, Diez Roux A, Poole C. Neighborhood characteristics associated with the location of food stores and food service places. *Am J Prev Med.* 2002;22(1):23–29.

50. Thomas J. Nutrition intervention in ethnic minority groups. *Proc Nutr Soc.* 2002;61(4):559–567.
51. Brownell KD, Cohen LR. Adherence to dietary regimens. 1: an overview of research. *Behav Med.* 1995;20(4):149–154.
52. de Castro JM, de Castro ES. Spontaneous meal patterns of humans: influence of the presence of other people. *Am J Clin Nutr.* 1989;50(2): 237–247.
53. Christakis NA, Fowler JH. The spread of obesity in a large social network over 32 years. *N Engl J Med.* 26 2007;357(4):370–379.
54. The Management of Overweight and Obesity Working Group. VA/DOD clinical practice guideline for screening and management of overweight and obesity. Vol 1.0. Washington, DC: Department of Veterans Affairs, Department of Defense; 2006 http://www.healthquality.va.gov/obesity/obe06_final1.pdf.
55. Puhl RM, Heuer CA. The stigma of obesity: a review and update. *Obesity (Silver Spring).* 2009;17(5):941–964.
56. Kaminsky J, Gadaleta D. A study of discrimination within the medical community as viewed by obese patients. *Obes Surg.* 2002;12(1):14–18.
57. Schwartz MB, Chambliss HO, Brownell KD, Blair SN, Billington C. Weight bias among health professionals specializing in obesity. *Obes Res.* 2003;11(9):1033–1039.
58. Klein D, Najman J, Kohrman AF, Munro C. Patient characteristics that elicit negative responses from family physicians. *J Fam Pract.* 1982;14(5): 881–888.
59. McTigue KM, Harris R, Hemphill B, et al. Screening and interventions for obesity in adults: summary of the evidence for the U.S. Preventive Services Task Force. *Ann Intern Med.* 2003;139(11):933–949.
60. Wadden TA, Foster GD. Behavioral treatment of obesity. *Med Clin North Am.* 2000;84(2):441–461, vii.
61. Digenio AG, Mancuso JP, Gerber RA, Dvorak RV. Comparison of methods for delivering a lifestyle modification program for obese patients: a randomized trial. *Ann Intern Med.* 2009;150(4):255–262.
62. U.S. Preventive Services Task Force. Screening for obesity in adults: recommendations and rationale. *Ann Intern Med.* 2003;139(11):930–932.
63. Wylie-Rosett J, Swencionis C, Ginsberg M, et al. Computerized weight loss intervention optimizes staff time: the clinical and cost results of a controlled clinical trial conducted in a managed care setting. *J Am Diet Assoc.* 2001;101(10):1155–1162; quiz 1163–1154.
64. Urban N, White E, Anderson GL, Curry S, Kristal AR. Correlates of maintenance of a low-fat diet among women in the Women's Health Trial. *Prev Med.* 1992;21(3):279–291.
65. Tinker LF, Perri MG, Patterson RE, et al. The effects of physical and emotional status on adherence to a low-fat dietary pattern in the Women's Health Initiative. *J Am Diet Assoc.* 2002;102(6):789–800, 888.
66. Schmid TL, Jeffery RW, Onstad L, Corrigan SA. Demographic, knowledge, physiological, and behavioral variables as predictors of compliance

with dietary treatment goals in hypertension. *Addict Behav.* 1991;16(3–4): 151–160.

67. Jeffery RW, Bjornson-Benson WM, Rosenthal BS, Lindquist RA, Kurth CL, Johnson SL. Correlates of weight loss and its maintenance over two years of follow-up among middle-aged men. *Prev Med.* 1984;13(2):155–168.

68. Boutelle KN, Kirschenbaum DS. Further support for consistent self-monitoring as a vital component of successful weight control. *Obes Res.* 1998;6(3):219–224.

69. Wing RR, Hill JO. Successful weight loss maintenance. *Annu Rev Nutr.* 2001;21:323–341.

70. Fujimoto K, Sakata T, Etou H, et al. Charting of daily weight pattern reinforces maintenance of weight reduction in moderately obese patients. *Am J Med Sci.* 1992;303(3):145–150.

71. Klem ML, Wing RR, McGuire MT, Seagle HM, Hill JO. A descriptive study of individuals successful at long-term maintenance of substantial weight loss. *Am J Clin Nutr.* 1997;66(2):239–246.

72. Levitsky DA, Garay J, Nausbaum M, Neighbors L, Dellavalle DM. Monitoring weight daily blocks the freshman weight gain: a model for combating the epidemic of obesity. *Int J Obes (Lond).* 2006;30(6):1003–1010.

73. McCann BS, Retzlaff BM, Dowdy AA, Walden CE, Knopp RH. Promoting adherence to low-fat, low-cholesterol diets: review and recommendations. *J Am Diet Assoc.* 1990;90(10):1408–1414, 1017.

74. Pearce JW, LeBow MD, Orchard J. Role of spouse involvement in the behavioral treatment of overweight women. *J Consult Clin Psychol.* 1981;49(2):236–244.

75. Rosenthal B, Allen GJ, Winter C. Husband involvement in the behavioral treatment of overweight women: initial effects and long-term follow-up. *Int J Obes.* 1980;4(2):165–173.

76. Black DR, Lantz CE. Spouse involvement and a possible long-term follow-up trap in weight loss. *Behav Res Ther.* 1984;22(5):557–562.

77. Dubbert PM, Wilson GT. Goal-setting and spouse involvement in the treatment of obesity. *Behav Res Ther.* 1984;22(3):227–242.

78. Glenny AM, O'Meara S, Melville A, Sheldon TA, Wilson C. The treatment and prevention of obesity: a systematic review of the literature. *Int J Obes Relat Metab Disord.* 1997;21(9):715–737.

79. Wing RR, Jeffery RW. Benefits of recruiting participants with friends and increasing social support for weight loss and maintenance. *J Consult Clin Psychol.* 1999;67(1):132–138.

80. Renjilian DA, Perri MG, Nezu AM, McKelvey WF, Shermer RL, Anton SD. Individual versus group therapy for obesity: effects of matching participants to their treatment preferences. *J Consult Clin Psychol.* 2001;69(4): 717–721.

81. Lowe MR, Miller-Kovach K, Phelan S. Weight-loss maintenance in overweight individuals one to five years following successful completion of a commercial weight loss program. *Int J Obes Relat Metab Disord.* 2001;25(3):325–331.

82. Gosselin C, Cote G. Weight loss maintenance in women two to eleven years after participating in a commercial program: a survey. *BMC Womens Health.* 2001;1(1):2.

83. Heshka S, Anderson JW, Atkinson RL, et al. Weight loss with self-help compared with a structured commercial program: a randomized trial. *JAMA.* 2003;289(14):1792–1798.

84. Tsai AG, Wadden TA, Womble LG, Byrne KJ. Commercial and self-help programs for weight control. *Psychiatr Clin North Am.* 2005;28(1):171–192, ix.

85. Womble LG, Wadden TA, McGuckin BG, Sargent SL, Rothman RA, Krauthamer-Ewing ES. A randomized controlled trial of a commercial internet weight loss program. *Obes Res.* 2004;12(6):1011–1018.

86. Gold BC, Burke S, Pintauro S, Buzzell P, Harvey-Berino J. Weight loss on the web: a pilot study comparing a structured behavioral intervention to a commercial program. *Obesity (Silver Spring).* 2007;15(1):155–164.

87. Brehm J. *A theory of psychological reactance.* New York: Academic; 1966.

88. Williams GC, Grow VM, Freedman ZR, Ryan RM, Deci EL. Motivational predictors of weight loss and weight-loss maintenance. *J Pers Soc Psychol.* 1996;70(1):115–126.

89. Mendonca P, Brehm S. Effects of choice on behavioral treatment of overweight children. *J Soc Clin Psychol.* 1983;1(4):343–358.

90. Sbrocco T, Nedegaard RC, Stone JM, Lewis EL. Behavioral choice treatment promotes continuing weight loss: preliminary results of a cognitive-behavioral decision-based treatment for obesity. *J Consult Clin Psychol.* 1999;67(2):260–266.

91. Nordmann AJ, Nordmann A, Briel M, et al. Effects of low-carbohydrate vs low-fat diets on weight loss and cardiovascular risk factors: a meta-analysis of randomized controlled trials. *Arch Intern Med.* 2006;166(3):285–293.

92. Brinkworth GD, Noakes M, Buckley JD, Keogh JB, Clifton PM. Long-term effects of a very-low-carbohydrate weight loss diet compared with an isocaloric low-fat diet after 12 mo. *Am J Clin Nutr.* 2009;90(1):23–32.

93. Gardner CD, Kiazand A, Alhassan S, et al. Comparison of the Atkins, Zone, Ornish, and LEARN diets for change in weight and related risk factors among overweight premenopausal women: the A TO Z Weight Loss Study: a randomized trial. *JAMA.* 2007;297(9):969–977.

94. Dansinger ML, Gleason JA, Griffith JL, Selker HP, Schaefer EJ. Comparison of the Atkins, Ornish, Weight Watchers, and Zone diets for weight loss and heart disease risk reduction: a randomized trial. *JAMA.* 2005;293(1):43–53.

95. Stern L, Iqbal N, Seshadri P, et al. The effects of low-carbohydrate versus conventional weight loss diets in severely obese adults: one-year follow-up of a randomized trial. *Ann Intern Med.* 2004;140(10):778–785.

96. Stubbs J, Ferres S, Horgan G. Energy density of foods: effects on energy intake. *Crit Rev Food Sci Nutr.* 2000;40(6):481–515.

97. Johnson RK. Dietary intake – how do we measure what people are really eating? *Obes Res.* 2002;10(Suppl 1):63S–68S.

98. Schoeller DA, Bandini LG, Dietz WH. Inaccuracies in self-reported intake identified by comparison with the doubly labelled water method. *Can J Physiol Pharmacol.* 1990;68(7):941–949.

99. Bandini LG, Schoeller DA, Cyr HN, Dietz WH. Validity of reported energy intake in obese and nonobese adolescents. *Am J Clin Nutr.* 1990;52(3): 421–425.

100. Livingstone MB, Prentice AM, Strain JJ, et al. Accuracy of weighed dietary records in studies of diet and health. *BMJ.* 1990;300(6726):708–712.

101. Black AE, Prentice AM, Goldberg GR, et al. Measurements of total energy expenditure provide insights into the validity of dietary measurements of energy intake. *J Am Diet Assoc.* 1993;93(5):572–579.

102. Schoeller DA. How accurate is self-reported dietary energy intake? *Nutr Rev.* 1990;48(10):373–379.

103. Schoeller DA. Measurement of energy expenditure in free-living humans by using doubly labeled water. *J Nutr.* 1988;118(11):1278–1289.

104. Prentice AM, Black AE, Coward WA, et al. High levels of energy expenditure in obese women. *Br Med J (Clin Res Ed).* 1986;292(6526): 983–987.

105. Briefel RR, Sempos CT, McDowell MA, Chien S, Alaimo K. Dietary methods research in the third National Health and Nutrition Examination Survey: underreporting of energy intake. *Am J Clin Nutr.* 1997;65(4 Suppl): 1203S–1209S.

106. Lichtman SW, Pisarska K, Berman ER, et al. Discrepancy between self-reported and actual caloric intake and exercise in obese subjects. *N Engl J Med.* 1992;327(27):1893–1898.

107. Poppitt SD, Swann D, Black AE, Prentice AM. Assessment of selective under-reporting of food intake by both obese and non-obese women in a metabolic facility. *Int J Obes Relat Metab Disord.* 1998;22(4): 303–311.

108. Vitolins MZ, Rand CS, Rapp SR, Ribisl PM, Sevick MA. Measuring adherence to behavioral and medical interventions. *Control Clin Trials.* 2000;21(5 Suppl):188S–194S.

109. Forster JL, Jeffery RW, VanNatta M, Pirie P. Hypertension prevention trial: do 24-h food records capture usual eating behavior in a dietary change study? *Am J Clin Nutr.* 1990;51(2):253–257.

110. Jonnalagadda SS, Mitchell DC, Smiciklas-Wright H, et al. Accuracy of energy intake data estimated by a multiple-pass, 24-hour dietary recall technique. *J Am Diet Assoc.* 2000;100(3):303–308; quiz 309–311.

111. Sacks FM, Svetkey LP, Vollmer WM, et al. Effects on blood pressure of reduced dietary sodium and the Dietary Approaches to Stop Hypertension (DASH) diet. DASH-Sodium Collaborative Research Group. *N Engl J Med.* 2001;344(1):3–10.

112. Westman EC. A review of very low carbohydrate diets. *J Clin Outcomes Manage.* 1999;6:36–40.

113. Isaksson B. Urinary nitrogen output as a validity test in dietary surveys. *Am J Clin Nutr.* 1980;33(1):4–5.

114. Bingham SA, Day NE. Using biochemical markers to assess the validity of prospective dietary assessment methods and the effect of energy adjustment. *Am J Clin Nutr.* 1997;65(4 Suppl):1130S–1137S.

115. Bingham SA, Cummings JH. Urine nitrogen as an independent validatory measure of dietary intake: a study of nitrogen balance in individuals consuming their normal diet. *Am J Clin Nutr.* 1985;42(6):1276–1289.

116. Le Marchand L, Hankin JH, Carter FS, et al. A pilot study on the use of plasma carotenoids and ascorbic acid as markers of compliance to a high fruit and vegetable dietary intervention. *Cancer Epidemiol Biomarkers Prev.* 1994;3(3):245–251.

117. Boden G, Sargrad K, Homko C, Mozzoli M, Stein TP. Effect of a low-carbohydrate diet on appetite, blood glucose levels, and insulin resistance in obese patients with type 2 diabetes. *Ann Intern Med.* 2005;142(6):403–411.

118. Sarkkinen ES, Agren JJ, Ahola I, Ovaskainen ML, Uusitupa MI. Fatty acid composition of serum cholesterol esters, and erythrocyte and platelet membranes as indicators of long-term adherence to fat-modified diets. *Am J Clin Nutr.* 1994;59(2):364–370.

119. van Staveren WA, Deurenberg P, Katan MB, Burema J, de Groot LC, Hoffmans MD. Validity of the fatty acid composition of subcutaneous fat tissue microbiopsies as an estimate of the long-term average fatty acid composition of the diet of separate individuals. *Am J Epidemiol.* 1986;123(3):455–463.

120. Streja DA, Boyko E, Rabkin SW. Predictors of outcome in a risk factor intervention trial using behavior modification. *Prev Med.* 1982;11(3):291–303.

121. Dolecek TA, Milas NC, Van Horn LV, et al. A long-term nutrition intervention experience: lipid responses and dietary adherence patterns in the Multiple Risk Factor Intervention Trial. *J Am Diet Assoc.* 1986;86(6): 752–758.

Chapter 4
Medication Adherence

Hayden B. Bosworth

> *Drugs don't work in patients who don't take them.*
>
> US Surgeon General, C. Everett Koop MD

A key component in the management of health-care conditions is the use of prescribed medications. The effectiveness of medications and their long-term benefits depends on adherence to the prescriber's instructions [1]. Adherence is defined as the extent to which people follow the instructions they are given for prescribed treatments [2]; it involves consumer choice and is intended to be non-judgmental, unlike compliance, which reinforces patient passivity and blame. On the other hand, concordance refers to an emerging consultative and consensual partnership between the consumer and their doctor [2]. Medication adherence behavior has been divided into two main concepts, namely adherence and persistence. Although conceptually similar, adherence refers to the intensity of drug use during the duration of therapy, whereas persistence refers to overall duration [3]. Medication non-adherence includes delaying prescription fills, failing to fill prescriptions, cutting dosages, and reducing the frequency of administration.

H.B. Bosworth (✉)
Center for Health Services Research in Primary Care, Durham Veterans Affairs Medical Center; Departments of Medicine, Psychiatry and Behavioral Sciences, School of Nursing, Duke University Medical Center, Durham, NC, USA
e-mail: hayden.bosworth@duke.edu

H. Bosworth (ed.), *Improving Patient Treatment Adherence*,
DOI 10.1007/978-1-4419-5866-2_4,
© Springer Science+Business Media, LLC 2010

Patients frequently do not adhere to essential medications, with substantial consequences to public health [4]. Medication non-adherence is an enormous burden to the world's health-care system. Half of the 3.2 billion annual prescriptions dispensed in the United States are not taken as prescribed [5]. Numerous studies have shown that patients with chronic conditions adhere only to 50–60% of medications as prescribed despite the evidence that medication therapy improves life expectancy and quality of life [6, 7]. These patterns of medication non-adherence are observed in most developed countries [1, 8]. Across different definitions of non-adherence, approximately 50% of patients do not take their prescribed medication as recommended [9–12]. The true rate of non-adherence may be higher as patients with a history of non-adherence are likely underrepresented in outcomes research.

The recognition of the importance of medication adherence has been increasing. A recent World Health Organization report states that because the magnitude of medication non-adherence and the scope of this sequelae are so alarming, more health benefits worldwide would result from improving adherence to existing treatments than any developing new medical treatments [4]. Interventions that stimulate better adherence to essential medications, even slightly, may meaningfully improve public health.

Cost of Medication Non-adherence

Poor adherence leads to considerable morbidity, mortality, and avoidable health-care costs [13–17]. Approximately 125,000 deaths per year in the United States are linked to medication non-adherence [18]. Between 33 and 69% of medication-related hospital admissions in the USA are due to poor adherence [5], with total cost estimates for non-adherence ranging from $100 to 300 billion each year including both direct and indirect costs [13, 16, 19–21]. These trends also apply worldwide [4]. As an example of the cost–benefit of medication adherence, for every additional dollar spent on adhering to a prescribed medication, medical costs would be reduced by $7 for people with diabetes, $5.10 for people with high cholesterol, and $3.98 for people with high blood pressure [1].

In addition to more obvious costs such as health-care expenses, non-adherence may lead to other undesirable outcomes, including patient and physician frustration, misdiagnoses, and in more extreme situations, unnecessary treatment and exacerbation of disease or fatality [22]. In fact, failure to identify and remediate poor adherence often results in intensified pharmacotherapy with increased doses of medication – thus increasing the overall cost of treatment as well as escalating the risk of adverse effects. Moreover, with the rise of performance measures that reward quality based on attainment of treatment targets, such as blood pressure, this reinforces the import of longitudinal medication adherence.

It is important to point out that what seems like a straightforward behavior – taking a pill on a regular schedule – is actually a complex endeavor. Successful pharmacological treatment of any medical condition requires patient adherence in a multiple-step pathway that includes (1) keeping a scheduled appointment with a provider; (2) accepting a prescription for a medication; (3) filling the prescription at a pharmacy; (4) taking the medication as prescribed; (5) maintaining an adequate supply of the medication by refilling the prescription in a timely manner; and (6) returning to the provider for on-going monitoring [5].

Ways to Measure Medication Adherence

Clinicians must frequently rely on their own judgment, but unfortunately demonstrate no better than chance accuracy in predicting the adherence of their patients [23]. Thus, alternative methods for assessing medication adherence other than relying on physicians' recognition are needed. Medication adherence is commonly measured in one of three ways: patient self-report, pharmacy refill records, or use of electronic lids (MEMS caps). These measures are limited by the degree of separation between the time and place of the measurement process from actual behavior. For example, self-report measures of medication adherence rely on patients' perception of their behavior and are subject to recall and reporting bias. Prescription refill records provide the prescribed medication quantity, but do not verify actual dosing or taking of medications [24, 25]. The approach using an electronic device to capture a dosing event and time is often considered the reference (i.e., gold) standard for measuring adherence, but electronic devices may not always precisely capture when or how much of the medication was ingested [24, 26]. Further, the electronic lids may be impractical in clinical practice or research studies because they are expensive.

Clinicians may conduct pill counts or review pharmacy records if available. The former method of assessing patient medication adherence is potentially problematic because apart from being intrusive, it does not give any indication of when the medication was taken or whether it was thrown away and thus may result in overestimation of adherence. Pharmacy refill records may provide a reliable and non-intrusive longitudinal measure of medication adherence. However, it is necessary that all patients obtain their medication from a centralized pharmacy such as the Veterans Administrations or a health maintenance organization in order to keep track of medication refills. In addition, this method of assessing medication adherence requires extensive data-tracking programs.

Data suggest that these measures of medication adherence may be assessing different, but related, concepts that may influence medication adherence. In one study, agreement between medication acquisition as assessed by centralized pill refill and a commonly used four-item measure of self-reported medication adherence (Morisky self-report measure) [27] indicated a significant, but a poor agreement ($\kappa = 0.19$, $p < 0.001$) in a sample of primary care patients with hypertension. However, both pill acquisition (undersupply and oversupply) and self-reported non-adherence were all independently associated with decreased likelihood of blood pressure control after adjusting for each other and patient factors [28]. Thus, measures of pill refill (i.e., medication acquisition) and self-reported adherence appear to provide distinct, complementary information about patients' medication-taking behavior.

A clinically based cut-point of 80% is commonly used to differentiate medication adherence, although skepticism exists about such cut-points because there are very few medications in which a clinically relevant cut-point has been empirically studied [29]. In addition, for some medications such as highly active antiretroviral therapy (HAART), adherence levels need to exceed 80%. Hansen et al. demonstrated that the commonly used cut-point of 80% had a reasonable balance between sensitivity and specificity in studies of adherence in patients with heart failure or hypertension. In addition, they reported that all measures provided similar estimates of overall adherence, although refill and electronic measures were in highest agreement [30].

In general, patients tend to overestimate their medication adherence [31] and unless a patient is not responding to therapy, it may be extremely difficult to identify poor medication adherence. Asking patients about their medication use is often the most practical means of ascertainment, but it is prone to inaccuracy. A key validated question is "Have you missed any pills in the past week?" and any indication of having missed one or more pills signals a problem with low adherence [32]. Compared to pill counts as the reference standard, asking non-responders about their medication adherence using this single question will detect 55% of those with less than complete adherence, with a specificity of 87% [LR+ 4.3 (95% CI 3.1–6.1); LR– 0.51 (95% CI 0.44–0.58)] [23]. The Morisky scale is a commonly used, validated, 4-item self-reported adherence measure that has been shown to be predictive of medication adherence [27, 33]. Other practical measures to assess adherence include watching for those who do not respond to increments in treatment intensity and patients who fail to attend appointments. Additional practical methods include review of pill bottles, and when available, checking on fill dates and pill counts. Finally, simply asking the patients to describe their medication regimen, such as when they take their medication and what they are for, can often be very informative.

Another practical method for identifying poor medication adherence involves awareness of timing. Patient adherence is greatest 5 days prior and 5 days post-appointment with health-care provider and usually tapers off significantly within 30 days – the so-called "white coat adherence" [5]. Physicians should have a heightened awareness of the possibility of poor adherence, but even patients in whom these indicators are absent miss taking medications as prescribed. Thus, poor adherence should always be considered when a patient's condition is not responding to therapy.

A simple and practical method for assessing medication adherence is for physicians to ask patients nonjudgmentally how often they miss doses. Patients generally want to please their physicians and will often say what they think their doctor wants to hear. It can be reassuring to the patient when the physician tells them, "I know it must be difficult to take all your medications regularly. How often do you miss taking them?" This approach makes most patients feel comfortable in telling the truth and facilitates the identification of poor adherence. A patient who admits to poor adherence is generally being candid [34]. Patients should also be asked whether they are having any side effects of their medications, whether they know why they are taking their medications, and what the benefits of taking them are, since these questions can often expose poor adherence to a regimen [27].

Predictors of Medication Non-adherence

The reasons for poor medication adherence are often multifactorial. Non-adherence to medications can be intentional or nonintentional. Intentional non-adherence is an active process whereby the patient chooses to deviate from the treatment regimen [35]. This may be a rational decision procession in which the individual weighs the risks and benefits of treatment against any adverse effects. Unintentional non-adherence is a passive process in which the patient may be careless or forgetful about adhering to the treatment regimen.

Adhering to a medication regimen in the case of a chronic illness like hypertension is a complex behavior. Patients must understand and recall instructions for taking medication, acquire and maintain an appropriate supply of prescribed agents, and take medication in line with instructions on a daily basis. Breakdowns in adherence may occur with any of these steps, be intentional or unintentional [35], and be influenced by myriad of patient, regimen, provider, and health system factors [36–38]. Most of the factors associated with adherence to medication regimens for chronic illness fit within the typology: characteristics of the patient, clinician factors including the patient–provider relationship, health-care factors, and environmental factors.

Patient Factors

Key reasons for non-adherence include adverse effects or other problems with medications, such as poor instructions, poor memory, inability to pay for medications, and poor relationships between patients and health-care providers [2]. Other reasons for non-adherence include polypharmacy, low literacy, depression, and substance abuse. A lack of confidence in the effectiveness of the treatment, being unconvinced of need for treatment because of a denial of the condition or belief that the need for medication went away (e.g., cured), and cost have also been found to be predictors of medication non-adherence [38]. In addition, disease factors such as symptom prominence, response to treatment and treatment regimen factors such as pill burden, regimen complexity, side effects, duration of needed treatment, and dosing are related to medication adherence [39].

Many review and clinical articles have included suggestions to reduce the complexity of the regimen, usually by decreasing the number of doses per day [40, 41]. In some literature, including diabetes, hypertension, and HIV/AIDS, there is strong, consistent evidence that increases in dose frequency and regimen complexity (multiple medications, multiple doses, specific dietary or time requirements) are related to poorer adherence [42]. Adherence is significantly higher among patients taking medications with a once-daily dosing schedule compared to thrice or more frequent dosing. Richter concluded that drugs with a long duration of action and without increasing side effects due to daily dosing are good candidates for a daily dosing schedule based on these drug characteristics. When symptom control is the target of medications, when non-adherence poses a threat due to disease progression or development of drug resistance, or when multiple tablets for disease are required per day, these factors may merit consideration for improved medication adherence and may include the use of fixed combinations of once-daily dosing formulations [43].

The presumed advantages of fixed dose combinations (FDC) are the following: (1) simpler dosage schedule improves adherence and therefore improves treatment outcomes; (2) reduction of inadvertent medication errors; (3) prevents and/or lowers the attainment of antimicrobial resistance by eliminating monotherapy (one drug is never in circulation by itself); (4) reduced drug shortages by simplifying drug handling and therefore lowering the risk of being "out of stock"; (5) procurement, management, and handling of drugs are simplified; and (6) side effects may be reduced by using one drug of the combination for the purpose [44]. The presumed disadvantages of fixed dose combinations are the following: (1) they are sometimes more expensive than separate tables, although not invariably so; (2) there are potential quality problems when medications are combined; and (3) dosing is inflexible and cannot easily be regulated to patients' needs as each patient has unique characteristics such as weight, age, pharmacogenetics, comorbidities [44].

Poor medication adherence is more likely to occur in certain contexts. Medication problems are common in the transition period from hospital discharge to the outpatient setting and often begin at the point of hospital discharge. Makaryus et al. found that less than 50% of patients were able to list all of their medications and even fewer could recount the purpose of their medications at hospital discharge [45]. In addition, Coleman et al. found that medication discrepancies were common, occurring ~15% of the time, and patients with medication discrepancies were two times more likely to be re-hospitalized within 30 days of discharge [46].

Poor adherence is also tied to health inequalities. Even in a national health system, socioeconomically disadvantaged patients are at 3–15 times increased odds for not redeeming a medication that they are prescribed for the first time compared to more socioeconomically advantaged peers [47].

Health literacy, defined as the "ability to understand and act on health information" [48], is one of the primary determinants of comprehension and potentially significant predictor of medication nonadherence. However, over 90 million adult Americans, 39% of the adults in United States, lack the literacy skills to effectively function in the current health-care environment [49] – a number that has not changed significantly in the past 10 years [50]. Low health literacy is found in many different health-care settings [51, 52] and is most common in older patients, those with lower education levels, immigrants, and racial/ethnic minorities [53]. Numeracy, or the ability to understand numbers, is especially critical in the health domain, where understanding or not understanding what numbers mean may have life-altering consequences. Numerical competence is needed to understand and weigh the risks and benefits of treatment, to decipher survival and mortality curves, and to navigate medical insurance forms and informed consent documents [54].

Patients are required to read medical information and comprehend what to do and when to do it. Patients may be required to perform numeric tasks including calculating the number of tablets for a single dose of medicine. They are expected to monitor themselves for both beneficial and adverse effects, know what to do if they miss a dose of medication, and master when, if, and how to obtain refills of their medication [55]. Chronic illnesses often require following an intensive and complex medical regime (medications, daily monitoring, routine physician visits, tests, etc.) such that the adverse consequences of low health literacy may be particularly pronounced and require serious consideration [56]. Methods for screening for health literacy include a number of measures as well as asking patients if they have a problem understanding the written health material.

Clinician Factors

Patients' confusion about a medical regimen and lack of knowledge of their disease state are among the many factors that adversely affect adherence [57, 58]. Ideally, patients would receive necessary information about safe and appropriate medication use when communicating with physicians or pharmacists, but studies indicate that those discussions are often incomplete [59, 60], and frequently forgotten. As a result, patients likely receive some of their education about how to administer and use a medication from the label on the medication bottle [61], which requires a high level of literacy.

Clinician factors such as clear communication and time spent on explaining the disease and the treatment help improve medication adherence. As providers see more patients in less time due to workforce and economic issues [62], the opportunity for effective patient education in the clinic is diminished. For some diseases such as diabetes, it has been shown that patients may be more receptive to education about their disease in a nonclinical setting [63, 64].

Additional clinical factors include patient–clinician relationship factors, such as trust, have been found to be related to medication adherence. Lastly, medication side effects and cost issues that may lead to non-adherence are frequently not discussed with physicians, a communication gap with important quality and safety implications [11, 12].

Health-Care Factors

Health-care delivery factors such as the wait for appointments or medications and convenience of the pharmacy and clinic influence patients' adherence [39]. The WHO report found that the main barriers to adherence related to regimen factors were dose frequency and side effects and emphasized the need for the health system to develop less frequent dosing and to mitigate side effects [65].

Higher drug copayments and three-tier pharmacy plans have been found to reduce adherence to drugs for management of such chronic conditions as diabetes, hypercholesterolemia, hypertension, and schizophrenia [66, 67]. Surveys find cost to be the leading reason why at least elderly patients do not fill prescriptions, skip doses, or take smaller doses, followed by other causes, such as medication adverse effects and beliefs about whether drugs improve health [68].

Environmental Factors

Recent attention has focused on environmental factors as being predictors of medication adherence. Such environmental factors include weather, social support, poverty, migration, and homelessness which have been considered as factors affecting adherence [69, 70].

Review of Successful Interventions to Improve Medication Adherence

A brief overview of successful interventions is provided given that there have been a number of reviews focusing on medication adherence. In the most recent update on the Cochrane review, articles were included if they reported an unconfounded random clinical trial (RCT) involving an intervention to improve adherence with prescribed medications, measured both medication adherence and treatment outcome, with at least 80% follow-up of each group studied and, for long-terms treatments, at least 6-month follow-up for studies with positive findings [71]. For short-term treatments, 4 of 10 interventions reported in nine RCTs showed an effect on both adherence and at least one clinical outcome, while one intervention reported in one RCT significantly improved patient adherence, but did not enhance the clinical outcome. For long-term treatments, 36 of 83 interventions reported in 70 RCTs were associated with improvements in adherence, but only 25 interventions led to improvement in at least one treatment outcome. Almost all of the interventions that were effective for long-term care were complex, including combinations of more convenient care, information, reminders, self-monitoring, reinforcement, counseling, family therapy, psychological therapy, crisis intervention, manual telephone follow-up, and supportive care. Even the most effective interventions did not lead to large improvements in adherence and treatment outcomes.

A review of articles published between 1998 and 2007 examining medication adherence and chronic illness found surprisingly few of these articles concerned with (1) chronic treatment, (2) regimen factors such as dosing, pill burden, and regimen complexity, and (3) adherence measured in a clear manner [42]. A suggestive pattern of the importance of regimen factors, especially dose frequency and regimen complexity, emerged from this review.

In another review of medication adherence in chronic medical conditions that included trials from 1967 to 2004, 37 trials were identified (including 12 informational, 10 behavioral, and 15 combined informational, behavioral, and/or social investigations), 20 reported a significant improvement in at least one adherence measure [72]. Adherence increased most consistently with behavioral interventions that reduced dosing demands (three of three studies with large effect sizes 0.90–1.20) and those involving monitoring and feedback (three of four studies, small to large effect sizes 0.27–0.81). Adherence also improved in six multisession informational trials (small to large effect sizes 0.35–1.13) and eight combined interventions (small to large effect sizes 0.43–1.20). Eleven studies (four informational, three behavioral, and four combined) demonstrated improvement in at least one clinical outcome, but effects were variable (very small to large effect sizes 0.17–3.41) and not consistently related to changes in adherence. The authors concluded that several types of interventions are effective in improving medication adherence in chronic medical conditions, but few significantly affected clinical outcomes.

In a recent meta-analysis investigating the effectiveness of interventions to improve medication adherence in older adults, the investigators identified 33 randomized controlled trials representing 11,827 participants. Interventions significantly improved medication adherence (mean effect size = 0.33), knowledge (effect size = 0.48), and health services utilization (effect size = 0.16). Moderator analyses showed larger adherence effect sizes for interventions employing special medication packaging, dose modification, participant monitoring of medication effects and side effects, succinct written instructions, and standardized (not tailored) interventions. Larger effects were observed for participants taking 3–5 medications and when pill count adherence was measured [73].

As Haynes, McKibbon, and Kanani commented as early as 1996, one would think that studies on the nature of non-adherence and on the effectiveness of strategies to help patients overcome would flourish. On the contrary, little has been published and there are limited recommendations available to improve medication adherence, beyond simplifying patients' regimens when possible. Thus, compared with the many thousands of trials for individual drugs, there are only a handful of rigorous trials of adherence intervention and these provide little evidence that medication adherence can be improved consistently.

In general, there have been reviews of medication adherence, but many of the interventions for long-term medications were exceedingly complex and labor intensive, and there are questions of how these interventions would be carried out in non-research settings, particularly in the current era of cost containment and staff reductions. However, given that the factors influencing medication adherence are many and varied, multifaceted, tailored interventions are necessary to improve self-administration of medication [74, 75]. Interventions are needed to enhance patient education, improve patients' self-treatment behaviors and skills, facilitate the identification and self-administration of patients' medications, and improve monitoring of their medication use [74]. In addition, to these patient-based interventions, other improvements may facilitate the medication use process, such as documentation of patients' adherence patterns and better communications among providers about these adherence patterns.

Evidence does not clearly support one single intervention to optimize medication adherence. In general, educational interventions do not consistently improve medication adherence in adults. Among the educational interventions, tailored interventions that involved ongoing contact with health-care professionals, pharmacists, or lay health mentors as well as an interactive computer-based educational session seemed more effective than interventions with mailed patient educational materials or brief interactions. Interventions that used memory aids and provided cues to improve adherence are somewhat effective, but studies were few in number and additional research is needed. While some strategies, such as time-specific blister packs, could be easily implemented, other strategies involving newer computer-based technologies need to be replicated to be generalizable [76–78]. Interventions that involve monitoring and feedback, as well as informational interventions delivered over multiple sessions, are probably also effective [72].

Methods for Improving Medication Adherence

Methods that can be used to improve adherence can be grouped into four general categories: patient education and behavioral programs, improved dosing schedules, improved communication between physicians and patients, and organizational issues such as increased hours when the clinic is open (including evening hours) and therefore shorter wait times.

Education and Behavioral Programs

Medication adherence in the context of chronic diseases is in many ways three steps. The first step is initiation, followed by adjustment, and then maintenance. Medication adherence management starts with instructing the patient at the initiation of treatment with careful monitoring and support during the early treatment [79, 80]. For patients who require more than one medication, whenever possible, all should be prescribed to be taken at the same time if this is consistent with therapeutic activity. Negotiating a therapy that the patient is able to follow should be a first priority. Besides simplifying the dosing regimen, some examples of ways to tailor the therapy to the individuals' needs include exploring the patients' schedule, beliefs, and preferences, altering the administration route, and using adherence aids [9, 81]. Less attention has been given to the evaluation of strategies that might be effective at maintaining adherence. The maintenance-directed intervention strategies used most consistently have been educational or behavioral in nature.

Adherence problems encountered at the start of treatment or during the course of treatment can be addressed by a five-step problem-solving approach: (1) specifying the problem in concrete terms, (2) identifying possible solutions, (3) developing a plan for implementing the solutions, (4) trying out the solutions, and (5) evaluating the results [80]. The five most common strategies of adherence problems have been identified and clinical management procedures developed for them: (1) the patient lacks knowledge of the disease and its treatment; (2) the patient rejects the diagnosis; (3) the patient rejects the prescribed drug; (4) the patient lacks the skills to establish self-medication as a habit; and (5) the patient engages in frequent self-debate decision to follow prescribed regimen [79].

Educational interventions involving patients, their family members, or both can be effective in improving adherence [82]. Decades of research have confirmed that the social context influences morbidity and mortality [83–85], in part because social support enhances treatment adherence [85–92]. Social support for chronic disease management includes both emotional support (i.e., the provision of empathy, feedback, trust, and love) and instrumental support (i.e., physical care, transportation, finances, and help with errands). Social support includes the involvement of others (family, friends, or coworkers) in the knowledge and treatment of the condition. Social support may be especially important for the self-management of chronic disease, as studies have found marriage is associated with medication adherence [93]. Encouraging patients to access social support can play a significant role in the successful initiation of medication regimen. The goal of social support strategies is to develop an ally who can help ease the behavioral change, reduce obstacles to maintenance, and be supportive during failures and successes. Social support is also crucial to long-term treatment plans that require continuous action on the part of the patient.

Combined use of written and verbal instruction may enhance treatment adherence [94]. Written instructions about the medication regimen should be a core part of every interaction with the patient. Written instructions should use short words and general terms (rather than medical jargon), simple sentence structure, active voice, avoidance of abstract concepts, and use of concrete suggestions.

Return demonstration of information (i.e., how to take pills) is a method to ensure patients understand relevant information. Package inserts are important to individuals for risk/benefit information but often fail to provide benefits of treatment and have little effect on self-reported behavior [95]. It is better to provide limited amounts of materials and these materials should relate to and reinforce what is covered in the visit [96]. Educational programs should be based on an appraisal of each individual's needs rather than relying upon general information for all. Providers must establish what is known before offering the patient new knowledge. Providers should use concrete examples to support or explain concepts.

Behavioral strategies, including self-monitoring, cueing, chaining (associating new behaviors with established ones), positive reinforcement, and patient contracting, have been used to enhance medication adherence [97, 98]. A contingency contract is wherein both providers and patients set forth a treatment goal and the specific obligations of each in attempting to accomplish this goal and a time limit for its achievement. Beyond increasing the likelihood of adherence to medication therapy, contracts offer a written outline of the expected behavior, the involvement of the patient in the decision-making process concerning the regimen and the opportunity to discuss potential problems and solutions with the provider, a formal commitment to the problem from the patient, and rewards which create incentives for adherence goals. Additional strategies include developing prompts and reminder systems, identifying a potential relapse into old behavior, setting appropriate and realistic goals, and rewarding achievement of new behaviors. Maintenance of most behaviors declines over time; constant questioning and follow-up are essential to ensure adequate adherence [31].

Some specific behavior recommendations for medication adherence include (1) using medication-reminder cues and placing medication-taking in their habitual daily routine. The cues can be activities, such as personal toilet, meals, coffee, or bedtime. An example of a physical cue is the medication container placed prominently by one's toothbrush; every time an individual may brush their teeth at night, they will be reminded to take their simvastatin. (2) Patients should receive a written medication description with instructions on starting the prescription.

This includes the drug's name, strength, and form; medical condition treated or purpose; number of doses per day and their time of day; the relationship to food, beverages, and other medications; and any special instructions as potential drug–drug interactions. (3) Patients should be encouraged to maintain a daily medication record of each dose taken or missed with relevant comments. The clinician or health-care extender can review with the patient this medication diary over the telephone or at the next clinic visit.

Goal setting must be implemented as part of the initiation of the treatment regimen. Working toward a goal that is specific, attainable, and proximal in time heightens self-efficacy and promotes behavioral change. A time frame should be included in the goals (e.g., in 2 weeks or at the time of the next visit in 4 weeks). Telephone contacts may be used to review progress toward the goal when the patient is not seen on a frequent basis. When the goal is attained, reinforcement is provided for the success, and the next level of the goals is set. When the patient is unsuccessful in attaining the behavior, the provider can encourage the patient to continue.

Several ethical issues must be addressed when considering and attempting to improve patient adherence to medication regimens [99]. First, the treatment being prescribed must be of known efficacy for this diagnosis and appropriate for the patient's circumstances. Second, methods for helping the patient to follow the treatment must be of established effectiveness. Third, in the end, the patient's right to refuse treatment must be respected.

Dosing Schedules

Strategies to improve dosing schedules include the use of pillboxes to organize daily doses, simplifying the regimen to daily dosing, and cues to remind patients to take medications. There is increasing number of products being introduced into the market to assist individuals with organizing their medications. A fundamental component of all these devices is the knowledge of how to initially organize their medications. Thus, for those with cognitive impairments or children, pillboxes may not be appropriate. In addition, newer medications are coming onto the market that are either combination medications or require less frequently using because of longer half lives. However, typically these medications are more costly and less likely to be covered by insurance. In terms of the combination medications there is also a need to be cautious regarding over medicating.

Patient–Provider Communication

Enhancing communication between the physician and the patient is a key and effective strategy in boosting the patient's ability to follow a medication regimen [100, 101]. However, education and training of medical personnel in adherence diagnosis and management is not always readily available in the current medical education. Authoritative text books on general medicine, medical therapies, pharmacology, and patient interviewing do not typically address adherence and its management. Drug industry publications for health-care professionals occasionally have brief descriptions of the rudiments of adherence management. Most clinicians learn adherence management by self-instruction from clinical experience. A variety of medical-care personnel can be trained to assist clinicians as effective adherence counselors, including nurses, physician's assistants, dietitians, psychologists, and non-degreed office staff.

Behaviors such as a provider making direct eye contact, transmitting interest in what the patient says, explaining recommendations thoroughly and clearly, praising treatment adherence and problem solving, and expressing willingness to modify the treatment plan in accordance with the patient's concerns have been demonstrated as ways to promote adherence [102]. Additional methods to improve the interaction of the provider with patients include expressing empathy and acceptance through the use of active listening and reflective responses. Providers should also resist entering into conflict with the patient and avoid the imposition of values or beliefs onto the patient.

Patients should be provided with a clear rationale for the necessity of a particular treatment and their concerns should be elicited and addressed. To ensure that the necessary information has been understood, key instructions should be provided both verbally and in written form, asking the patients to verify that they understand the instructions [103]. Common misperceptions should be anticipated and avoided, including that the medication can be stopped when the prescription runs out or the condition comes under control, that different medications cannot be taken together at the same time of the day, and that symptoms are guides to when to take the medication. In addition, use of medical jargon is likely to leave patients feeling disengaged and devoid of responsibility for their care.

Organizational Issues

Missing appointments is correlated with lower adherence rates to prescribed regimens and is the first sign of dropping out of care entirely, the most severe form of non-adherence. Appointment reminders by letter or telephone provide a relatively easy method to overcome this problem, by contacting patients to keep appointments and by contacting patients immediately if appointments are missed. Calling patients who miss appointments is logically the most important method of helping patients adhere to prescribed regimens, because reminding or recalling patients is effective and relatively inexpensive [104] and dropping out of care results in total non-adherence to prescribed medications. Additional organizational factors include making follow-up visits convenient and efficient for the patient. Delays in seeing patients and problems with transportation and parking can undermine a patient's willingness to adhere with a medication regimen and to keep follow-up appointments.

For health-care systems in which pharmacy records are readily available, a review of the refill frequency and the date of the last refill may also help identify non-adherence. Once medication non-adherence is recognized, care providers and patients can work collaboratively to develop patient-specific solutions to address non-adherence barriers.

Conclusion

While medication non-adherence is prevalent and a significant barrier to quality health care, enhancing medication adherence requires a combination of appropriate educational, behavioral, and communication strategies. The notion that the provider is solely responsible for the patient's behavior and outcome is no longer tenable in the United States health-care system.

Anticipating the most common adverse events as well as when they are likely to occur and what can be done to ameliorate them can also improve medication adherence. It is useful to ask patients what they already know and believe about the medications before and after explaining these points. The simplest adherence management available to clinician is a time efficient, problem-solving process based on questioning the patient. The process aims to determine if an adherence problem is present, to define the problem, and to design and test a solution by collaborative negotiation with the patient. Asking the patient open-ended questions to describe their adherence practices starts the process and the search for adherence problems. The questions must be asked in a manner that is non-judgmental and non-threatening to gain the patient's trust and truthfulness. Usually the patient's answers provide information which quickly makes the next logical question obvious to the clinician. The major obstacle to adherence management is getting the process started. To facilitate the start, some suggested questions directed to the patient are frequently cited: "Please describe for me how you remember to take your medicine." "Many patients find it difficult to take their medicine regularly. Do you ever miss or forget to take your medicine?" "What do you think you could do to solve the problem of missing doses?" "Are there any future events that may interfere with taking your medication, and how do you plan to cope?"

Medication treatment adherence must be addressed on several levels, including the patient, the provider, and the health-care system. Patients need the knowledge, attitude, and skills to follow an appropriately prescribed regimen [74]. Similarly, providers need to follow established guidelines in prescribing regimen; ensure that patients understand the reason for the prescribed drugs and possible side effects, the interactions with other agents, and the manner in which the drug is to be taken; and ensure that the recommended regimen is as simple as possible. Finally, the system or organization within which providers work needs to provide resources and set policies that support optimal practices, particularly prevention-oriented activities [105].

The importance of recognizing and improving medication adherence continues to draw more attention as the cost of medications continues to increase, advances in medication treatment for various diseases continues, and the use of these medications increases as the population ages (Table 4.1).

Table 4.1 Summary of medication adherence recommendations

Recommendations	
Patient	Patient education on the disease and treatment is essential as well as understanding the methods for taking the medication, contraindications, and side effects
	Identifying medication non-adherence – key validated question is "Have you missed any pills in the past week?" and any indication of having missed one or more pills signals a problem with low adherence [32].
	Combined use of written and verbal instruction may enhance treatment adherence
	Behavioral strategies, including self-monitoring, cueing, chaining, positive reinforcement, patient contracting, goal setting
Provider	Improving training of health-care providers to identify and treat medication non-adherence
	Focus on methods for communication (e.g., clear communication, development of treatment plan, make direct eye contact)
	Provide clear rationale for treatment and assess concerns
	Instructions should be provided verbally and written – "teach back" methods should be considered
	Common misperceptions should be anticipated and avoided
	Medication adherence involves three steps: initiation, alteration, maintenance
	Shared decision making
	Simplify medication regimen whenever possible
	Involve family members when ever possible
Organizational	Missed appointments is a clear indicator of poor adherence
	Review of the refill frequency and the date of the last refill if centralized medical records
	Use of team approach and/or health-care extenders related to improved medication adherence

References

1. Sabate E. *Adherence to long-term therapies: Evidence for action.* Geneva, Switzerland: World Health Organization; 2003.
2. Haynes RB, Yao X, Degani A, Kripalani S, Garg A, McDonald HP. Interventions to enhance medication adherence. *Cochrane Database Syst Rev.* 2005;4:CD000011.

3. Cramer JA, Roy A, Burrell A, Fairchild CJ, Fuldeore MJ, Ollendorf DA, et al. Medication compliance and persistence: terminology and definitions. *Value Health*. 2008;11(1):44–47.

4. World Health Organization. *Adherence to long-term therapies: Evidence for action*. Geneva: World Health Organization; 2003.

5. Osterberg L, Blaschke T. Adherence to medication. *N Engl J Med*. 2005;353(5):487–497.

6. Benner JS, Glynn RJ, Mogun H, Neumann PJ, Weinstein MC, Avorn J. Long-term persistence in use of statin therapy in elderly patients. *JAMA*. 2002;288(4):455–461.

7. Avorn J, Monette J, Lacour A, Bohn RL, Monane M, Mogun H, et al. Persistence of use of lipid-lowering medications: a cross-national study. *JAMA*. 1998;279(18):1458–1462.

8. Balkrishnan R. The importance of medication adherence in improving chronic-disease related outcomes: what we know and what we need to further know. *Med Care*. 2005;43(6):517–520.

9. Feldman R, Bacher M, Campbell N, Drover A, Chockalingam A. Adherence to pharmacologic management of hypertension. *Can J Public Health*. 1998;89(5):I16–I18.

10. Flack J, Novikov, SV, Ferrario CM. Benefits of adherence to antihypertensive drug therapy. *Eur Soc Cardiol*. 1996;17(Suppl A):16–20.

11. Mallion JM, Baguet JP, Siche JP, Tremel F, de Gaudemaris R. Compliance, electronic monitoring and antihypertensive drugs. *J Hypertens Suppl*. 1998;16(1):S75–S79.

12. Haynes RB, McKibbon KA, Kanani R. Systematic review of randomised trials of interventions to assist patients to follow prescriptions for medications. *Lancet*. 1996;348(9024):383–386.

13. McDonnell PJ, Jacobs MR. Hospital admissions resulting from preventable adverse drug reactions. *Ann Pharmacother*. 2002;36(9):1331–1336.

14. Rodgers PT, Ruffin DM. Medication nonadherence–Part I: the health and humanistic consequences. *Manag Care Interface*. 1998;11(8):58–60.

15. Schiff GD, Fung S, Speroff T, McNutt RA. Decompensated heart failure: symptoms, patterns of onset, and contributing factors. *Am J Med*. 2003;114(8):625–630.

16. Senst BL, Achusim LE, Genest RP, Cosentino LA, Ford CC, Little JA, et al. Practical approach to determining costs and frequency of adverse drug events in a health care network. *Am J Health Syst Pharm*. 2001;58(12):1126–1132.

17. Ho PM, Rumsfeld JS, Masoudi FA, McClure DL, Plomondon ME, Steiner JF, et al. Effect of medication nonadherence on hospitalization and mortality among patients with diabetes mellitus. *Arch Intern Med*. 2006;166(17):1836–1841.

18. McCarthy R. The price you pay for the drug not taken. *Bus Health* 1998;16:27–33.

19. National Council on Patient Information and Education. Enhancing prescription medication adherence: a national action plan http://www.talkaboutrx. org/documents/enhancing_prescription_medicine_adherence.pdf. Accessed 6/2/2008.

20. Berg JS, Dischler J, Wagner DJ, Raia JJ, Palmer-Shevlin N. Medication compliance: a healthcare problem. *Ann Pharmacother*. 1993;27(9 Suppl): S1–S24.
21. Levy G, Zamacona MK, Jusko WJ. Developing compliance instructions for drug labeling. *Clin Pharmacol Ther*. 2000;68(6):586–591.
22. DiMatteo MR, Giordani PJ, Lepper HS, Croghan TW. Patient adherence and medical treatment outcomes: a meta-analysis. *Med Care*. 2002;40(9): 794–811.
23. Stephenson BJ, Rowe BH, Haynes RB, Macharia WM, Leon G. Is this patient taking the treatment as prescribed? *JAMA*. 1993;269(21): 2779–2781.
24. Choo PW, Rand CS, Inui TS, Lee ML, Cain E, Cordeiro-Breault M, et al. Validation of patient reports, automated pharmacy records, and pill counts with electronic monitoring of adherence to antihypertensive therapy. *Med Care*. 1999;37(9):846–857.
25. Steiner JF, Prochazka AV. The assessment of refill compliance using pharmacy records: methods, validity, and applications. *J Clin Epidemiol*. 1997;50(1):105–116.
26. Rosen MI, Rigsby MO, Salahi JT, Ryan CE, Cramer JA. Electronic monitoring and counseling to improve medication adherence. *Behav Res Ther*. 2004;42(4):409–422.
27. Morisky E, Green, LW, Levine, DM. Concurrent and predictive validity of a self-reported measure of medication adherence. *Med Care*. 1986;24:67–74.
28. Thorpe C, Bryson CL, Maciejewski, ML, Bosworth, HB. Medication acquisition and self-reported adherence in veterans with hypertension. *Med Care*. 2009;47(4): 474–481.
29. Morgan AL, Masoudi FA, Havranek EP, Jones PG, Peterson PN, Krumholz HM, et al. Difficulty taking medications, depression, and health status in heart failure patients. *J Card Fail*. 2006;12(1):54–60.
30. Hansen RA, Kim MM, Song L, Tu W, Wu J, Murray MD. Comparison of methods to assess medication adherence and classify nonadherence. *Ann Pharmacother*. 2009;43(3):413–422.
31. Dunbar-Jacob J, Dwyer K, Dunning EJ. Compliance with antihypertensive regimen: a review of the research in the 1980s. *Ann Behav Med*. 1991;13(1):31–39.
32. Haynes RB, McDonald HP, Garg AX. Helping patients follow prescribed treatment: clinical applications. *JAMA*. 2002;288(22):2880–2883.
33. Shalansky SJ, Levy AR, Ignaszewski AP. Self-reported Morisky score for identifying nonadherence with cardiovascular medications (September). *Ann Pharmacother*. 2004;38(9):1363–1368.
34. Stephenson BJ, Rowe BH, Haynes RB, Macharia WM, Leon G. The rational clinical examination. Is this patient taking the treatment as prescribed? *JAMA*. 1993;269(21):2779–2781.
35. Lowry KP, Dudley TK, Oddone EZ, Bosworth HB. Intentional and unintentional nonadherence to antihypertensive medication. *Ann Pharmacother*. 2005;39(7–8):1198–1203.

36. Bosworth HB, George LK, Hays JC, Steffens DC. Psychosocial and clinical factors as predictors of the outcome of unipolar depression. *Int J Geriatr Psychiatry.* 2002;17(3):238–246.

37. Bosworth HB, Olsen MK, Oddone EZ. Improving blood pressure control by tailored feedback to patients and clinicians. *Am Heart J.* 2005;149(5): 795–803.

38. Bosworth HB. Medication adherence. In: Bosworth HB. OE, Weinberger M, eds. *Patient treatment adherence: Concepts, interventions, and measurement.* Mahwah, NJ: Lawrence Erlbaum Associates; 2006.

39. Ickovics JR, Meisler AW. Adherence in AIDS clinical trials: a framework for clinical research and clinical care. *J Clin Epidemiol.* 1997;50(4):385–391.

40. Haynes RB, McDonald H, Garg AX, Montague P. Interventions for helping patients to follow prescriptions for medications. *Cochrane Database Syst Rev.* 2002;2:CD000011.

41. McDonald HP, Garg AX, Haynes RB. Interventions to enhance patient adherence to medication prescriptions: scientific review. *JAMA.* 2002;288(22):2868–2879.

42. Ingersoll KS, Cohen J. The impact of medication regimen factors on adherence to chronic treatment: a review of literature. *J Behav Med.* 2008;31(3):213–224.

43. Richter A, Anton SE, Koch P, Dennett SL. The impact of reducing dose frequency on health outcomes. *Clin Ther.* 2003;25(8):2307–2335; discussion 6.

44. Seedat YK. Fixed drug combination in hypertension and hyperlipidaemia in the developing world. *Cardiovasc J Afr.* 2008;19(3):124–126.

45. Makaryus AN, Friedman EA. Patients' understanding of their treatment plans and diagnosis at discharge. *Mayo Clin Proc.* 2005;80(8):991–994.

46. Coleman EA, Mahoney E, Parry C. Assessing the quality of preparation for posthospital care from the patient's perspective: the care transitions measure. *Med Care.* 2005;43(3):246–255.

47. Wamala S, Merlo J, Bostrom G, Hogstedt C, Agren G. Socioeconomic disadvantage and primary non-adherence with medication in Sweden. *Int J Qual Health Care.* 2007;19(3):134–140.

48. McCray AT. Promoting health literacy. *J Am Med Inform Assoc.* 2005;12:152–163.

49. Institute of Medicine. *Health literacy. A prescription to end confusion.* Washington, DC: National Academies Press; 2004.

50. United States Department of Education. *National assessment of adult literacy: A first look at the literacy of America's adults in the 21st century.* Washington, DC: National Center for Education Statistics; 2005.

51. Gazmararian JA, Baker DW, Williams MV, Parker RM, Scott TL, Green DC, et al. Health literacy among Medicare enrollees in a managed care organization. *JAMA.* 1999;281(6):545–551.

52. Williams M, Parker, RM., Baker, DW, et al. Inadequate functional health literacy among patients at two public hospitals. *J Am Med Assoc.* 1995;274(21):1677–1682.

53. Wilson FL, Racine E, Tekieli V, Williams B. Literacy, readability and cultural barriers: critical factors to consider when educating older African Americans about anticoagulation therapy. *J Clin Nurs.* 2003;12(2):275–282.

54. Nelson W, Reyna VF, Fagerlin A, Lipkus I, Peters E. Clinical implications of numeracy: theory and practice. *Ann Behav Med.* 2008;35(3):261–274.

55. Gazmararian JA, Williams MV, Peel J, Baker DW. Health literacy and knowledge of chronic disease. *Patient Educ Couns.* 2003;51(3):267–275.

56. Parker RM, Gazmararian JA. Health literacy: essential for health communication. *J Health Commun.* 2003;8(Suppl 1):116–118.

57. Mehta S, Moore RD, Graham NM. Potential factors affecting adherence with HIV therapy. *AIDS.* 1997;11(14):1665–1670.

58. Isaac IM, Tamblyn RM. Compliance and cognitive function: a methodological approach to measuring unintentional errors in medication compliance in the elderly. *Gerontologist.* 1993;33:772–781.

59. Tarn DM, Heritage J, Paterniti DA, Hays RD, Kravitz RL, Wenger NS. Physician communication when prescribing new medications. *Arch Intern Med.* 2006;166(17):1855–1862.

60. Svarstad BL, Bultman DC, Mount JK. Patient counseling provided in community pharmacies: effects of state regulation, pharmacist age, and busyness. *J Am Pharm Assoc* 2004;44(1):22–29.

61. Shrank WH, Avorn J. Educating patients about their medications: the potential and limitations of written drug information. *Health Aff (Millwood).* 2007;26(3):731–740.

62. Lee PP, Hoskins HD, Jr., Parke DW, 3rd. Access to care: eye care provider workforce considerations in 2020. *Arch Ophthalmol.* 2007;125(3):406–410.

63. Simmons D, Rush E, Crook N. Development and piloting of a community health worker-based intervention for the prevention of diabetes among New Zealand Maori in Te Wai o Rona: Diabetes Prevention Strategy. *Public Health Nutr.* 2008;11(12):1318–1325.

64. Simmons D, Voyle J, Rush E, Dear M. The New Zealand experience in peer support interventions among people with diabetes. *Fam Pract.* 2009:1–9.

65. Organization WH. *Adherence to long-term therapies: Evidence for action.* Geneva: World Health Organization; 2003.

66. Paez KA, Zhao L, Hwang W. Rising out-of-pocket spending for chronic conditions: a ten-year trend. *Health Aff (Millwood).* 2009;28(1):15–25.

67. Solomon MD, Goldman DP, Joyce GF, Escarce JJ. Cost sharing and the initiation of drug therapy for the chronically ill. *Arch Intern Med.* 2009;169(8):740–748; discussion 8–9.

68. Safran DG, Neuman P, Schoen C, Kitchman MS, Wilson IB, Cooper B, et al. Prescription drug coverage and seniors: findings from a 2003 national survey. *Health Aff (Millwood).* 2005; Suppl Web Exclusives:W5-152-W5-66.

69. Balint S, O'Donnell R. Beyond compliance. *Occup Health Saf* (Waco, Tex.) 2007;76(6):104, 6–7.

70. Misra A, Ganda OP. Migration and its impact on adiposity and type 2 diabetes. *Nutrition* (Burbank, Los Angeles County, California). 2007;23(9):696–708.

71. Haynes RB, Ackloo E, Sahota N, McDonald HP, Yao X. Interventions for enhancing medication adherence. *Cochrane Database Syst Rev.* 2008(2):CD000011.
72. Kripalani S, Yao X, Haynes RB. Interventions to enhance medication adherence in chronic medical conditions: a systematic review. *Arch Intern Med.* 2007;167(6):540–550.
73. Conn VS, Hafdahl AR, Cooper PS, Ruppar TM, Mehr DR, Russell CL. Interventions to improve medication adherence among older adults: meta-analysis of adherence outcomes among randomized controlled trials. *Gerontologist.* 2009;49(4):447–462.
74. Miller N, Hill, MN, Kottke T, Ockene IS. The multilevel compliance challenge: recommendations for a call to action. A statement for healthcare professionals. *Circulation.* 1997;95:1085–1090.
75. Hill MN, Miller NH. Compliance enhancement. A call for multidisciplinary team approaches. *Circulation.* 1996;93(1):4–6.
76. Schlenk EA, Bernardo LM, Organist LA, Klem ML, Engberg S. Optimizing medication adherence in older patients: a systematic review. *J Clin Outcomes Manag.* 2008;15(12):595–606.
77. Russell CL, Conn VS, Jantarakupt P. Older adult medication compliance: integrated review of randomized controlled trials. *Am J Health Behav.* 2006;30(6):636–650.
78. van Eijken M, Tsang S, Wensing M, de Smet PA, Grol RP. Interventions to improve medication compliance in older patients living in the community: a systematic review of the literature. *Drugs Aging.* 2003;20(3):229–240.
79. Russel M. *Behavioral counseling in medicine: Strategies for modifying at-risk behavior.* New York, NY: Oxford; 1986.
80. Taylor CB, Miller, NH. The behavioral approach. In: Wenger NK, Weinstein HK, eds. *Rehabilitation of the coronary patient.* New York, NY: Churchill Livingstone; 1992:461–471.
81. Heyscue BE, Levin GM, Merrick JP. Compliance with depot antipsychotic medication by patients attending outpatient clinics. *Psychiatr Serv.* 1998;49(9):1232–1234.
82. Patton K, Meyers J, Lewis BE. Enhancement of compliance among patients with hypertension. *Am J Manag Care.* 1997;3(11):1693–1698.
83. Berkman LF. Assessing the physical health effects of social networks and social support. *Ann Rev Public Health.* 1984;5:413–432.
84. Cohen S. Social relationships and health. *Am Psychol.* 2004;59(8):676–684.
85. DiMatteo MR. Social support and patient adherence to medical treatment: a meta-analysis. *Health Psychol.* 2004;23(2):207–218.
86. McCann BS, Retzlaff BM, Dowdy AA, Walden CE, Knopp RH. Promoting adherence to low-fat, low-cholesterol diets: review and recommendations. *J Am Diet Assoc.* 1990;90(10):1408–1414.
87. Bovbjerg VE, McCann BS, Brief DJ, Follette WC, Retzlaff BM, Dowdy AA, et al. Spouse support and long-term adherence to lipid-lowering diets. *Am J Epidemiol.* 1995;141(5):451–460.

88. Catz SL, Kelly JA, Bogart LM, Benotsch EG, McAuliffe TL. Patterns, correlates, and barriers to medication adherence among persons prescribed new treatments for HIV disease. *Health Psychol*. 2000;19(2):124–133.

89. Sherbourne CD, Hays RD, Ordway L, DiMatteo MR, Kravitz RL. Antecedents of adherence to medical recommendations: results from the medical outcomes study. *J Behav Med*. 1992;15(5):447–468.

90. Ogedegbe G, Harrison M, Robbins L, Mancuso CA, Allegrante JP. Barriers and facilitators of medication adherence in hypertensive African Americans: a qualitative study. *Ethn Dis*. 2004;14(1):3–12.

91. Molassiotis A, Nahas-Lopez V, Chung WY, Lam SW, Li CK, Lau TF. Factors associated with adherence to antiretroviral medication in HIV-infected patients. *Intern J STD AIDS*. 2002;13(5):301–310.

92. Voils C, Steinhauser K, McCant F, Oddone E, Bosworth HB. *Understanding adherence to blood pressure-lowering regimens: A qualitative study of facilitators and barriers*. Baltimore, MD: Health Services Research and Development National Meeting; 2005.

93. Kopjar B, Sales AE, Pineros SL, Sun H, Li YF, Hedeen AN. Adherence with statin therapy in secondary prevention of coronary heart disease in veterans administration male population. *Am J Cardiol*. 2003;92(9):1106–1108.

94. Pratt J, Jones, JJ. Noncompliance with therapy: an ongoing problem in treating hypertension. *Prim Cardiol*. 1995;21:34–38.

95. Urquhart J. Correlates of variable patient compliance in drug trials: relevance in the new health care environment. *Adv Drug Res*. 1995;26:237–257.

96. Sivarajan ES, Newton KM, Almes MJ, Kempf TM, Mansfield LW, Bruce RA. Limited effects of outpatient teaching and counseling after myocardial infarction: a controlled study. *Heart Lung*. 1983;12(1):65–73.

97. Haynes R, Sackett DL, Gibson ES, Taylor DW, Hackett BC, Roberts RS, Johnson AL. Improvement of medication compliance in uncontrolled hypertension. *Lancet*. 1976;1:1265–1268.

98. Bailey WC, Richards JM, Jr., Brooks CM, Soong SJ, Windsor RA, Manzella BA. A randomized trial to improve self-management practices of adults with asthma. *Arch Intern Med*. 1990;150(8):1664–1668.

99. Levine RJ. Monitoring for adherence: ethical considerations. *Am J Respir Crit Care Med*. 1994;149(2 Pt 1):287–288.

100. Ciechanowski PS, Katon WJ, Russo JE, Walker EA. The patient-provider relationship: attachment theory and adherence to treatment in diabetes. *Am J Psychiatry*. 2001;158(1):29–35.

101. Alexander SC, Sleath B, Golin CE, Kalinowski CT. Patient-provider communication. In: Bosworth HB, Oddone EZ, Weinberger M, eds. *Patient treatment adherence: Concepts, interventions, and measurement*. Mahwah, NJ: Lawrence Erlbaum Associates; 2006:329–372.

102. Bender BG. Overcoming barriers to nonadherence in asthma treatment. *J Allergy Clin Immunol*. 2002;109(6 Suppl):S554–S559.

103. Horne R. Patients' beliefs about treatment: the hidden determinant of treatment outcome? *J Psychosom Res*. 1999;47(6):491–495.

104. Yusuf S, Sleight P, Pogue J, Bosch J, Davies R, Dagenais G. Effects of an angiotensin-converting-enzyme inhibitor, ramipril, on cardiovascular events in high-risk patients. The heart outcomes prevention evaluation study investigators. *N Engl J Med*. 2000;342(3):145–153.
105. Haynes RB, Montague P, Oliver T, McKibbon KA, Brouwers MC, Kanani R. Interventions for helping patients to follow prescriptions for medications. *Cochrane Database Syst Rev*. 2000;2:CD000011.

Chapter 5
Smoking Cessation and Adherence

Lesley Rohrer, Brigid Lynn, Mike Hill, Laura J. Fish, and Lori A. Bastian

Introduction

This chapter addresses the problem of adherence to smoking cessation. Several types of interventions targeting smokers have been successful at promoting cessation. In this review, we will provide examples of successful interventions for primary and secondary prevention and provide recommendations to improve adherence to smoking cessation among patients in their clinical practice.

Statement of the Problem

Cigarette smoking is the leading cause of preventable death in the USA. It is known to cause cancer, heart disease, peripheral vascular disease, and chronic pulmonary disease. According to estimates, 25% of adults in the USA continue to smoke despite awareness of the causal association between smoking and disease [1]. Smoking cessation

L.A. Bastian (✉)
Center for Health Services Research in Primary Care, Durham Veterans Affairs Medical Center; Cancer Prevention, Detection and Control Research Program, Duke Comprehensive Cancer Center, Duke University Medical Center; Department of Medicine, Duke University Medical Center, Durham, NC, USA
e-mail: basti001@mc.duke.edu

H. Bosworth (ed.), *Improving Patient Treatment Adherence*,
DOI 10.1007/978-1-4419-5866-2_5,
© Springer Science+Business Media, LLC 2010

confers appreciable reductions in risk for cancer and cardiovascular disease, with risk reduced to that of a nonsmoker within 12 months post-cessation [1, 2]. Thus, encouraging smoking cessation is necessary to reduce incidence rates of cancer and other smoking-related health outcomes.

Smoking cessation has also been shown to reduce disease severity in patients diagnosed with cardiovascular disease and cancer. Among patients with coronary heart disease, a meta-analysis has found a 36% reduction in mortality for those who quit smoking compared to those who continued to smoke [3]. For patients who have been smokers and who experience a cardiac event, quitting reduces the risk of a recurrent event by 50% [4]. Yet, only 42% of current smokers hospitalized with heart disease report receiving counseling about smoking cessation [5].

Similarly, quitting smoking after cancer diagnosis decreases the number and severity of complications as well as risk for tumor progression and the development of a second primary cancer [6]. Patients with cancer who stop smoking have improved survival and quality of life [7]. This relationship holds true even for late stage cancer patients [8]. Although some clinicians may presume that smoking cessation may be an unreasonable burden for cancer patients [9], stopping smoking contributes to improved physical functioning and increased quality of life and enhances oncology treatment for these patients [10, 11].

Some patient populations are motivated to stop smoking and are reasonably successful. A cardiovascular event such as a myocardial infarction, bypass surgery, or stroke among smokers is associated with significant cessation rates immediately after hospitalization but adherence rates are less impressive. Studies have shown 50–60% quit rates at 6 months for patients who are advised to quit after having a heart attack [12, 13]. Among smokers hospitalized for heart disease, a stepped-care intervention that included starting with a low-intensity intervention and then exposing treatment failures to successively more intense intervention demonstrated cessation rates of 53% compared to 42% for the minimal intervention group [14]. However, this differential effect was not statistically significant at the 1-year follow-up survey (39 vs. 36% cessation rates). Even among smokers admitted to a hospital for serious heart disease events, up to 70% start smoking again within a year [15].

The prevalence of smoking and cessation rates are notably different by socioeconomic indicators. In fact, smoking prevalence rates are increasing in low-income, less educated, minority, and adolescent populations [16]. Smoking prevalence is almost three times higher among women who have only 9–11 years of education (33%) than among women with college graduation or more years of education (11%) [17]. Finally, blacks may begin smoking at a later age and are less likely to quit smoking than whites [18].

Despite the highest prevalence of smoking occurring among patients with substance abuse [19], schizophrenia [19], and alcoholism [20], these individuals have low rates of cessation. Compared with non-alcoholics, individuals with a history of alcoholism report higher levels of nicotine dependence and are generally less likely to stop smoking following cessation interventions [21, 22]. Several have proposed that this is related to the comorbidity of alcohol dependence and depression [23]. Schizophrenic patients also have high rates of smoking (58–88%) and are often nicotine-dependent smokers who have great difficulty with cessation [24]. These groups require more pharmacotherapy-based research.

A meta-analysis was performed to examine whether history of depression is associated with failure to quit smoking [25]. No difference in either short-term or long-term abstinence was observed between smokers with or without a history of depression [26]. These results are in contrast to smokers with current depression. Glassman et al. reported a quit rate of 14% for study subjects meeting criteria for major depression, whereas 31% of subjects without depression successfully quit [27]. Depressed smokers appear to experience more withdrawal symptoms on quitting, are less likely to be successful at quitting, and are more likely to relapse [28]. Nicotine replacement therapy (NRT) may be particularly important prior to initiating a quit attempt among individuals with depression.

To review, an estimated 70% of adult smokers want to quit smoking [29] yet adherence to smoking cessation (abstinence rates) is relatively low in the general population and very low in special populations that have very high rates of smoking. Overall, rates of 6- and 12-month abstinence are 8–27% in the more successful interventions and 0–19% for control groups [30]. Although relapse is the most frequent outcome of cessation, with reported rates as high as 83–89% depending on the intervention, understanding the factors associated with relapse is complicated.

Interventions

Examples of Methods Used in Successful Programs

Interventions that combine physician recommendation, generic self-help guides, tailored print materials, telephone counseling, and pharmacotherapy have been shown to increase the likelihood of smoking cessation when compared to control groups or generic self-help guides alone [31]. Quit rates for these programs are modest, ranging from 6 to 26%, with multi-component interventions achieving the highest cessation rates.

Physician Recommendation

The unique role of the primary care physician in enhancing smoking cessation is obvious. More than 75% of smokers have contact with their physician each year [32]. Thus physicians have enormous potential opportunities to counsel their patients regarding cessation. And, it has been well established that physicians can have a significant effect on the smoking behavior of their patients [33, 34]. Simple advice by one's physician to stop smoking is more effective than no advice at all, and the effectiveness of physicians' advice increases with the "dose" of the intervention (ranging from 50 s to 15 min of counseling) [35, 36]. A single 3-min physician counseling session produces a cessation rate of about 10% at 1 year [35]. Involving two or more health-care providers (e.g., physician, nurse, pharmacist) can raise the cessation rate to about 20% [35]. Follow-up phone calls from office staff and individualized letters signed by a physician have been shown to improve cessation rates [35].

In 2000 (and revised in 2008), the US Public Health Service released a clinical practice guideline for promoting smoking cessation that called on health-care providers to follow a 5A protocol: *A*sk about smoking at every visit; *A*dvise all tobacco users to quit; *A*ssess willingness to make a quit attempt; *A*ssist the patient in quitting (i.e., helping set a quit date, referring to a special program, and prescribing pharmacotherapy tailored to their addiction level and habits); and *A*rrange a follow-up contact within 1 week after quit date to provide further assistance [31, 35]. Although the majority of smokers are identified at clinic visits and report receiving advice during these visits, effective smoking cessation assistance such as counseling and pharmacotherapy are generally underutilized [37]. In a recent study of 4,000 smokers in nine HMOs, smokers were more often offered Advice (77%) than Assist (33–41%) and Arrange (13%) [38]. In this study, smokers who used classes/counseling or pharmacotherapy (Assist) were twice as likely to quit compared with smokers not using these services.

Because the 5A protocols are not highly utilized in primary care, several modified protocols have been recommended [39]. Clinics could implement standardized 5A protocols that do not rely on physicians and can be administered by nursing or administrative staff. For example, at check in, a patient could receive Ask, Advise, and Refer [40]. A member of the health-care team could send an e-mail to the patient with links to Internet-based smoking cessation programs or offer to provide ongoing e-mail support [41].

Generic Self-Help Guides

Self-help cessation programs that can include printed cessation guides and nicotine replacement therapies are used and preferred by the majority of smokers who are trying to quit [42]. These modalities enable individuals to engage in the cessation process at their own pace and to avoid the logistical barriers of group-based programs. Additionally, these modalities can be proactively provided to smokers who are not motivated to quit and likely would not seek assistance to do so [43]. Self-help guides can offer information and specific skills needed to quit smoking and be developed to be appropriate for specific target groups (e.g., those with low reading levels, older smokers, African Americans) [44]. Thus, self-help interventions are recommended for widespread dissemination by the Agency for Healthcare Research and Quality (AHRQ).

The majority of smokers quit on their own, without the help of a physician or therapist [45]. Therefore, smoking cessation materials that smokers can use on their own have the potential to reach a large number of smokers in a cost-effective manner. The purpose of self-help interventions is to provide a structured approach to smoking cessation without the need for person to person contact. Self-help interventions, in the form of written materials, videotapes, audiotapes, or

Web-based programs, have the potential to bridge the gap between the clinical approach to smoking cessation oriented toward individuals and public health approaches that target populations [43]. Self-regulatory skills required to withstand the urge to smoke, however, may be better learned and retained through face-to-face contact than through the simple modeling offered by self-help materials [46].

Self-Help Interventions with Tailoring

There is increasing evidence that tailoring self-help materials to individual characteristics increase the effectiveness of the materials [47]. According to Skinner et al., "tailored print communications have demonstrated an enhanced ability to attract notice and readership ... are more effective than non-tailored communications for influencing health behavior change ... (and) can be an important adjunct to other intervention components" [48].

"Tailoring" begins with the development of message objectives, the translation of those objectives into message elements (e.g., text, illustrations, and graphic design characteristics) and assignment of the elements to participant variables (e.g., relationship to patient, stage of readiness to quit). Individual responses to questionnaires are used to select relevant message elements from the computer-based library of possible text and graphical pieces. Using word processing packages, clip art, and a high-grade color printer, these graphics and text are placed into a graphical layout to yield a highly customized printed health communication.

Etter et al. conducted a randomized trial among a sample of 2,000 daily smokers in French-speaking Switzerland to test the effectiveness of a computer-tailored smoking cessation program as compared to a usual care control group [49]. The outcome measure was self-reported abstinence (no puff of tobacco in the last 4 weeks) at 7 months after enrollment. The intervention consisted of an eight-page tailored counseling letter, tailored to the stage of readiness for smoking cessation, level of nicotine dependence, attitudes toward smoking, self-efficacy, and previous quit experience, and two 16-page booklets corresponding to the stage of readiness for smoking cessation. Self-reported abstinence was 2.6 times greater in the intervention group than in the control group (5.8 vs. 2.2%, $p < 0.001$). In multivariate analysis, significant predictors of cessation were participation in the program, a previous quit attempt in the past year, greater level of stage of readiness to quit, and nicotine dependence. The authors concluded that the program was effective among smokers in a general population, including smokers typically resistant to change such as pre-contemplators and heavy smokers [49].

Shiffman et al. evaluated the efficacy of the Committed Quitters Program (CQP), a computer-tailored set of printed behavioral support materials offered free to purchasers of the NicoDerm CQ patches, which comes with a users' guide and audiotape [50]. Callers to the CQP enrollment were randomized to either receive the users' guide or CQP. CQP consisted of 3–5 mailings over a 10-week period. The materials included a calendar booklet, two tri-fold brochures, a newsletter, and an award certificate. The materials were tailored on demographics, smoking history, motives for quitting, expected difficulties quitting, and potential high-risk situations. Abstinence and use of program materials were assessed by telephone interview at 6 and 12 weeks. Overall, abstinence rates did not differ significantly between the two groups. However, participants who reported using the program materials (80% of the sample) were more likely to report quitting at 6 weeks (38.8 vs. 30.7%) and 12 weeks (18.2 vs. 11.1%) than the users' guide group. The authors concluded that the CQP program was an effective behavioral treatment, improving quit rates over nicotine replacement therapy and brief non-tailored materials.

Strecher reviewed 10 trials that examined the effectiveness of tailored print communications as compared to standard materials for smoking cessation [51]. In the majority of studies, tailored materials had a significant impact ($p < 0.01$) and an additional study found significant improvements in cessation rates for light and moderate smokers. Among pre-contemplators, significant positive movement through stages of readiness was noted.

Telephone Counseling

Telephone counseling is a cost-effective intervention that broadens the reach of health interventions by efficiently providing individual assistance to a large population, including those in isolated communities [52, 53]. Telephone counseling may be proactive, in which one or more calls are initiated by the counselor, or it may be reactive in which a smoker calls a quit-line or a help-line. Smokers may access proactive counseling by calling a help-line and scheduling calls with a counselor who will contact them at an established time [54]. Telephone counseling may serve as the main intervention or as an adjunct to face-to-face counseling or nicotine replacement therapy [54].

A meta-analysis of trials comparing proactive counseling as the main intervention or as a supplement to self-help materials to a less intensive intervention found telephone counseling increases quit rates by 60% [54]. Proactive counseling is particularly effective when it supplements self-help materials as it encourages the use of self-help materials and recommended quitting strategies [52–56]. Orleans et al. found that telephone counseling increased quit rates and adherence to the quitting protocol included in the self-help materials given to the smokers [56]. The counseling had a long-term effect on smoking cessation that was evident at both an 8-month and a 16-month follow-up. Counseling also increased the number of serious quit attempts made, and non-quitters reported a greater mean reduction in daily nicotine intake. Borland et al. also found that telephone counseling facilitated smoking cessation as compared to those who only received self-help materials [52]. The counseling increased quit attempts and reduced the rate of relapse for those who did quit.

Multiple telephone calls are more effective than single telephone counseling calls, and the flexibility of telephone counseling allows for the counseling calls to be scheduled according to the needs of the recipient [53, 54]. Zhu et al. examined the effectiveness of multiple and single session phone calls to a control group that received a smoking quit kit [57]. Multiple session counseling calls had higher quit rates than single session calls, and both counseling interventions had higher abstinent rates than the control group. The phone calls for the multiple session intervention were structured so that three of the five calls occurred during the first week post-quit attempt. This relapse-sensitive schedule fostered accountability and provided additional social support for the quitter when needed the most. Zhu et al. also found a dose–response relation between the number of calls and abstinence rates which was achieved by reducing the relapse rates [57]. It may be beneficial to exploit the flexibility of telephone counseling calls and schedule calls when the risk of relapse is highest and the needs of the quitter may be the greatest [52, 54, 57, 58].

Proactive telephone counseling is most effective as a main intervention. The calls encourage use of self-help materials, adherence to quitting protocols, and they initiate changes [53]. Successful interventions involve multiple phone calls that take advantage of the flexibility of telephone counseling and schedule the calls when they are most needed [54].

Nicotine Replacement Therapy (NRT)

Pharmacotherapy is a safe and effective treatment for nicotine dependence [35, 59]. It is recommended that NRT be considered a part of treatment for every smoker unless pregnant or breastfeeding, the smoker is an adolescent or smokes less than 10 cigarettes a day, or there is a medical contraindication such as uncontrolled high blood pressure or prior allergic reaction to the product [35]. By replacing the nicotine from cigarettes, NRT effectively relieves withdrawal symptoms and reduces the urge to smoke, which facilitates behavior modification [17, 59]. The US Department of Health and Human Services identifies nicotine gum, nicotine inhaler, nicotine lozenge, nicotine nasal spray, nicotine patch, bupropion SR, and varenicline as first-line medications in the treatment of nicotine dependence [31].

A meta-analysis of the effectiveness of the gum, patch, nasal spray, nasal inhaler, and nicotine lozenges found all forms of NRT to be significantly more effective than placebo in achieving abstinence [59]. NRT increased long-term quit rates 1.5- to 2-fold [59]. The 2 mg nicotine gum (nicotine polacrilex) improves long-term abstinence rates 30–80% compared to placebo [35]. For the most dependent smokers, the 4 mg gum is more effective than the 2 mg gum [17, 59]. Meta-analysis of the transdermal nicotine patch found that smokers who used the patch were more than twice as likely to quit smoking as were those who wore a placebo patch [60]. The nicotine inhaler and nicotine nasal spray both double the long-term abstinence rates when compared to placebo [35]. Abstinence rates after 12 months for smokers using nasal spray and inhaler were 24 and 17%, respectively [59]. Compared to placebo, use of nicotine lozenges to stop smoking resulted in 2.1–3.7 greater odds of being abstinent after 6 weeks and abstinence was maintained 1 year after quitting [61]. Silagy et al. found 20% of smokers who used the lozenge were abstinent after 12 months [59].

Sustained release bupropion is the first non-nicotine medication approved by the FDA for smoking cessation [35]. Studies examining the effectiveness of bupropion indicate that bupropion increases 12-month smoking abstinence twofold compared to placebo [62]. Results from one study associates bupropion with higher quitting rates than the nicotine patch [63]. Bupropion is considered an effective therapy for relapsed smokers and for smokers with a history of depression, as well as preventative treatment in smokers who have successfully quit [62, 63]. In an actual practice setting (Group Health Cooperative) the combination of bupropion and minimal or moderate counseling was associated with 1-year quit rates of 24 and 33% [64]. In one study, bupropion combined with NRT increased quit rates compared to single therapies [65].

Varenicline stimulates dopamine release which reduces nicotine cravings and withdrawal symptoms. The drug also blocks nicotine receptors which may reduce the pleasurable effects of continued nicotine usage. The pooled results of two identically designed randomized double blind studies showed varenicline resulted in significantly higher abstinence rates at the end of 12 weeks of treatment compared to both placebo and bupropion SR [66]. The increased rate of abstinence remained present at a 52-week follow-up. These results demonstrated the odds of quitting smoking using varenicline increased almost four-fold compared to placebo, and twofold compared to bupropion SR [66]. A new warning was recently added to the varenicline label noting an increased risk of neuropsychiatric symptoms associated with the usage of varenicline [67]. These neuropsychiatric symptoms include agitation, depressed mood, suicidal ideation and behavior, and worsening of preexisting psychiatric conditions [67].

A comparison of the nicotine gum, patch, spray, and inhaler found no difference in effects on withdrawal symptoms or abstinence rates [68]. Abuse liability of the NRTs plus the lozenge is also demonstrated to be low [69]. The nicotine patch diffuses nicotine through the skin at a constant rate and it is recognized as the easiest form of NRT to use [17, 59, 68]. The patch is effective whether worn 16 or 24 h/day, and there is no evidence that weaning from treatment is better than abrupt withdrawal [60]. Hajek et al. found that the patch had the highest adherence rates compared to the gum, spray, and inhaler which were used less than the recommended amount [68]. The nasal spray has the fastest nicotine delivery; however, 75–100% of smokers who use the spray experience adverse effects [61, 68]. For smokers who prefer acute oral administration of nicotine, but find the spray and inhaler irritating or feel uncomfortable with chewing gum, the lozenge may also be an effective form of NRT [61]. Table 5.1 summarizes currently approved first-line medications for treating tobacco use [31, 70–72].

Examples of Novel Intervention Methods

Family Support Interventions

The initiation, maintenance, and cessation of smoking are strongly influenced by family members and close contacts [73]. Several studies have shown that support from the spouse or a friend is predictive of smoking cessation [74–77]. In particular, positive support, such as expressing pleasure at the smoker's efforts to quit, predicts cessation [76, 78]. Unfortunately, negative behaviors, such as complaining about smoking, are predictive for smoking relapse [79, 80]. Positive behaviors can be taught and have been successfully incorporated in telephone-based interventions [81, 82]. In a recent meta-analysis of support interventions [73, 83], interventions that enhance positive partner support were most effective when implemented with live-in or married partners. In an observational study of patients with head and neck cancers, positive family member support was associated with smoking cessation [84]. This finding suggests that the effectiveness of a smoking cessation intervention in chronically ill patients may be enhanced if it also involves the patient's relatives in the smoking cessation program.

Internet Interventions

The Internet can be accessed 24 h a day from almost anywhere including home, work, libraries, and even coffee shops and airports. The easy access from anywhere and by anyone makes the Internet a cost-effective and efficient method to provide smoking cessation information to large numbers of smokers. Numerous smoking cessation programs are available on the Internet today including sites supported

Table 5.1 First-line medications for treating tobacco use

Pharmacologic therapy	Advantages	Disadvantages	Possible side effects	Dose and cost[a]
Nicotine patch	Available over the counter and by prescription May reduce morning cravings when worn overnight Few side effects	No method available to temporarily increase nicotine delivery to deal with cravings	Skin irritation Dizziness Tachycardia Insomnia Headache Nausea Vomiting Muscle aches and stiffness	7 mg patch, $37 per box 14 mg patch, $47 per box 21 mg patch, $48 per box
Nicotine gum	Sold over the counter Flexible dosing schedule Faster nicotine delivery compared to the patch	Frequent use is required (under dosing is common)	Bad taste Mouth/throat irritation Hiccups Nausea Jaw pain Tachycardia	2 mg gum, $48 per box of 100–170 4 mg gum, $63 per box of 100–110

Table 5.1 (continued)

Pharmacologic therapy	Advantages	Disadvantages	Possible side effects	Dose and cost[a]
Nicotine lozenge	Sold over the counter Flexible dosing schedule Faster nicotine delivery compared to the patch	Frequent use is required (under dosing is common)	Sleep problems Nausea Hiccups Heartburn Coughing Headache Flatulence	2 mg lozenge, $34 per box of 72 lozenges 4 mg lozenge, $39 per box of 72 lozenges
Nicotine inhaler	Flexible dosing schedule Faster nicotine delivery compared to the patch Mimics hand to mouth action of smoking	Frequent use is required (under dosing is common) Available only by prescription	Coughing Throat irritation Upset stomach	10 mg cartridges $196 per box of 168 cartridges
Nicotine nasal spray	Flexible dosing schedule Fastest delivery of nicotine among NRTs	NRT with highest potential for habit forming use Frequent use is required (under dosing is common) Available only by prescription	Nasal/throat irritation Runny nose Watery eyes Sneezing Coughing	$49 per bottle (approximately 100 doses)

Table 5.1 (continued)

Pharmacologic therapy	Advantages	Disadvantages	Possible side effects	Dose and cost[a]
Varenicline	Reduces pleasure associated with smoking Reduces withdrawal symptoms	Available only by prescription May exacerbate existing psychiatric illnesses	Headache Nausea Vomiting Insomnia Unusual dreams Changes in taste Flatulence Depressed mood Suicidal ideation Suicide Changes in behavior	1 mg $131 per month
Bupropion SR	Can be used alone or with nicotine replacement therapy	Available only by prescription Contraindicated in patients with history of seizure, eating disorder, and those taking an MAO inhibitor	Insomnia Dry mouth	150 mg twice a day $97 per month (generic); $197 to $210 per month (brand name)

[a]Except where indicated, rate of use determines how long supplies will last

by the American Lung Association (www.lungusa.org), the National Cancer Institute (smokefree.gov), and the US Department of Health and Human Services Office on Women's Health (www.4woman. gov/QuitSmoking). These Web-based smoking cessation programs, as well as the many others that are available, may be comprised of a step-by-step cessation guide, instant messaging, support communities, links to other online resources, and information regarding local, state, and national telephone quitlines. Enrollment in these programs is easy and anonymous, and smokers are allowed to progress at their own rate and visit the intervention site as often or as little as they like. Multiple contacts can be made with the smoker via email and assistance may be personalized to meet the needs of the smoker [85].

Despite the numbers of Web-based smoking cessation programs available today, there is little information about the effectiveness of these programs [85–87]. Bessell et al. systematically reviewed 10 health-related comparative studies that used the Internet to deliver an intervention [88]. One smoking cessation program was included in the review. While there was evidence that the Internet may be a useful and cost-effective intervention method, they concluded that considerable research needs to be done to determine the impact of Internet use on health outcomes [88]. Both Feil et al. and Lenert et al. developed and evaluated an Internet smoking cessation program and both found encouraging results in the behavior of the smokers that suggest that the Internet may be useful in smoking cessation programs [85, 87]. Lenert et al. suggest that e-mail may be used to supplement and enhance Web-based materials [85]. Future Internet interventions may examine the impact of tailoring e-mail messages to promote smoking cessation.

There are several problems inherent in evaluating the Web-based smoking cessation programs. The anonymity of the Internet-based programs may be part of the appeal to smokers; however, it makes it challenging to track participants; requesting specific identification from smokers may influence the decision to participate and thus bias the sample [87]. E-mail may be used to assist with tracking participants; however, it is easy to change an e-mail address as well as to ignore messages [85, 87]. The anonymity of participants as well as the ease of using the Internet may pose a problem to a thorough evaluation of Web-based programs as it is difficult to verify that participants are not utilizing other alternative Web sites or obtaining additional information elsewhere [87].

Telephone Quitlines

Telephone smoking cessation programs called quitlines (such as the ones available in the USA by calling 1-800-QUIT-NOW) have recently been implemented and are being evaluated [31]. Smoking cessation services such as the ones provided by 1-800-QUIT-NOW include working with a trained counselor to develop a personalized quit smoking plan, coping strategies, information, and support. The services are free to use and are available to anyone with access to a telephone [89]. At least some contacts are initiated by quitline counselors, including call-back counseling [31].

Proactive quitlines are shown to be effective in increasing abstinence rates compared to little or no intervention [31, 90, 91]. There is evidence of dose–response, with odds of quitting increasing with three or more sessions [90]. Quitlines used in conjunction with medication are more effective than using medication alone [31].

Clinical and Research Implications

As expressed throughout the chapter, smoking cessation adherence is difficult and physicians play an important role in the smoking cessation process. Physicians often work in high-demand situations with time constraints and, consequently, may hesitate to engage in a more in-depth smoking cessation intervention [92]. The 5As are a quick and effective resource to help physicians facilitate the smoking cessation process [31].

While the 5As are a great technique for patients interested in quitting, not every smoker may be interested in giving quitting a try. Motivational interviewing (MI) techniques may be particularly helpful and beneficial for physicians when patients express hesitation or reluctance to quit smoking.

The guiding principle behind MI is that each individual possesses both the potential for change and the resourcefulness to accomplish that change. Individuals often feel ambivalent about change and can become trapped in a cycle of harmful behavior. The role of the motivational interviewer is to help the individual overcome his/her ambivalence about change through a collaborative approach so that natural change processes can occur [93].

Motivational interviewing often has a large impact in a small amount of time [93]. Most smokers have thought about quitting and motivational interviewing focuses on these behavior change thoughts. Using a few basic motivational interviewing techniques has the potential to shift the patient's focus from continuing to smoke to arguing for smoking cessation. The focus shift may lead to increased motivation and self-efficacy and therefore increasing smoking cessation attempts and adherence. Table 5.2 outlines practical ways a physician may combine the 5As techniques with motivational interviewing to address smoking cessation with a patient [31, 71].

Summary

Stopping smoking prolongs life and reduces morbidity. With one-quarter of the population continuing to smoke and rising rates of smoking initiation in adolescents, more interventions need to be developed and disseminated broadly. Research is needed to evaluate both short-term and long-term cessation rates and to better understand the factors contributing to relapse. The presence of multiple smokers in a household not only contributes to relapse but also exposes vulnerable children to passive smoking [94, 95]. From a public health perspective, more emphasis needs to be placed on the negative effects of passive smoking.

To date, the most successful interventions (cessation rates over 50%) incorporate multiple components (tailored print materials, telephone counseling, and NRT) and target special populations such as those with a recent diagnosis of heart disease or cancer [13, 96, 97]. Future interventions can attempt to promote cessation among specific target groups by utilizing multi-component interventions.

Clearly, physicians and other health-care providers play an important role in the campaign against smoking. Despite this enormous potential many physicians do not follow clinical recommendations to counsel based on the 5A model [38]. Time and lack of reimbursement are major obstacles to integrating smoking cessation services. Novel ways to provide these services in a busy office practice are being explored and may include the use of federally funded centralized counseling services (quitlines) such as those provided by the American Cancer Society and National Cancer Institute.

Table 5.2 Practical uses of 5 A's and motivational interviewing for physicians

5 A's defined	Example questions and statements
Ask – screen all patients for tobacco use	*"Do you currently smoke cigarettes?"*
Advise – to quit	*"Because of your medical history, it is important that you quit smoking."*
Assess – willingness to quit	**Assess motivation to quit:** • The assessment of motivation can be completed during an office visit using a motivation scale: *"On a scale from 0 to 10 where 0 is not motivated at all and 10 is extremely motivated, how motivated are you to quit smoking?"* **Goals of "Assess" for a patient willing to quit smoking with MI-based examples:** • *Counseling (include information on NRT and self-help resources):* *"You rated yourself a … on the scale, quitting must be important to you. What is motivating you to quit smoking?"* *"You said … is a big motivator for you to quit smoking and you rated your motivation as high. What do you think about getting some information that might help you out with the quitting process?"* • *Schedule follow-up:* *"Based on our conversation today it seems like you are motivated and ready to take some action and move forward in your quitting process. We covered a lot of information today, so let's make an appointment to talk again in the next 2 weeks to check in and see what is working best for you."* **Goals of "Assess" for a patient unwilling to quit smoking with MI-based examples:** • *Explore unwillingness to quit smoking:* Likes/dislikes: *"You rated yourself a … on the motivation scale, quitting smoking right now seems like it would be a tough challenge for you to take on. What are some of the things you like about smoking? You mentioned you like … now what are a few things you don't like about smoking?"*

Table 5.2 (continued)

5 A's defined	Example questions and statements
	Advantages/disadvantages: "*What are some of the good things about smoking? Some of the good things about smoking are ... now tell me some of the less good things about smoking.*"
	"*Based on our brief conversation, it sounds like smoking is integrated into your life and it would be tough to quit. At the same time there are some things you don't like about smoking. Next time we see each other we will check in again and see what has been influencing your smoking behavior.*"
Assist – with quitting	**Setting a quit date:**
	• Within 2 weeks of the office visit or counseling sessions
	Goals of "Assist" with MI-based examples:
	• Check in on motivation and smoking cessation information from previous "*Assess*" appointment
	"*It has been a little while since we last talked, what has happened with your quitting process since then?*"
	• *Explore support/encouragement*
	"*Support from family and friends is often helpful for people during the quitting process and also for staying quit. What do the people around you do that you find most supportive and encouraging?*"
	• *Identify triggers/alternatives to smoking*
	"*As we have already discussed, some aspects of quitting are challenging. When do you find it most challenging to not smoke? What do you do to get past a particularly tough craving for a cigarette?*"
	• *Discuss benefits and side effects of NRT and non-nicotine medication for smoking cessation*
	"*You mentioned that sometimes you . . . to get past a tough craving to smoke. How has the NRT you chose to try out working? What about the NRT works best for you? What reactions have you had while using the NRT, both good and bad?*"

Table 5.2 (continued)

5 A's defined	Example questions and statements

Arrange – follow-up contact within 1 week	**Follow-up:**
	• Within the first week or two of the quit date
	• A second follow-up a month later
	• Follow-ups can be completed via telephone, email, or in person
	Goals of "Arrange" with MI-based examples:
	• *Assess progress:*
	  "Tell me what's been going on with your quitting process since last time we talked."
	
	• *Congratulate success:*
	  "Quitting is a process, often a difficult one, and any progression forward is a big step as far as quitting is concerned. You have been extremely successful by . . . which takes a great deal of strength and hard work."
	
	• *Difficult situations, relapse, and moving forward:*
	  "What have you found most difficult in your quitting process? . . . has been challenging for you, what have you previously done to make it more or less difficult? What do you think would help you take on this particular challenge in your quitting process?"
	
	• *NRT:*
	  "What has been your experience thus far using (NRT type)? It sounds like . . . is working well? It sounds like . . . is not working well, tell me more about what has been going on. We have . . . as other NRT options. What might work best for you?"

References

1. ACS. *Facts and figures 2000*. Atlanta, GA: American Cancer Society; 2000.
2. Peto R, Darby S, Deo H, et al. Smoking, smoking cessation, and lung cancer in the UK since 1950: combination of national statistics with two case-control studies. *Br Med J*. 2000;321:323–329.
3. Critchley J, et al. Smoking cessation for the secondary prevention of coronary heart disease. [Update in *Cochrane Database Syst Rev*. 2004;1:CD003041; PMID: 14974003]. *Cochrane Database Syst Rev*. 2003;4:CD003041.
4. Miller M, et al. *The practice of coronary disease prevention*. Baltimore, MD: Williams & Williams; 1996.
5. Houston TK, et al. Post-myocardial infarction smoking cessation counseling: associations with immediate and late mortality in older Medicare patients. *Am J Med*. 2005;118(3):269.
6. Lerman C, et al. Treating tobacco dependence: state of the science and new directions. *J Clin Oncol*. 2005;23(2):311–323.
7. Garces YI, et al. The relationship between cigarette smoking and quality of life after lung cancer diagnosis.[see comment]. *Chest*. 2004;126(6):1733–1741.
8. Ebbert JO, et al. Duration of smoking abstinence as a predictor for non-small-cell lung cancer survival in women. *Lung Cancer*. 2005;47(2):165–172.
9. Davison AG, et al. Smoking habits of long-term survivors of surgery for lung cancer. *Thorax*. 1982;37:331–333.
10. Gritz ER, et al. Smoking cessation in cancer patients: never too late to quit. In: Given B, Given CW, Champion V, et al., eds. *Evidence-based Cancer Care and Prevention*. New York, NY: Springer; 2003.
11. Gritz ER, et al. Smoking, The missing drug interaction in clinical trials: ignoring the obvious. *Cancer Epidemiol Biomarkers Prev*. 2005;14(10):2287–2293.
12. DeBusk R, Houston M, Superko H, et al. A case management system for coronary risk factor modification after acute MI. *Ann Intern Med*. 1994;120: 721–729.
13. Ockene J, Kristeller J, Goldberg R, et al. Smoking cessation and severity of disease: the coronary artery smoking intervention study. *Health Psychol*. 1992;11:119–126.
14. Reid R, Pipe A, Higginson L, et al. Stepped-care approach to smoking cessation in patients hospitalized for CAD. *J Cardiopulm Rehabil*. 2003;23: 176–182.
15. Rigotti NA, Singer DE, Mulley AG, et al. Smoking cessation following admission to a cardiac care unit. *J Gen Intern Med*. 1991;6:305–311.
16. Watson JM, Scarinci IC, Klesges RC, et al. Relationships among smoking status, ethnicity, socioeconomic indicators, and life style variables in a biracial sample of women. *Prev Med*. 2003;37:138–147.
17. U.S. Department of Health and Human Services. *Reducing tobacco use: A report of the surgeon general*. Atlanta, GA: U.S. Department of Health and Human Services, Centers for Disease Control and Prevention, National Center for Chronic Disease Prevention and Health Promotion, Office on Smoking and Health; 2000.

18. Kiefe CI, Williams OD, Greenlund KJ, et al. Health care access and seven year change in cigarette smoking. *Am J Prev Med.* 1998;47:229–233.

19. Gariti P, Alterman AI, Mulvaney FD, et al. The relationship between psychopathology and smoking cessation treatment response. *Drug Alcohol.* 2000;60:267–273.

20. Hurt RD, Eberman KM, Croghan KP, et al. Nicotine dependence treatment during in-patient treatment for other addictions: a prospective intervention trial. *Alcohol Clin Exp Res.* 1994;18:867–872.

21. Hays JT, Offord KP, Croghan It, et al. Smoking cessation rates in active and recovering alcoholics treated for recovering nicotine dependence. *Ann Behav Med.* 1999;21:1–8.

22. Hymowitz N, Cummings KM, Hyland A, et al. Predictors of smoking cessation in a cohort of adult smokers followed for five years. *Tobac Control.* 1997;6:S57–S62.

23. Patten CA, Drews AA, Myers MG, et al. Effects of depressive symptoms on smoking abstinence and treatment adherence among smokers with a history of alcohol dependence. *Psychol Addict Behav.* 2002;16:135–142.

24. George TP, Vessicchio JC, Termine A, et al. A placebo controlled trial of Buproprion for smoking cessation in schizophrenics. *Biol Psychol.* 2002;52:53–61.

25. Hitsman B, Borrelli B, McCharque DE, et al. History of depression and smoking cessation outcome: a meta-analysis. *J Consult Clin Psychol.* 2003;71: 657–663.

26. Ginsberg JP, Klesges RC, Johnson KC, et al. The relationship between a history of depression and adherence to a multi component smoking-cessation program. *Addict Behav.* 1997;22:783–787.

27. Glassman AH, Helzer JE, Covey LS, et al. Smoking, smoking cessation, and major depression. *JAMA.* 1990;264:1546–1549.

28. Hall SM, Munoz RF, Reus VI, et al. Nicotine, negative affect, and depression. *J Consult Clin Psychol.* 1993;61:761–767.

29. Centers for Disease Control and Prevention. Cigarette smoking among adults – United States, 2000. In *Morb Mortal Wkly Rep.* 2002;51(29):642–645.

30. Lawrence D, Graber JE, Mills Sl, et al. Smoking and intervention in U.S. racial/ethnic minority populations: an assessment of the literature. *Prev Med.* 2003;36:204–216.

31. Fiore MC, Jaén CR, Baker TB, et al. *Treating tobacco use and dependence: 2008 update. Quick Reference Guide for Clinicians.* Rockville, MD: U.S. Department of Health and Human Services. Public Health Service; April 2009.

32. Davis RM. Uniting physicians against smoking: the need for a coordinated national strategy. *JAMA.* 1988;259:2900–2901.

33. Russell M, Wilson C, Taylor C, Baker C. Effects of general practitioners' advice against smoking. *Br Med J.* 1979;2:231–235.

34. Ockene JK, Zapka JG. Physician-based smoking intervention: a rededication to a five-step strategy to smoking research. *Addict Behav.* 1997;22: 835–848.

35. Fiore MC, Bailey WC, Cohen SJ et al. *Treating tobacco use and dependence. A clinical practice guideline.* AHRQ publication No. 00-0032. Rockville, MD: US Dept of Health and Human Services; 2000.

36. Hollis J, Lichenstein E, Vogt T, et al. Nurse-assisted counseling for smokers in primary care. *Ann Intern Med.* 193;118:521–525.

37. National Institutes of Health state-of-the-science conference statement: tobacco use: prevention, cessation, and control. *Ann Intern Med.* 2006;145:839–844.

38. Quinn VP, Hollis JF, Smith KS, Rigotti NA, Solberg SI, Hu W, Stevens VJ. Effectiveness of the 5-As Tobacco Cessation Treatments in Nine HMOs. *J Gen Intern Med.* 2009:24:149–154.

39. Bastian LA. If it is as simple as AAAAA B C, Why don't we do it?_J *Gen Intern Med.* 2009:24(2):284–285.

40. Schroeder SA. What to do with a patient who smokes. *JAMA.* 2005;294: 482–487.

41. Krist AH, Woolf SH, Frazier CO, Johnson RE, Rothemich SF, Wilson DB, Devers KJ, Kerns JW. An electronic linkage system for health behavior counseling: effect on delivery of the 5A's. *Am J Prev Med.* 2008;35(5S):S350–S358.

42. AHCPR. Smoking cessation clinical practice guideline. *JAMA.* 1996;275: 1270–1280.

43. Curry SJ. Self-help interventions for smoking cessation. *J Consult Clin Psychol.* 1993;61:790–803.

44. Resnicow K, Vaughan R, Futterman R, et al. A self-help smoking cessation program for inner-city African Americans: results from the Harlem Health Connection Project. *Health Educ Behav.* 1997;24:201–217.

45. Fiore MC, Novotny TE, Pierce JP, et al. Methods used to quit smoking in the United States. Do cessation programs help? *JAMA.* 1990;263(20):2760–2765, 1990 May 23–30.

46. Killen JD, Fortman SP, David L, et al. Nicotine patch and self-help video for cigarette smoking cessation. *J Consult Clin Psychol.* 1997;65:663–672.

47. Lancaster T, Stead LF. Self-help interventions for smoking cessation. *Cochrane Database of Systematic Reviews* 2005, Issue 3. Art. No.: CD001118. DOI: 10.1002/14651858.CD001118.pub2.

48. Skinner CS, Campbell MK, Rimer BK, et al. How effective is tailored print communication? *Ann Behav Med.* 1999;21:290–298.

49. Etter J, Perneger TV. Effectiveness of a computer tailored smoking cessation intervention. *Arch Intern Med.* 2001;161:2596–2601.

50. Shiffman S, Paty JA, Rohay JM, et al. The efficacy of a computer-tailored smoking cessation materials as a supplement to nicotine patch therapy. *Drug Alcohol Depend.* 2001;64:35–46.

51. Strecher VJ. Computer-tailored smoking cessation materials: a review and discussion. *Patient Educ Couns.* 1999;36:107–117.

52. Borland R, Segan C, Livingston P, et al. The effectiveness of callback counselling for smoking cessation: a randomized trial. *Addiction.* 2001;96: 881–889.

53. McBride C, Rimer B. Using the telephone to improve health behavior and health service delivery. *Patient Educ Couns*. 1999;37:3–18.
54. Stead LF, Perera R, Lancaster T. Telephone counselling for smoking cessation. *Cochrane Database of Systematic Reviews* 2006, Issue 3. Art. No.: CD002850. DOI: 10.1002/14651858.CD002850.pub2.
55. Curry SJ, McBride C, Grothaus L, et al. A randomized trial of self-help materials, personalized feedback, and telephone counseling with nonvolunteer smokers. *J Consult Clin Psychol*. 1995;63(6):1005–1014.
56. Orleans CT, Shoenbach V, Wagner E, et al. Self-help quit smoking interventions: effects of self-help materials, social support instructions, and telephone counseling. *J Consult Clin Psychol*. 1991;59(3):439–448.
57. Zhu SH, Stretch, V, Balabanis M, et al. Telephone counseling for smoking cessation: effects of single-session and multiple-session interventions. *J Consult Clin Psychol*. 1996;64(1):202–211.
58. Miller CE, Ratner PA, Johnson JL. Reducing cardiovascular risk: identifying predictors of smoking relapse. *Can J Cardiovasc Nurs*. 2003;13:7–12.
59. Stead LF, Perera R, Bullen C, Mant D, Lancaster T. Nicotine replacement therapy for smoking cessation. *Cochrane Database of Systematic Reviews* 2008, Issue 1. Art. No.: CD000146. DOI: 10.1002/14651858.CD000146.pub3.
60. Fiore M, Smith S, Jorenby D, et al. The effectiveness of the nicotine patch for smoking cessation: a meta-analysis. *JAMA*. 1994;271(24):1940–1947.
61. Shiffman S, Dresler C, Hajek P, et al. (2002). Efficacy of a nicotine lozenge for smoking cessation. *Arch Intern Med*. 2002;162:1267–1276.
62. Jorenby D. Clinical efficacy of bupropion in the management of smoking cessation. *Drugs*. 2002;62(Suppl 2):25–35.
63. Holm K, Spencer C. Bupropion a review of its use in the management of smoking cessation. Drugs. 2000;59(4):1007–1024.
64. Swan GE, McAfee T, Curry SJ, et al. Effectiveness of bupropion SR for smoking cessation in a health care setting. *Arch Intern Med*. 2003;163:2337–2344.
65. Jorenby DE, Leischow SJ, Nides MA, et al. A controlled trial of sustained-release buproprion, a nicotine patch, or both for smoking cessation. *N Engl J Med*. 1999;340:685–691.
66. Nides M, Glover ED, Reus VI, et al. Varenicline versus Bupropion SR or Placebo for smoking cessation: a pooled analysis. *Am J Health Behav*. 2008;32(6):664–675.
67. FDA Public Health Advisory. Food and Drug Administration Website. http://www.fda.gov/cder/drug/advisory/varenicline.htm. Accessed April 18; 2009.
68. Hajek P, West R, Foulds J, et al. Randomized comparative trial of nicotine polacrilex, a transdermal patch, nasal spray, and an inhaler. *Arch Intern Med*. 1999;159:2033–2038.
69. Houtsmuller E, Henningerfield J, Stitzer M. Subjective effects of the nicotine lozenge: assessment of abuse liability. *Psychopharmacology*. 2003;167: 20–27.
70. ACS Guide to Quitting Smoking. American Cancer Society web site. http://www.cancer.org/docroot/PED/content/PED_10_13X_Guide_for_Quitting_Smoking.asp. Accessed January 23; 2009.

71. Okuyemi KS, Nollen NL, Ahluwalia, JS. Interventions to facilitate smoking cessation. *Am Fam Phys*. 2006;74(2):262–271.

72. American Lung Association Web site. Nicotine Replacement Therapy (NRT) and Other Medications Which Aid Smoking Cessation. http://www.lungusa.org/site/pp.asp?c=dvLUK9OOE&b=33566. July 2006. Accessed April 19; 2009.

73. Park EW, et al. Does enhancing partner support and interaction improve smoking cessation? A meta-analysis. *Ann Fam Med*. 2004;2(2): 170–174.

74. Ockene JK, et al. Relationship of psychosocial factors to smoking behavior change in an intervention program. *Prev Med*. 1982;11(1):13–28.

75. Gulliver SB, et al. An investigation of self-efficacy, partner support and daily stresses as predictors of relapse to smoking in self-quitters. *Addiction*. 1995;90(6):767–772.

76. Coppotelli HC, et al. Partner support and other determinants of smoking cessation maintenance among women. *J Consult Clin Psychol*. 1985;53(4): 455–460.

77. Morgan GD, et al. Abstinence from smoking and the social environment. *J Consult Clin Psychol*. 1988;56(2):298–301.

78. Mermelstein R, et al. Partner support and relapse in smoking-cessation programs. *J Consult Clin Psychol*. 1983;51(3):465–466.

79. Cohen S, et al. Partner behaviors that support quitting smoking. *J Consult Clin Psychol*. 1990;58(3):304–309.

80. Roski J, et al. Long-term associations of helpful and harmful spousal behaviors with smoking cessation. *Addict Behav*. 1996;21(2):173–185.

81. Patten CA, et al. Training support persons to help smokers quit: a pilot study. *Am J Prev Med*. 2004;26(5):386–390.

82. McBride CM, et al. Prenatal and postpartum smoking abstinence a partner-assisted approach. *Am J Prev Med*. 2004;27(3):232–238.

83. Park EW, Schultz JK, Tudiver FG, Campbell T, Becker LA. Enhancing partner support to improve smoking cessation. *Cochrane Database of Systematic Reviews* 2004, Issue 3. Art. No.: CD002928. DOI: 10.1002/14651858.CD002928.pub2.

84. Schnoll RA, et al. Correlates of tobacco use among smokers and recent quitters diagnosed with cancer. *Patient Educ Couns*. 2002;46(2):137–145.

85. Lenert L, Munoz R, Stoddard J, et al. Design and pilot evaluation of an Internet smoking cessation program. *J Am Med Inform Assn*. 2003;10:16–20.

86. Curry S, Ludman E, McClure J. Self-administered treatment for smoking cessation. *J Clin Psychol*. 2003;59(3):305–319.

87. Feil E, Noell J, Lichtenstein E, et al. Evaluation of an Internet-based smoking cessation program: lessons learned from a pilot study. *Nicotine Tob Res*. 2003;5:189–194.

88. Bessell T, McDonald S, Silagy C, et al. Do internet interventions for consumers cause more harm than good? A systematic review. *Health Expect*. 2002;5:28–37.

89. 1-800-QuitNow Frequently Asked Questions page. US Department of Health and Human Services, National Institutes of Health, and National Cancer

Institute Contracted Web Site. http://1800quitnow.cancer.gov/faq.aspx. Accessed February 2; 2009.

90. Stead LF, Perera R, Lancaster T. Telephone counselling for smoking cessation. *Cochrane Database Syst Rev.* 2006;(3). Art. No.: CD002850. DOI: 10.1002/14651858.CD002850.pub2.

91. Zhu SH, Anderson CM, Tedeschi GJ, et al. Evidence of real-world effectiveness of a telephone quitline for smokers. *N Engl J Med.* 2002;347(14): 1087–1093.

92. Manfredi C, LeHew CW. Why implementation processes vary across the 5A's of the smoking cessation guideline: administrators' perspectives. *Nicotine Tob Res.* 2008;10(11):1597–1607.

93. Miller WR, Rollnick S. *Motivational interviewing: Preparing people for change. 2nd Ed.* New York, NY: Guilford; 2002:9–41.

94. Stoddard JJ, Gray B. Maternal smoking and medical expenditures for childhood respiratory illness. *Am J Public Health.* 1997;87:205–209.

95. Aligne CA, Stoddard JJ. Tobacco and children. An economic evaluation of the medical effects of parental smoking. *Arch Pediatr Adolesc Med.* 1997;151:648–653.

96. Schnoll RA, Malstrom JC, Rothman RL, et al. Longitudinal predictors of continued tobacco use among patients diagnosed with cancer. *Ann Behav Med.* 2003;25:214–222.

97. Haustein KO. What can we do in secondary prevention of cigarette smoking? *Eur J Cardiovasc Prev Rehabil.* 2003;10:476–485.

Chapter 6
Cancer Screening Adherence

Jennifer M. Gierisch and Lori A. Bastian

Cancer is a devastating and debilitating disease. Each year more than 1.4 million people are diagnosed with non-skin cancers and 565,650 lives are lost in the United States [1]. Primary prevention of cancer through behavioral modifications in risk factors such as tobacco use, sun exposure, obesity, physical inactivity, unhealthy diet, and alcohol consumption can reduce the burden of cancer tremendously [2, 3]. However, beyond the small proportion of cancers linked to genetic mutations, many cancers are sporadic. Early detection via evidence-based screening tests (i.e., secondary prevention) remains an effective option for controlling the burden of cancer [4].

The purpose of this chapter is to provide an overview of the issue related to cancer screening adherence and to identify evidence-based or promising interventions for addressing non-adherence. We focus on screening adherence issues related to two of the most common cancers for which there is widespread agreement on the efficacy of screening, breast and colorectal cancers [5, 6].

J.M. Gierisch (✉)
General Internal Medicine, Duke University Medical Center, Durham, NC, USA
e-mail: j.gierisch@duke.edu

H. Bosworth (ed.), *Improving Patient Treatment Adherence*,
DOI 10.1007/978-1-4419-5866-2_6,
© Springer Science+Business Media, LLC 2010

Burden of Breast Cancer and Mammography Adherence

Breast cancer is the second most common cancer in women in the USA with an estimated 182,460 diagnosed cases and 40,480 deaths in 2008 [1]. Breast cancer incidence varies across race and ethnic groups. It ranges from 69.8 cases per 100,000 per year in American Indian and Alaskan Native women to 132.5 cases per 100,000 per year in white women [1]. Secondary prevention via mammography is an effective way to reduce morbidity and mortality from breast cancer. Use of mammography can lead to early diagnosis of breast cancer when tumors are smaller and patients may have more treatment options [5, 7].

Estimates of mammography use vary widely due to broad variation in sampling frames, inconsistent definitions of mammography adherence, and differences in mammography screening measurement [8]. Although there has been a recent push to standardize operational definitions of mammography use, none have been widely adopted at this time [8–11]. Lack of consensus is largely based on disagreement among scientific organizations on the recommended intervals between screenings. While some organizations recommend women be screened every 1–2 years (e.g., National Cancer Institute [12], US Preventive Services Task Force [5]), other organizations recommend every year (e.g., American Cancer Society [13]). Irrespective of how the interval is defined, most medical organizations in the USA now recommend mammography screening for women aged 40 and older.

Mammography use has been disseminated widely in the USA [14]. Currently, about 85% of age-appropriate women have had at least one mammogram [15], and 66% of US women report a recent mammogram (e.g., within the last 2 years) [16]. While ever and recent screening rates have increased dramatically over the last 20 years [17], rates of repeat mammography screening (i.e., minimally, two consecutive screening mammograms at specified intervals) are much less encouraging. In a weighted analysis across 37 studies, only 38% (on an annual interval screening) to 46% (on a biennial screening interval) of women aged 50 and older obtained a repeat screening [8]. To achieve the full benefits of mammography, women should be screened regularly [7, 18, 19]. Increased rates of regular screening at annual intervals could reduce breast cancer deaths by 22% each year [20]; however, current reports show a decline in the historically high rates of mammography use [16, 21, 22].

Burden of Colorectal Cancer and Use of Screening Tests

Colorectal cancer is the second leading cause of cancer deaths and the third most common cancer in men and women in the USA. The American Cancer Society estimates 49,960 deaths and 148,810 cases in 2008 [1]. Overall, colorectal cancer incidence is higher in men than in women. Incidence rates range from 42.1 per 100,000 per year in American Indian and Alaskan Native men to 72.6 per 100,000 per year in African American men. In women, it ranges from 32.9 per 100,000 per year in Hispanics to 55 per 100,000 per year in African Americans.

Regular screening leads to the early detection of colorectal cancers [6] and, in some instances, the detection and removal of precancerous colorectal polyps [1]. As such, colorectal cancer screening can lead to reductions in both mortality and incidence via screening. If detected in an early stage, colorectal cancer has a 90% 5-year survival rate [23]. The American Cancer Society, US Multisociety Task Force on Colorectal Cancer, US Preventive Services Task Force, and the National Cancer Institute recommend that average risk men and women aged 50 years and older be screened for colorectal cancers [23, 24].

Many colorectal cancer screening tests are currently available. Recently revised colorectal cancer screening guidelines divide current screening test into two groups: test used to primarily detect cancer (e.g., stool tests) and test used to detect adenomatous polyps and cancer (e.g., flexible sigmoidoscopy, colonoscopy, double-contrast barium enema, and CT colonography) [23]. Notwithstanding multiple options for screening, colorectal cancer screening is underused. Less than half of age-eligible adults are up to date for screening [25–27]. As many as 9,632 deaths each year could be prevented with better uptake of and adherence to appropriate colorectal cancer screening and follow-up [28].

Risk Factors for Screening Non-adherence

Many studies have identified factors associated with mammography use and colorectal cancer screening. However, the majority of previous research was often retrospective and cross-sectional in nature or took place in the context of an intervention to prompt uptake of screening, with limited follow-up. Few studies have reviewed the literature systematically [29, 30]. Below we summarize some of the major findings as they pertain to factors associated with mammography and colorectal cancer screening adherence.

Factors Associated with Mammography Adherence

Sociodemographic, psychosocial, and behavioral correlates of mammography use have been documented extensively [10, 29–34]. Poor mammography adherence is associated with not being married [10, 30], low income/money concerns [10, 30, 35–37], and low educational attainment [10, 30, 37]. Being a smoker [10, 30, 38], overweight/obesity [39], drinking alcohol [30], reporting poor health status [40], and no family history of breast cancer [30, 35] are also associated with mammography non-adherence.

Mammography use also varies across age groups [29]. Overall, women aged 50–65 years are more likely to be screened as compared to women in their forties [19, 33, 38] or women older than 65 years [34, 37, 41, 42]. Mammography screening barriers (e.g., cost, comorbidities) likely vary among women of different age groups. Additionally, shifting medical recommendations on the frequency and efficacy of mammography screening may contribute to non-adherence, especially for women in their forties [43–45].

Many studies have explored race and ethnicity as correlates of mammography use [40, 46]. However, race and ethnicity were not significant predictors of mammography adherence across two systematic reviews of mammography use [29, 30]. Much of the racial and ethnic disparity in screening rates may be accounted for by other factors such as educational attainment, income, insurance status, and physician recommendation [46–48]. However, barriers to mammography adherence vary across racial and ethnic groups. For example, barriers related to the cost of obtaining mammograms, pain, and the safety of receiving mammograms may be stronger barriers for Latina and African American women [30, 49] as compared to other ethnic groups.

A variety of psychosocial variables are correlated with mammography non-adherence such as no/low intentions to seek a mammogram [29, 50], ambivalence toward mammography [33, 51], perceiving barriers to seeking a mammogram [30, 52, 53], and low(er) perceived risk of getting breast cancer [54, 55]. Breast health beliefs such as poor knowledge of screening guidelines [30, 33, 52], embarrassment/modesty [30], and thinking mammograms are only needed when there are symptoms [30] are also correlated with mammography non-adherence.

Rates of mammography adherence also vary across patients' past mammography experiences, previous patterns of use, and health care-related factors. Having a history of breast problems [30] or false-positive mammograms [56], prior mammography use [29, 40, 50, 57] or attending other cancer screening tests [30], and satisfaction with past mammography experience [58, 59] are predictive of mammography adherence. Health-care variables such as having a usual source of medical care [10, 30, 37, 40], having health insurance [10, 19, 30, 37, 47], and receiving a provider recommendation to get a mammogram [30, 33, 35, 57] are consistently associated with mammography screening adherence.

Factors Associated with Colorectal Cancer Screening Adherence

The uptake of colorectal cancer screening lags far behind other evidence-based cancer screenings such as mammography and pap tests [60]. Some of the reasons for lack of uptake pertain to the screening tools themselves. There are multiple options for colorectal cancer screening and many types of health-care providers are involved in delivering colorectal cancer screenings (e.g., primary care, gastroenterology, diagnostic radiology). Each testing option has its own set of barriers and benefits related to costs, convenience, and patient/provider preferences [23, 24]. The tests have different guidelines for adherence and some tests are recommended at different intervals by various health organizations. In addition, unlike other screening tools, many colorectal cancer screening tests involve a high level of patient participation and time commitment, ranging from collection of multiple home stool samples and dietary restrictions for fecal occult blood testing to bowel preparation and the need for patients to coordinate transportation after sedation for testing via colonoscopy. It is important to consider patient burden and preferences for screening tests because experiences with past screening modalities influence patients' future colorectal cancer screening adherence [61, 62].

Many patient-level factors are associated with colorectal cancer screening adherence. Patients who are of older age [29, 63], male [63, 64], and have higher incomes [26] are more likely to be up to date with colorectal cancer screenings. Having health insurance [65, 66], a usual source of care [63, 65, 66], seeking other types of preventive services [60, 67, 68], and having a routine doctor visit in the past year [26, 68, 69] are also associated with colorectal cancer screening adherence. Poor self-reported health or difficulties with activities of daily living [29, 69] and low literacy skills [70, 71] are associated with non-adherence. Being of non-white race/ethnicity, especially Hispanic ethnicity [26, 69], has also been associated with colorectal cancer screening non-adherence.

Certain patient perceptions, beliefs, and attitudes are also associated with colorectal cancer adherence. Patients' lack of awareness of colorectal cancer and available screening options is one of the most robust and persistent barriers [26, 66, 72–74]. Other psychosocial correlates such as intentions to be screened [75], perceived benefits [29, 76] and barriers to obtaining a screening test [27, 29, 76–78], and self-efficacy (i.e., confidence) to obtaining a screening test [75] are positively associated with colorectal cancer screening adherence.

Provider recommendation of screening has been a powerful and consistent predictor of colorectal cancer screening adherence [26, 63, 72, 74]. However, patient reported rates of provider recommendations of colorectal cancer screening are relatively low when compared to other cancer screening tests [73]. In a nationally representative sample of US adults, only 10% of age-eligible patients not current with testing and who had a doctor visit in the past year reported receiving a colorectal cancer screening recommendation [74].

There are several reasons that health-care providers do not recommend, offer, or order cancer screening tests. Prior patient refusal of screening [79] and patient comorbidities [79], provider forgetfulness [79, 80], provider knowledge, and attitudes toward screening [79, 80] all influence recommendation rates. Competing demands such as attending to acute complaints and managing ongoing health issues also make it difficult to provide or counsel on the importance of cancer screening [79, 81, 82]. Klabunde and colleagues (2006) explored predictors of receiving a physician recommendation for colorectal cancer among Medicare consumers. They reported that being aged 50–64 years, white race, having greater than a high school education, higher colorectal cancer risk, having one or more chronic medical conditions, and attending a routine or preventive care visit in the past 12 months predicted physician recommendation of a colorectal cancer screening test [72]. Notwithstanding multiple barriers, increasing provider recommendation of screening offers a potentially powerful tool for increasing colorectal cancer screening adherence.

Behavioral Adherence Interventions

Increasing use of colorectal cancer screening and mammography at recommended intervals and targeting intervention efforts at populations less likely to be screened are essential components of reducing the burden of these cancers [65]. Multiple evidence reviews have isolated intervention strategies to enhance adherence to mammography [29, 83–98]. Far fewer reviews have evaluated colorectal cancer screening interventions, most focused exclusively on screening via fecal occult blood testing (FOBT) [88, 89, 95–97].

Drawing conclusions across multiple evidence reviews is difficult; most reviews vary in the intervention typologies used. Therefore, we base our categorization of intervention strategies, in part, on the typology used by the Task Force on Community Preventive Services (Task Force) (http://www.thecommunityguide.org/) [95, 96, 99]. Below we summarize the finding from the Task Force and other evidence reviews in order to identify strategies for increasing adherence to mammography and colorectal cancer screening that may be of particular interest to clinicians. Table 6.1 summarizes effective intervention strategies and corresponding evidence.

Table 6.1 Interventions to enhance mammography and colorectal cancer screening adherence

Intervention strategy	Target of strategy	Intervention example	Evidence review support (Author, publication year)
Patient-directed communication strategies:			
Reminders	Patient	Tailored or generic print reminders to make an appointment Direct invitation via telephone or personal contact with fixed or flexible appointment time Physician's recommendation to get screened	[a]Baron et al. (2008) [1] [c]Bonfill et al. (2001) [2] [c]Denhaerynck et al. (2003) [3] [a]Jepson et al. (2000) [4] [c]Legler et al. (2002) [5] [a]Shea et al. (1996) [6] [c]Sohl and Moyer (2007) [7] [a]Stone et al. (2002) [8] [c]Wagner (1998) [9] [c]Yabroff and Mandelblatt (1999) [10] [c]Yabroff et al. (2001) [11]
Individual education	Patient	Telephone counseling tailored on barriers to screening adherence One-on-one instruction delivered via lay health advisor or health-care worker	[c]Baron et al. (2008) [1] [a]Jepson et al. (2000) [4] [c]Legler et al. (2002) [5] [c]Sohl and Moyer (2007) [7] [a]Stone et al. (2002) [8] [c]Yabroff and Mandelblatt (1999) [10] [c]Yabroff et al. (2001) [11]

Table 6.1 (continued)

Intervention strategy	Target of strategy	Intervention example	Evidence review support (Author, publication year)
Small media	Patient	Audio-visual materials Print materials (brochures, pamphlets, newsletters)	[a]Baron et al. (2008) [1] [c]Bonfill et al. (2001) [2] [c]Sohl and Moyer (2007) [7] [a]Stone et al. (2002) [8]
Patient-directed access-enhancing strategies:			
Reducing out-of-pocket costs	Patient	Reducing co-payments Vouchers to subside out-of-pocket expenses	[c]Bailey et al. (2005) [12] [c]Baron et al. (2008) [13] [a]Jepson et al. (2000) [4] [c]Legler et al. (2002) [5] [a]Stone et al. (2002) [8]
Reducing structural barriers	Patient	Extending facility hours Mobile mammography vans Providing FOBT kits	[c]Bailey et al. (2005) [12] [a]Baron et al. (2008) [13] [c]Legler et al. (2002) [5]

Table 6.1 (continued)

Intervention strategy	Target of strategy	Intervention example	Evidence review support (Author, publication year)
Provider-directed strategies:			
Assessment and feedback	Provider	Evaluate providers' performance in delivering/offering screening Supply providers with information on rates of service delivery	[a]Jepson et al. (2000) [4] [a]Sabatino et al. (2008) [14] [a]Snell and Buck (1996) [15] [a]Stone et al. (2002) [8]
Reminders	Provider	Flow chart or checklist to remind providers to recommend/offer screening	[b]Guide to Community Preventive Services (2008) [16] [c]Jepson et al. (2000) [4] [c]Mandelblatt and Yabroff (1999) [17] [c,d]Shea et al. (1996) [6] [a]Snell and Buck (1996) [15] [a]Stone et al. (2002) [8]
Education	Provider	In-person detailing Individual education session Workshops and lectures	[c]Mandelblatt and Yabroff (1999) [17] [a]Stone et al. (2002) [8]

Table 6.1 (continued)

Intervention strategy	Target of strategy	Intervention example	Evidence review support (Author, publication year)
Changes in work processes	Provider and organization	Nonmedical staff identify patients in need of screening Nurse staff deliver/recommends screening service Separate prevention visits	[b]Mandelblatt and Yabroff (1999) [17] [a]Stone et al. (2002) [8]
Combined strategies: Multicomponent strategies	Multiple targets	Combination of any of the above intervention strategies: • Patient reminders + vouchers • Prevention visits + individual education • Telephone counseling + extending facility hours	[a]Baron et al. (2008) [1] [c]Bailey et al. (2005) [12] [c]Bonfill et al. (2001) [2] [c]Legler et al. (2002) [5] [a]Jepson et al. (2000) [4] [c]Yabroff et al. (2001) [11]

[a]Study provides evidence in support of intervention to enhance mammography adherence and colorectal cancer screening via fecal occult blood testing

[b]Study provides evidence in support of intervention to enhance mammography adherence and colorectal cancer screening via fecal occult blood testing and flexible sigmoidoscopy

[c]Study provides evidence in support of intervention to enhance mammography adherence

[d]Study included colorectal cancer screening via rectal exam, fecal occult blood testing, and sigmoidoscopy. Results were not separated by each screening modality

Patient-Directed Communication Strategies

Extensive evidence supports the use of patient-directed communications such as reminders, small media (e.g., letters, brochures, newsletters), and individual education (e.g., telephone counseling, one-on-one instruction) to promote mammography adherence [29, 83, 84, 90, 92, 97, 99]. For colorectal cancer screening via FOBT, multiple evidence reviews support the use of patient reminders to increase adherence [29, 79, 89, 97, 99]. Fewer evidence reviews support the use of individual education [29, 89] and small media [89, 99] to promote colorectal cancer screening adherence.

Patient-directed communications come in multiple formats such as mailed letters, postcards, and automated or direct-contact telephone calls. Communications can originate from a variety of sources such as insurance providers, lay health educators, nurses, or mammography facilities. These communications can include fixed appointment times or a reminder to call for an appointment. The content of patient-directed communications can range from generic ("Women should get mammograms every year or two.") to tailored content that is meant for one specific individual ("<PATIENT NAME>, most medical organizations recommend that women your age should be screened for breast cancer via mammography once a year. You last received your mammogram on <DATE> and are due for your mammogram next month. Please call <FACILITY PHONE NUMBER> to schedule your appointment.")

While the terms tailored and targeted sometimes are used interchangeably, these terms connote different communication strategies. Targeted communications are developed to appeal to segments of the population divided into subgroups, based on characteristics such as race or gender. To create tailored communications, data are collected from individuals so that unique messages can be created or "tailored" for that individual. Communications can be tailored on multiple variables such as cultural preferences, personal barriers, beliefs, and past behaviors [100].

Tailored communications may be more relevant than untailored communications and, therefore, are more likely to be read and remembered [100]. Mammography promotion interventions that were tailored outperformed generic interventions, though effects were modest [29, 92].Tailored strategies coupled with physician recommendations [92] and those that were informed by behavioral theory [86, 91, 92] produced the strongest intervention effects.

Many steps are involved in developing tailored communications. First, data are collected about patients from interviews, claims data, health records, or other sources. Next, a "message library" is constructed that contains messages, images, or graphics corresponding to each value of variables that will be used to tailor communications. Then, a computer program is developed to select specific message elements based on values collected from or about an individual. Based on empirically derived decision rules, message algorithms are developed to combine elements from the message library into coherent, individualized communications [100].

Patient-Directed Access-Enhancing Strategies

Patient-directed intervention efforts may also target access-related barriers. Such intervention strategies reduce patient burden associated with obtaining health services and broadly fall into two categories: reducing out-of-pocket cost and reducing structural barriers [96]. Interventions that reduce out-of-pocket cost include a wide variety of strategies that seek to overcome the economic barriers associated with obtaining cancer screenings such as reducing co-payments, providing payment vouchers, or other financial subsides paid to reduce the costs associated with screening (e.g., travel, childcare) [96]. Interventions aimed at reducing structural barriers seek to alleviate the noneconomic impediments to obtaining cancer screenings [96]. These interventions seek to facilitate greater access to screening services by simplifying administrative procedures (e.g., scheduling assistance), offering services at more convenient times or locations, providing transportation to screening facilities or translation services, and reducing the time needed for appointment completion.

Evidence supports the use of access-enhancing interventions to improve mammography adherence [29, 84, 89, 96, 98]. For women with historically lower rates of mammography use (e.g., older, poorer, less formal education), access-enhancing intervention strategies produced the highest adherence rates compared to other types of interventions [84]. Across evidence reviews, mobile mammography units and vouchers were some of the most common access-enhancing strategies used [84, 96], especially for low-income women [98]. Providing patient financial incentives for mammography screening was also a common and effective access-enhancing intervention compared to patient-directed communications and provider-directed strategies [89].

Colorectal cancer screening adherence via FOBT also benefits from patient-directed access-enhancing strategies [29, 89, 96]. For colorectal cancer screening, mailing/providing FOBT kits with return postage was the most common and effective intervention to reduce structural barriers [96]. Patient financial incentives also improved colorectal cancer screening via FOBT; however, patient reminders and provider-directed intervention strategies outperformed patient financial incentive interventions [89]. It is important to note that while access-enhancing interventions are effective at improving mammography and colorectal cancer screening adherence, many access-enhancing intervention programs also included other types of secondary intervention supports [96, 98].

Provider-Directed Strategies

Intervention strategies frequently target health-care providers in order to improve cancer screening adherence. The goal of provider-directed intervention efforts is to facilitate and encourage health-care providers to deliver, order, or recommend health services, such as cancer screenings, at recommended intervals [95]. Provider-directed strategies broadly fall into four categories: performance assessment and feedback, incentives, provider reminders, and educational strategies.

Provider assessment and feedback and provider incentives strategies seek to influence providers' attitudes toward screening and increase screening discussions with patients. In turn, providers may offer, order, or recommend more screening tests [95]. Provider incentives are direct or indirect inducements to motivate health-care providers' referral or recommendation of screening services [95]. Insufficient evidence is available to assess the efficacy of provider incentives on mammography or colorectal cancer screening adherence [89, 95].

Multiple evidence reviews support the use of provider assessment and feedback intervention strategies to improve mammography and FOBT adherence [29, 88, 89, 95]. Assessment and feedback intervention strategies evaluate and provide measures of service delivery. Assessment and feedback can be specific to one health-care provider or an average for a practice. Rates of screening may be compared to internal goals set by providers or a standard set by quality or performance improvement agencies. Feedback may occur once or repeatedly over a course of several months. The optimal number and frequency of assessment and feedback loops needed to improve screening rates are not known.

Provider reminders systems improve mammography [29, 86, 88, 89, 97, 101] and colorectal cancer screening via FOBT [88, 89, 97, 101] and flexible sigmoidoscopy [101]. Analogous to patient reminders, provider reminders take many forms (e.g., flow charts, checklists, notations). The reminders can be electronically or manually generated and occur before, during, or after a clinic visit to cue providers that patients are due (reminder) or overdue (recall) for a screening. Computerized reminder systems may be particularly useful in promoting cancer screening adherence because of their ability to automate and routinize reminder systems [88, 97, 102]. While effective, computerized reminder systems may be difficult to implement in a clinic setting. Many computerized reminder systems are designed for the specific needs of particular practices and, thus, are not generalizable to other health-care practices [102]. Also technology capabilities of practices may impede implementation and maintenance of computerized reminder systems [102]. Despite these limitations, computerized reminder systems are a proven intervention strategy and work is ongoing to make such systems more available and sustainable.

Provider education presents another promising intervention strategy. Provider education takes many formats such as academic detailing, individual instruction, and workshops. The educational information can be delivered via multiple formats such as the Internet, in-person instruction, or mailings. Compared to other provider-directed strategies to improve mammography and colorectal cancer screening, far less evidence supports the use of provider educational strategies [86, 89]. Provider education may be more effective when combined with other intervention strategies, such as reminder systems or assessment and feedback [88].

Other Intervention Strategies

Changes in organizational work processes improve mammography and colorectal cancer screening adherence [86, 89]. These interventions include a wide variety of strategies that seek to change organizational processes such as clinical procedures, infrastructure, or job duties in order to facilitate service delivery. Mass media messaging (e.g., television, radio advertising, billboards), provider incentives (e.g., monetary rewards for performance, indirect compensation via CME credits), and patient-directed group education (e.g., classes and slideshows taught by health professionals or trained peer educators) do not have sufficient evidence to support these strategies as stand-alone interventions for improving colorectal cancer or mammography screening adherence [86, 89, 95, 96, 99]. These strategies may serve as secondary supports in multicomponent interventions.

Multicomponent interventions are successful in improving colorectal cancer and mammography adherence [29, 85, 91, 98], especially when there are numerous barriers to screening adherence. For example, access-enhancing strategies (e.g., mobile vans, facilitated scheduling, vouchers) coupled with individually directed intervention strategies (e.g., reminders, individual education) were the most effective interventions for women with historically lower rates of mammography adherence [84]. For physician-directed interventions, effect sizes were stronger for interventions that focused on a combination of visit-based (e.g., reminders, flowcharts) and outside of office visit strategies (e.g., education, audit with feedback) [88]. Specific combinations of intervention strategies depend on the particular screening behavior and target population.

Future Directions and New Technological Advances

While much is known about effective strategies to improve mammography and colorectal cancer screening, additional research is needed across a variety of areas. Cancer mortality and morbidity reductions are only realized through sustained and regular screening. However, a paucity of research has been conducted on maintenance of episodic behaviors. As such, long-term adherence of cancer screening continues to be a vexing problem, and future research will increasingly need to focus on maintaining adherence. In addition, researchers should aim to test evidence-based intervention strategies in diverse clinical practices (e.g., privately owned, rural, urban) and with traditionally underserved populations, such as recent immigrants or persons with low (health) literacy [99, 103]. Such research will expand what we know about effective interventions to such settings and populations. Assessing intervention strategies with insufficient evidence (e.g., provider incentives) [95] and testing effective FOBT intervention strategies with more invasive colorectal cancer screening modalities (e.g., colonoscopy) also are key gaps in intervention research.

Relatively simple patient interventions, such as reminders, are effective. Reminders are also less costly than other successful, but more intensive interventions, such as telephone counseling or tailored print materials. Some patients, however, may need more intensive interventions to become adherent. Adaptive interventions are well suited to evaluate optimal and minimal intervention components necessary to change behavior and sustain adherence. In adaptive interventions, varying dosages of intervention components are given to different individuals across time. Intervention dosage changes in response to the needs of individuals and progresses from minimal to more intensive intervention strategies [104]. Such stepped or adaptive interventions give the right "dose" of intervention to each person. Since less costly interventions are followed by more intensive interventions as needed, adaptive interventions may be more cost-effective than nonadaptive interventions. Future cancer screening interventions trials have been designed to test such adaptive interventions and results are forthcoming.

Tailored messages improve cancer screening adherence. However, targeted messages that are a "good fit" for individual characteristics may perform equally well [100]. More research is needed into which variables present the most powerful constructs on which to tailor or target health promotion communications. Also researchers are unclear if tailored communications sustain adherence at levels superior to non-tailored communications once intervention efforts are terminated. Therefore, researchers should test the *comparative* effectiveness of tailored and non-tailored intervention strategies on cancer screening adherence and maintenance.

Newer electronic and communication technologies are changing the way people receive information and offer promising alternative to traditional intervention channels. Communication technologies such as automated telephone or text messaging, Internet-based applications (e.g., e-mail reminders, online support groups, health education Web sites), and automated computer-controlled interactive telephone counseling may improve delivery and cost-effectiveness of proven intervention strategies. Also health promotion messages delivered via newer technologies may be superior in "cutting through the clutter" of information. Consequently, patients may attend more to health messages delivered via automated phone or Internet-based channels compared to traditional channels (e.g., mail). Little work has compared traditional print or person-delivered strategies with computerized or automated strategies although early results are promising [105].

Advances in screening technology also may improve initial uptake and adherence to mammography and colorectal cancer screening. Full-field digital mammography improves the ability to take, store, display, and manipulate images [106]. Digital mammography also has greater sensitivity, especially in younger, denser breast tissue [106]. Contrast-enhanced mammography and tomosynthesis are other promising technologies currently under study. Compared to film mammography, both of these techniques have superior sensitivity with dense breast tissue, thus reducing recall rates and increasing tumor detection. However, both tests are prone to motion artifacts and require higher doses of radiation than conventional mammography [106].

Several new colorectal cancer screening technologies are on the market or under evaluation. Two new noninvasive fecal test technologies, fecal immunochemical tests (FIT) and fecal DNA tests, present some advantages over guaiac-based FOBT. FIT detect human globin and have superior sensitivity to guaiac-based FOBT [107]. Also FIT requires only one or two stool samples (as compared to three samples for guaiac-based tests) and no medication or dietary restrictions, advantages that may increase patient testing satisfaction and adherence. Fecal DNA testing shows promise as another noninvasive test for colorectal cancer but has not received US Food and Drug Administration approval. Fecal DNA testing detects known colorectal cancer markers of genetic mutation. Similar to FIT, stool DNA testing offers the possibility to have superior sensitivity to guaiac-based tests [107].

CT colonography or "virtual colonoscopy" is another emerging screening test on the market. While CT colonography still requires bowel preparation, it does not require sedation, thus reducing the need for patients to coordinate transportation after testing. Also CT colonography does not have the risk of perforation and bleeding associated with performing a colonoscopy. Widespread use of CT colonography has some drawbacks. High-quality imaging is operator dependent and current professional capacity may not be adequate. Also CT colonography increase patients' radiation exposure and may not be able to detect flat or depressed lesions [107].

Clinical Implications of Cancer Screening

Clinicians are faced with multiple challenges when promoting cancer screening adherence. First, clinicians serve as important advocates in promoting cancer screenings to their patients [51]. As such, providers facilitate patient choice around evidence-based screening options. Each screening test presents benefits and drawback that may affect patient receptivity and, thus, adherence. Clinicians must be informed of testing cost, convenience, and predictive value trade-offs so they can assist patients' informed decision-making. Clinicians also are tasked with staying abreast of emerging screening technologies as patients may question the need or usefulness of conventional screening methods compared with emerging testing technologies.

Another implication of screening adherence is management of the clinical and emotional sequelae of abnormal screening results. Multiple types of clinicians are involved in diagnostic follow-up of abnormal results. Clinicians can play a key role in coordinating between the patient, other clinicians, and health-care organizations involved in diagnostic follow-up and, if disease is confirmed, treatment. An abnormal test result increases patients' level of anxiety and worry [108, 109]. Patients with a history of false-positive results may be prompted to sustain adherence or less likely to seek testing in the future [56, 110]. False-positive results also may erode trust in all preventive screening and other health services. In order to manage the deleterious effects of abnormal tests, clinicians can help clarify misperceptions about follow-up care, help reduce clinical barriers to receiving care, and manage harmful psychological fall-out from abnormal test results.

There are many evidence-based cancer screening adherence interventions. The cost associated with implementing both patient- and provider-directed intervention strategies, however, limits dose, duration, and dissemination of interventions. For patient-directed interventions strategies, the cost of producing and delivering patient reminders, small media, and individual education limits implementation. For provider-directed intervention strategies, limitations in staffing, facilities, and other intervention costs restrict intervention efforts, especially in smaller clinics with access to fewer resources. Also as new and more accurate tests become available, practices will have the added cost of purchasing new, potentially more expensive, equipment and modifying clinic procedures to accommodate new screening technologies.

Conclusions

Although certain groups appear to be at greater risk than others, cancer screening adherence remains at suboptimal levels across all age-eligible groups [19]. Substantial reductions in morbidity and mortality can only be achieved through sustained adherence to colorectal and breast cancer screenings. Clinicians can play a key role in promoting cancer screenings. Provider recommendation is a robust predictor of regular cancer screening as lack of awareness of colorectal cancer, ambiguity around mammography screening tests, and confusion around screening intervals persist [26, 51, 66, 72–74]. Also understanding the trade-offs of conventional and newer screening tests presents a significant challenge for health-care providers as they assist patients with making informed choices about how to screen for cancers of the colon and breast. Insurance coverage is necessary, but not sufficient, to obtain high levels of cancer screening at recommended intervals. Cost is still a strong predictor of adherence to cancer screenings and intervention efforts must target psychosocial, structural, and economic barriers to screening.

Many evidence-based cancer screening adherence interventions exist. Relatively simple interventions, such as patient or provider reminders, are able to increase mammography and colorectal cancer screening [99]. More intensive intervention efforts are needed for populations with significant access and economic barriers. Multicomponent intervention strategies that target key barriers are successful in sustaining behavior change. Cost and staff resources continue to be a major barrier to intervention implementation [99]. Use of evidence-based materials and messages may be one way to alleviate some of the costs associated with intervention implementation. The Web site Cancer Control PLANET provides a rich source of evidence-based programs and materials (http://cancercontrolplanet.cancer.gov/). Of the available evidence-based intervention, selection of specific intervention strategies should take into account the intended populations to be reached, barriers of said population, and organizational resources available to implement intervention strategies.

References

1. American Cancer Society. *Cancer facts and figures 2008.* Atlanta, GA: American Cancer Society; 2008.
2. Gandini S, Botteri E, Iodice S, et al. Tobacco smoking and cancer: a meta-analysis. *Intern J Cancer.* 2008;122:155–164.
3. Saladi RN, Persaud AN. The causes of skin cancer: a comprehensive review. *Drugs Today (Barc).* 2005;41:37–53.
4. Dumitrescu RG, Cotarla I. Understanding breast cancer risk – where do we stand in 2005? *J Cell Mol Med.* 2005;9:208–221.
5. Humphrey LL, Helfand M, Chan BK, et al. Breast cancer screening: a summary of the evidence for the U.S. preventive services task force. *Ann Intern Med.* 2002;137:347–360.
6. U.S. Preventive Services Task Force. Screening for colorectal cancer: U.S. preventive services task force recommendation statement. *Ann Intern Med.* 2008;149:627–637.
7. McCarthy EP, Burns RB, Freund KM, et al. Mammography use, breast cancer stage at diagnosis, and survival among older women. *J Am Geriatr Soc.* 2000;48:1226–1233.
8. Clark MA, Rakowski W, Bonacore LB. Repeat mammography: prevalence estimates and considerations for assessment. *Ann Behav Med.* 2003;26: 201–211.
9. Partin MR, Slater JS, Caplan L. Randomized controlled trial of a repeat mammography intervention: effect of adherence definitions on results. *Prev Med.* 2005;41:734–740.
10. Rakowski W, Breen N, Meissner H, et al. Prevalence and correlates of repeat mammography among women aged 55–79 in the Year 2000 National Health Interview Survey. *Prev Med.* 2004;39:1–10.

11. Boudreau DM, Luce CL, Ludman E, et al. Concordance of population-based estimates of mammography screening. *Prev Med.* 2007;45:262–266.
12. National Cancer Institute. NCI Statement on Mammography Screening. Available at: http://www.cancer.gov/newscenter/mammstatement31jan02. Accessed October 1; 2007.
13. Smith RA, Saslow D, Sawyer KA, et al. American Cancer Society guidelines for breast cancer screening: update 2003. *CA: Cancer J Clin.* 2003;53: 141–169.
14. Breen N, Wagener DK, Brown ML, et al. Progress in cancer screening over a decade: results of cancer screening from the 1987, 1992, and 1998 National Health Interview Surveys. *J Natl Canc Inst.* 2001;93:1704–1713.
15. Blackman DK, Bennett EM, Miller DS. Trends in self-reported use of mammograms (1989–1997) and Papanicolaou tests (1991–1997) – Behavioral Risk Factor Surveillance System. *MMWR Surveill Summ: Morb Mortal Wkly Rep.* 1999;48:1–22.
16. Breen N, Cronin K, Meissner HI, et al. Reported drop in mammography: is this cause for concern? *Cancer.* 2007;109:2405–2409.
17. Ghafoor A, Jemal A, Ward E, et al. Trends in breast cancer by race and ethnicity. *CA: Cancer J Clin.* 2003;53:342–355.
18. Michaelson J, Satija S, Moore R, et al. The pattern of breast cancer screening utilization and its consequences. *Cancer.* 2002;94:37–43.
19. Blanchard K, Colbert JA, Puri D, et al. Mammographic screening: patterns of use and estimated impact on breast carcinoma survival. *Cancer.* 2004;101:495–507.
20. Byers T, Mouchawar J, Marks J, et al. The American Cancer Society challenge goals. How far can cancer rates decline in the U.S. by the year 2015? *Cancer.* 1999;86:715–727.
21. Centers for Disease Control and Prevention. Use of mammograms among women aged ≥ 40 years – United States, 2000–2005. *MMWR Morb Mortal Wkly Rep.* 2007;56:49–51.
22. Feldstein AC, Vogt TM, Aickin M, et al. Mammography screening rates decline: a person-time approach to evaluation. *Prev Med.* 2006;43:178–182.
23. McFarland EG, Levin B, Lieberman DA, et al. Revised colorectal screening guidelines: joint effort of the American Cancer Society, U.S. Multisociety Task Force on Colorectal Cancer, and American College of Radiology. *Radiology.* 2008;248:717–720.
24. Whitlock EP, Lin JS, Liles E, Beil TL, Fu R. Screening for colorectal cancer: a targeted, updated systematic review for the U.S. Preventive Services Task Force. *Ann Intern Med.* 2008;149:638–658.
25. Peterson NB, Murff HJ, Ness RM, et al. Colorectal cancer screening among men and women in the United States. *J Women's Health.* 2007;16:57–65.
26. Seeff LC, Nadel MR, Klabunde CN, et al. Patterns and predictors of colorectal cancer test use in the adult U.S. population. *Cancer.* 2004;100: 2093–2103.
27. Farmer MM, Bastani R, Kwan L, et al. Predictors of colorectal cancer screening from patients enrolled in a managed care health plan. *Cancer.* 2008;112:1230–1238.

28. National Cancer Policy Board Institute of Medicine. *Fulfilling the potential of cancer prevention and early detection.* Washington, DC: The National Academies Press; 2003.

29. Jepson R, Clegg A, Forbes C, et al. The determinants of screening uptake and interventions for increasing uptake: a systematic review. *Health Technol Assess.* 2000;4:i–vii, 1–133.

30. Schueler KM, Chu PW, Smith-Bindman R. Factors associated with mammography utilization: a systematic quantitative review of the literature. *J Women's Health.* 2008;17:1477–1498.

31. Meissner HI, Breen N, Taubman ML, et al. Which women aren't getting mammograms and why? (United States). *Cancer Causes Control.* 2007;18:61–70.

32. Earp JA, Eng E, O'Malley MS, et al. Increasing use of mammography among older, rural African American women: results from a community trial. *Am J Public Health.* 2002;92:646–654.

33. Halabi S, Skinner CS, Samsa GP, et al. Factors associated with repeat mammography screening. *J Fam Pract.* 2000;49:1104–1112.

34. Rauscher GH, Hawley ST, Earp JA. Baseline predictors of initiation vs. maintenance of regular mammography use among rural women. *Prev Med.* 2005;40:822–830.

35. Calvocoressi L, Stolar M, Kasl SV, et al. Applying recursive partitioning to a prospective study of factors associated with adherence to mammography screening guidelines. *Am J Epidemiol.* 2005;162:1215–1224.

36. Kim J, Jang SN. Socioeconomic disparities in breast cancer screening among US women: trends from 2000 to 2005. *J Prev Med Public Health.* 2008;41:186–194.

37. Hiatt RA, Klabunde C, Breen N, et al. Cancer screening practices from National Health Interview Surveys: past, present, and future. *J Natl Canc Inst.* 2002;94:1837–1846.

38. Rakowski W, Meissner H, Vernon SW, et al. Correlates of repeat and recent mammography for women ages 45–75 in the 2002–2003 Health Information National Trends Survey (HINTS 2003). *Cancer Epidemiol, Biomarkers Prev.* 2006;15:2093–2101.

39. Cohen SS, Palmieri RT, Nyante SJ, et al. Obesity and screening for breast, cervical, and colorectal cancer in women: a review. *Cancer.* 2008;112: 1892–1904.

40. Bobo JK, Shapiro JA, Schulman J, et al. On-schedule mammography rescreening in the National Breast and Cervical Cancer Early Detection Program. *Cancer Epidemiol, Biomarkers Prev.* 2004;13: 620–630.

41. Champion V. Relationship of age to mammography compliance. *Cancer.* 1994;74:329–335.

42. Coughlin SS, Berkowitz Z, Hawkins NA, et al. Breast and colorectal cancer screening and sources of cancer information among older women in the United States: results from the 2003 Health Information National Trends Survey. *Prev Chronic Dis.* 2007;4:A57.

43. Armstrong K, Moye E, Williams S, et al. Screening mammography in women 40–49 years of age: a systematic review for the American College of Physicians. *Ann Intern Med.* 2007;146:516–526.

44. Calvocoressi L, Sun A, Kasl SV, et al. Mammography screening of women in their 40 s: impact of changes in screening guidelines. *Cancer.* 2008;112: 473–480.

45. Rimer BK, Halabi S, Strigo TS, et al. Confusion about mammography: prevalence and consequences. *J Women's Health Gend Based Med.* 1999;8:509–520.

46. Chagpar AB, Polk HC, Jr., McMasters KM. Racial trends in mammography rates: a population-based study. *Surgery.* 2008;144:467–472.

47. Sabatino SA, Coates RJ, Uhler RJ, et al. Disparities in mammography use among US women aged 40–64 years, by race, ethnicity, income, and health insurance status, 1993 and 2005. *Med Care.* 2008;46:692–700.

48. O'Malley MS, Earp JA, Hawley ST, et al. The association of race/ethnicity, socioeconomic status, and physician recommendation for mammography: who gets the message about breast cancer screening? *Am J Public Health.* 2001;91:49–54.

49. Purc-Stephenson RJ, Gorey KM. Lower adherence to screening mammography guidelines among ethnic minority women in America: a meta-analytic review. *Prev Med.* 2008;46:479–488.

50. Rutter DR. Attendance and reattendance for breast cancer screening: a prospective 3-year test of the theory of planned behaviour. *Br J Health Psychol.* 2000;5:1–13.

51. Han PK, Kobrin SC, Klein WM, et al. Perceived ambiguity about screening mammography recommendations: association with future mammography uptake and perceptions. *Cancer Epidemiol, Biomarkers Prev.* 2007;16: 458–466.

52. Russell KM, Champion VL, Skinner CS. Psychosocial factors related to repeat mammography screening over 5 years in African American women. *Cancer Nurs.* 2006;29:236–243.

53. Menon U, Champion V, Monahan PO, et al. Health belief model variables as predictors of progression in stage of mammography adoption. *Am J Health Promot.* 2007;21:255–261.

54. Katapodi MC, Lee KA, Facione NC, et al. Predictors of perceived breast cancer risk and the relation between perceived risk and breast cancer screening: a meta-analytic review. *Prev Med.* 2004;38:388–402.

55. McCaul KD, Branstetter AD, Schroeder DM, et al. What is the relationship between breast cancer risk and mammography screening? A meta-analytic review. *Health Psychol.* 1996;15:423–429.

56. Brewer NT, Salz T, Lillie SE. Systematic review: the long-term effects of false-positive mammograms. *Ann Intern Med.* 2007;146:502–510.

57. Mayne L, Earp JA. Initial and repeat mammography screening: different behaviors/different predictors. *J Rural Health.* 2003;19:63–71.

58. Somkin CP, McPhee SJ, Nguyen T, et al. The effect of access and satisfaction on regular mammogram and Papanicolaou test screening in a multiethnic population. *Med Care.* 2004;42:914–926.

59. Peipins LA, Shapiro JA, Bobo JK, et al. Impact of women's experiences during mammography on adherence to rescreening (United States). *Cancer Causes Control.* 2006;17:439–447.

60. Carlos RC, Fendrick AM, Patterson SK, et al. Associations in breast and colon cancer screening behavior in women. *Acad Radiol.* 2005;12:451–458.

61. Vernon SW. Participation in colorectal cancer screening: a review. *J Natl Canc Inst.* 1997;89:1406–1422.

62. Hawley ST, Volk RJ, Krishnamurthy P, et al. Preferences for colorectal cancer screening among racially/ethnically diverse primary care patients. *Med Care.* 2008;46:S10–S16.

63. Meissner HI, Breen N, Klabunde CN, et al. Patterns of colorectal cancer screening uptake among men and women in the United States. *Cancer Epidemiol, Biomarkers Prev.* 2006;15:389–394.

64. Chen X, White MC, Peipins LA, et al. Increase in screening for colorectal cancer in older Americans: results from a national survey. *J Am Geriatr Soc.* 2008;56:1511–1516.

65. Swan J, Breen N, Coates RJ, et al. Progress in cancer screening practices in the United States: results from the 2000 National Health Interview Survey. *Cancer.* 2003;97:1528–1540.

66. Shapiro JA, Seeff LC, Thompson TD, et al. Colorectal cancer test use from the 2005 National Health Interview Survey. *Cancer Epidemiol, Biomarkers Prev.* 2008;17:1623–1630.

67. Shapiro JA, Seeff LC, Nadel MR. Colorectal cancer-screening tests and associated health behaviors. *Am J Prev Med.* 2001;21:132–137.

68. McQueen A, Vernon SW, Meissner HI, et al. Are there gender differences in colorectal cancer test use prevalence and correlates? *Cancer Epidemiol, Biomarkers Prev.* 2006;15:782–791.

69. Ioannou GN, Chapko MK, Dominitz JA. Predictors of colorectal cancer screening participation in the United States. *Am J Gastroenterol.* 2003;98:2082–2091.

70. Dolan NC, Ferreira MR, Davis TC, et al. Colorectal cancer screening knowledge, attitudes, and beliefs among veterans: does literacy make a difference? *J Clin Oncol.* 2004;22:2617–2622.

71. Peterson NB, Dwyer KA, Mulvaney SA, et al. The influence of health literacy on colorectal cancer screening knowledge, beliefs and behavior. *J Natl Med Assoc.* 2007;99:1105–1112.

72. Klabunde CN, Schenck AP, Davis WW. Barriers to colorectal cancer screening among medicare consumers. *Am J Prev Med.* 2006;30:313–319.

73. Finney Rutten LJ, Nelson DE, et al. Examination of population-wide trends in barriers to cancer screening from a diffusion of innovation perspective (1987–2000). *Prev Med.* 2004;38:258–268.

74. Klabunde CN, Vernon SW, Nadel MR, et al. Barriers to colorectal cancer screening: a comparison of reports from primary care physicians and average-risk adults. *Med Care.* 2005;43:939–944.

75. McQueen A, Vernon SW, Myers RE, et al. Correlates and predictors of colorectal cancer screening among male automotive workers. *Cancer Epidemiol, Biomarkers Prev.* 2007;16:500–509.

76. Beydoun HA, Beydoun MA. Predictors of colorectal cancer screening behaviors among average-risk older adults in the United States. *Cancer Causes Control*. 2008;19:339–359.

77. Greiner KA, James AS, Born W, et al. Predictors of fecal occult blood test (FOBT) completion among low-income adults. *Prev Med*. 2005;41: 676–684.

78. James AS, Campbell MK, Hudson MA. Perceived barriers and benefits to colon cancer screening among African Americans in North Carolina: how does perception relate to screening behavior? *Cancer Epidemiol, Biomarkers Prev*. 2002;11:529–534.

79. Guerra CE, Schwartz JS, Armstrong K, et al. Barriers of and facilitators to physician recommendation of colorectal cancer screening. *J Gen Intern Med*. 2007;22:1681–1688.

80. Dulai GS, Farmer MM, Ganz PA, et al. Primary care provider perceptions of barriers to and facilitators of colorectal cancer screening in a managed care setting. *Cancer*. 2004;100:1843–1852.

81. Jaen CR, Stange KC, Nutting PA. Competing demands of primary care: a model for the delivery of clinical preventive services. *J Fam Pract*. 1994;38:166–171.

82. Crabtree BF, Miller WL, Tallia AF, et al. Delivery of clinical preventive services in family medicine offices. *Ann Fam Med*. 2005;3:430–435.

83. Bonfill X, Marzo M, Pladevall M, et al. Strategies for increasing women participation in community breast cancer screening. *Cochrane Database Syst Rev*. 2001:2CD002943.

84. Legler J, Meissner HI, Coyne C, et al. The effectiveness of interventions to promote mammography among women with historically lower rates of screening. *Cancer Epidemiol, Biomarkers Prev*. 2002;11:59–71.

85. Yabroff KR, Mandelblatt JS. Interventions targeted toward patients to increase mammography use. *Cancer Epidemiol, Biomarkers Prev*. 1999;8:749–757.

86. Mandelblatt JS, Yabroff KR. Effectiveness of interventions designed to increase mammography use: a meta-analysis of provider-targeted strategies. *Cancer Epidemiol, Biomarkers Prev*. 1999;8:759–767.

87. Ratner PA, Bottorff JL, Johnson JL, et al. A meta-analysis of mammography screening promotion. *Cancer Detect Prev*. 2001;25:147–160.

88. Snell JL, Buck EL. Increasing cancer screening: a meta-analysis. *Prev Med*. 1996;25:702–707.

89. Stone EG, Morton SC, Hulscher ME, et al. Interventions that increase use of adult immunization and cancer screening services: a meta-analysis. *Ann Intern Med*. 2002;136:641–651.

90. Wagner TH. The effectiveness of mailed patient reminders on mammography screening: a meta-analysis. *Am J Prev Med*. 1998;14:64–70.

91. Yabroff KR, O'Malley A, Mangan P, et al. Inreach and outreach interventions to improve mammography use. *J Am Med Women's Assoc*. 2001;56:166–173, 188.

92. Sohl SJ, Moyer A. Tailored interventions to promote mammography screening: a meta-analytic review. *Prev Med.* 2007;45:252–261.
93. Denhaerynck K, Lesaffre E, Baele J, et al. Mammography screening attendance: meta-analysis of the effect of direct-contact invitation. *Am J Prev Med.* 2003;25:195–203.
94. Mandelblatt J, Kanetsky PA. Effectiveness of interventions to enhance physician screening for breast cancer. *J Fam Pract.* 1995;40:162–171.
95. Sabatino SA, Habarta N, Baron RC, et al. Interventions to increase recommendation and delivery of screening for breast, cervical, and colorectal cancers by healthcare providers systematic reviews of provider assessment and feedback and provider incentives. *Am J Prev Med.* 2008;35:S67–S74.
96. Baron RC, Rimer BK, Coates RJ, et al. Client-directed interventions to increase community access to breast, cervical, and colorectal cancer screening a systematic review. *Am J Prev Med.* 2008;35:S56–S66.
97. Shea S, DuMouchel W, Bahamonde L. A meta-analysis of 16 randomized controlled trials to evaluate computer-based clinical reminder systems for preventive care in the ambulatory setting. *J Am Med Inform Assoc.* 1996;3:399–409.
98. Bailey TM, Delva J, Gretebeck K, et al. A systematic review of mammography educational interventions for low-income women. *Am J Health Promot.* 2005;20:96–107.
99. Baron RC, Rimer BK, Breslow RA, et al. Client-directed interventions to increase community demand for breast, cervical, and colorectal cancer screening a systematic review. *Am J Prev Med.* 2008;35:S34–S55.
100. Kreuter MW, Wray RJ. Tailored and targeted health communication: strategies for enhancing information relevance. *Am J Health Behav.* 2003;27(Suppl 3):S227–S232.
101. Guide to Community Preventive Services. Provider-Oriented Cancer Screening Interventions: Provider Reminders. Available at: www.thecommunityguide.org/cancer/screening/provider-reminders.htm. Accessed January 19; 2009.
102. Nease DE, Jr., Ruffin MTt, Klinkman MS, et al. Impact of a generalizable reminder system on colorectal cancer screening in diverse primary care practices: a report from the prompting and reminding at encounters for prevention project. *Med Care.* 2008;46:S68–S73.
103. Zapka J. Innovative provider- and health system-directed approaches to improving colorectal cancer screening delivery. *Med Care.* 2008;46: S62–S67.
104. Collins LM, Murphy SA, Bierman KL. A conceptual framework for adaptive preventive interventions. *Prev Sci.* 2004;5:185–196.
105. DeFrank JT, Rimer BK, Gierisch JM, et al. Impact of mailed and automated telephone reminders on receipt of repeat mammograms: a randomized controlled trial. *Am J Prev Med.* 2009;36(6):459–467.
106. Singh V, Saunders C, Wylie L, et al. New diagnostic techniques for breast cancer detection. *Future Oncol.* 2008;4:501–513.

107. Zauber AG, Levin TR, Jaffe CC, et al. Implications of new colorectal can-
     cer screening technologies for primary care practice. *Med Care*. 2008;46:
     S138–S146.
108. Lipkus IM, Halabi S, Strigo TS, et al. The impact of abnormal mammograms
     on psychosocial outcomes and subsequent screening. *Psychooncology*.
     2000;9:402–410.
109. Blanchard K, Colbert JA, Kopans DB, et al. Long-term risk of false-positive
     screening results and subsequent biopsy as a function of mammography use.
     Radiology. 2006;240:335–342.
110. Zheng YF, Saito T, Takahashi M, et al. Factors associated with intentions to
     adhere to colorectal cancer screening follow-up exams. *BMC Public Health*.
     2006;6:272.

Chapter 7
Hormonal Contraceptives and Adherence

Jeanette R. Chin, Geeta K. Swamy, Serina E. Floyd, and Lori A. Bastian

Introduction

Hormonal contraceptives are among the most widely used reversible methods of preventing pregnancy. In 2002, oral contraceptive pills (OCPs) were the most popular contraceptive method, used by 11.6 million women in the USA [1]. Unfortunately, for methods such as OCPs, which depend on adherence in order to be effective, there is a large difference in failure rates between perfect use and typical use. For example, the first year failure rate for OCPs with perfect use is only 0.3%, but with typical use it is 8% [2].

Problems with adherence frequently lead to unintended pregnancies. In 2001, the last year for which data are available, 3.1 million (49%) US pregnancies were unintended (unwanted or mistimed), a number essentially unchanged from 1994 [3]. Four out of ten (42%) of these pregnancies resulted in abortion [3]. The unintended pregnancy rate is particularly high among women of lower socioeconomic status, women who have not completed high school, minority women, and women aged 18–24 years [3]. In 2001, 28% of unintended conceptions occurred during a month when contraception was used. It is estimated

J.R. Chin (✉)
Center for Health Services Research in Primary Care, Durham Veterans Affairs Medical Center and Duke University, Durham, NC, USA
e-mail: jeanette.chin@duke.edu

H. Bosworth (ed.), *Improving Patient Treatment Adherence*,
DOI 10.1007/978-1-4419-5866-2_7,
© Springer Science+Business Media, LLC 2010

that just over 1 million of the unintended pregnancies each year are associated with OCP use, misuse, or discontinuation [4]. Unintended pregnancies are associated with adverse maternal behaviors such as late initiation of prenatal care and tobacco and alcohol use during pregnancy [5, 6]. Unintended pregnancies are also associated with adverse outcomes for children such as low birth weight, higher rates of death in the first year of life, and child abuse [6]. The direct medical costs of unintended pregnancies in this country are estimated at 5.0 billion dollars per year [7].

Because OCPs require daily adherence to be most effective, much of the research into contraceptive adherence has naturally focused on this method. Problems with adherence to OCPs include missing pills, taking pills out of order, sporadic use, starting a new package early or late, not using a back-up contraceptive method when indicated, and discontinuing OCPs without substituting an effective method. Almost half (47%) of OCP users miss one or more pills per cycle, and 22% miss two or more [8]. Discontinuation rates for OCPs are also high. An estimated 32% of new OCP users discontinue the method during the first year of use [9]. One administrative claims database study found that more than 35% of new OCP users aged 15–40 years did not refill their prescriptions at 3 months [10]. Another recent database study of nearly a million US women found that over 12 months only 16–34% of women consistently refilled their prescriptions for hormonal contraceptives [11].

Side effects (such as bleeding problems, nausea, and breast tenderness) are cited as the most frequent reasons for discontinuation of hormonal contraceptives in most studies [12–14]. It is important to note that irregular bleeding, for example, may be a consequence of non-adherence rather than a true medication side effect.

Access to contraception also plays an important role in adherence. A recent study of 1,716 women of primarily lower socioeconomic status found that 60% of subjects discontinued OCPs by the 6-month follow-up point, and that although 34% of them stopped the method due to side effects, 46% stopped because of problems obtaining OCPs or difficulties remembering to take them [15]. Addressing access issues must be a part of improving adherence, especially for those at greatest risk of encountering barriers.

Other factors associated with poor adherence to OCPs include not having an established routine for pill taking and not reading and understanding all the written information that comes with the pill package [8]. The patient–provider interaction and counseling play important roles in improving adherence. It is estimated that 7–27% of women stop using a contraceptive method during the first year for reasons that could be addressed through communication with a provider [16]. Satisfaction with OCPs as a method of birth control is lower among women who give their providers low counseling scores and among women unaware of the multiple non-contraceptive benefits of OCPs [8]. Some of the non-contraceptive benefits of combination (estrogen and progesterone) OCPs are listed in Table 7.1.

Table 7.1 Non-contraceptive benefits of combination OCPs

- Decreased risk of ovarian cancer, including among *BRCA 1* or *2* mutation carriers
- Decreased risk of endometrial cancer
- Decreased acne
- Decreased benign breast disease
- Decreased pelvic inflammatory disease (PID) in current users
- Decreased ectopic pregnancies
- Decreased dysmenorrhea and menorrhagia
- Effective treatment of polycystic ovarian syndrome (PCOS) symptoms such as hirsutism, acne, and irregular bleeding

OCPs, oral contraceptive pills
Source: Adapted from [128]

Clinicians should do everything possible to help women achieve their reproductive goals. Contraceptive counseling sessions should include an exploration of the patient's reproductive goals, background, beliefs, and concerns. Sessions should also identify risk factors for adherence problems and discuss efficacy, side effects, risks, myths, appropriate use, non-contraceptive benefits, and what to do in the case of missed or late doses. Providers may refer to the World Health Organization's (WHO) guidelines on what patients should do in cases of missed doses of various contraceptive methods [17]. Most importantly, the contraceptive counseling visit allows the establishment of a strong provider–patient relationship with promotion of close follow-up.

Interventions

Provider counseling has a positive impact on contraceptive knowledge, if not adherence. Gaudet et al. studied 649 Canadian women filling a prescription for OCPs [18]. Participants were asked about whether they had discussed 12 different topics regarding OCP side effects, non-contraceptive benefits, potential problems, and myths with their providers. Provider–patient discussion was associated with improved knowledge of these topics. Little et al. studied 636 women presenting for a checkup and for a refill of OCPs. They found that those women randomized to receive an educational leaflet and to be questioned regarding contraception by a provider had significantly improved knowledge of factors which contribute to pill failure, appropriate actions to take after pill failure, and emergency contraception [19]. Recently, Melnick et al. found that educational home visits by nurses improved women's contraceptive self-efficacy (a belief that one can prevent pregnancy by controlling sexual and contraceptive-use behavior) [20].

Multiple trials have studied the effectiveness of various types of interventions on reducing unintended pregnancies and sexually transmitted diseases (STDs). Petersen et al. randomized 764 North Carolina women, aged 16–44 years, who were not planning a pregnancy in the next year and were not using an IUD or sterilization as contraception, to either pregnancy and STD prevention counseling sessions (adapted from motivational interviewing) or a control group of general health counseling [21]. At 2 months of follow-up, the proportion of both intervention and control subjects who had improved their level of contraceptive use or maintained a high level of contraceptive use (as determined by effectiveness of the method and consistency of use) was significantly greater than at baseline. However, by 12 months of follow-up, these improvements were no longer seen and there were no differences between the intervention and control arms with regard to contraceptive use.

Peipert et al. evaluated an intervention aimed at increasing dual method (condoms in addition to another method) contraceptive use in order to prevent STDs and unintended pregnancies [22]. They enrolled 542 women aged 13–35 years who desired to avoid pregnancy for at least 24 months and were determined to be at high risk for STDs and unintended pregnancies. "High risk" was primarily defined as age <25 years or, if older than 25 years, a history of an unintended pregnancy or STD. The intervention was based on the transtheoretical model of behavior change and consisted of a computer-based system which administered a series of questions, with feedback tailored to the subject's readiness to change her contraceptive and condom-use behavior. The control group received computerized general contraceptive information. Although subjects in the intervention arm reported a 70% increase in dual method use, there was no difference in the rates of unintended pregnancies or incident STDs between the two groups and, in a reanalysis of the data, women with a past unplanned pregnancy were not more likely to use contraception than those without a prior unplanned pregnancy [23]. These results indicate that achieving consistency in behavior change may be particularly challenging and that the relationship between unplanned pregnancy and contraception is complex.

Boyer et al. randomized 2,157 female Marine recruits, aged 17 years or older, to an experimental intervention aimed at preventing STDs and unintended pregnancies or a control intervention aimed at preventing physical training injuries and cancer [24]. The experimental intervention consisted of four, 2-h group sessions conducted during the 13-week recruit training period. These sessions used a cognitive-behavioral approach, focusing on key elements of the informational–motivation–behavioral skills model, a conceptualization which has shown efficacy as a part of interventions aimed at changing HIV risk behavior. A higher proportion of women in the control group had either a post-intervention STD or an unintended pregnancy during an average of 14 months of follow-up. However, there was no significant difference between the groups when only unintended pregnancies were evaluated as an outcome.

Pregnancy/Postpartum

Several investigators have focused interventions aimed at improving contraceptive adherence among women who are pregnant or postpartum. Traditionally, it has been felt that these women might be more motivated to use contraception and avoid an unintended pregnancy. This assumption has been questioned, however, with regard to postpartum women [25]. A 2002 Cochrane review assessing the effects of postpartum education on contraceptive use identified only three trials (from Lebanon, Peru, and Nepal) [26]. The authors' conclusions were that the effectiveness of postpartum education on contraceptive use has not yet been established in RCTs. They found that postpartum education might be effective in increasing contraceptive use in the short term, but data are limited with regard to preventing unplanned pregnancies. In 2004, Gilliam et al. reported the results of a multi-component postpartum intervention aimed at young (mean age 19 years) Black women which involved counseling, a videotape, and written material covering OCPs [27]. Although the study was limited by small sample size, the intervention did not result in an increase in OCP adherence or decrease in repeat pregnancies at 1 year of follow-up.

Currently, the data are limited with regard to which strategies are most likely to improve adherence to hormonal contraception. A recent Cochrane review on this topic found little evidence from RCTs that supports the hypothesis that counseling improves contraceptive adherence. More research with larger sample sizes, improved follow-up, and high-quality interventions is needed [28].

Adolescents

Most interventions aimed at improving contraceptive adherence and preventing unintended pregnancies target the adolescent population. According to the most recent data, each year in the USA 7.5% of female adolescents aged 15–19 years become pregnant [29] and about 28% of these pregnancies end in abortion [30]. Although the teenage pregnancy rate in this country continues to decline [31], it remains well above rates in other developed countries [32]. The overwhelming majority of these pregnancies are unintended [33], indicating a problem with obtaining and/or using contraception. Adolescents who become pregnant are more likely to be Black or Hispanic, to come from single-parent homes of lower socioeconomic status, to have older male partners, to live in the southern states, and to be themselves children of mothers with limited schooling and a history of teenage pregnancy [34, 35]. Children born to teenage mothers are at a higher risk of being low birth weight, suffering neglect and abuse, performing poorly in school, and becoming teenage parents themselves than children born to adult mothers [35, 36]. Society and the taxpayers bear the cost of adolescent childbearing in multiple ways, including welfare support to young mothers, lost tax revenue due to these mothers' reduced employability and earnings, and foster care [36].

According to the 2002 National Survey of Family Growth (NSFG), three out of four teens used a method of contraception at their first intercourse and 83% of female adolescents used a method at their most recent intercourse [33]. Condoms, OCPs, and depot medroxyprogesterone acetate (DMPA) remain the most popular methods among sexually active adolescents [37]. Although most sexually active adolescents may be using some type of contraception, this use is inconsistent and adherence is particularly problematic in this population. Analysis of Ohio Medicaid claims data of 12- to 19-year olds identified as being at high risk for pregnancy found that only 20% of those teens using any type of prescribed contraceptive were adherent for a full year [38]. High discontinuation rates for both DMPA and OCPs in adolescents are primarily due to side effects and/or trouble remembering injections or pills [39].

A diverse range of types of interventions have been studied to improve contraceptive use and reduce pregnancies in adolescents. In one of the earliest studies, Jay et al., in 1984, randomized 57 females aged 14–19 years from lower socioeconomic backgrounds to either a peer counseling or a nurse counseling program aimed at improving contraceptive adherence. Subjects in both arms received OCPs at the initial visit as well as at 1-, 2-, and 4-month follow-up visits. Adherence with OCPs was measured by a composite of avoidance of pregnancy, appointment adherence, pill count, and urinary fluorescence for riboflavin (to monitor use of the OCP/riboflavin combination). At the 2-month follow-up, adolescents counseled by a peer had significantly lower non-adherence levels than those counseled by a nurse. But at the 4-month follow-up, there was no difference between the two study arms with regard to adherence.

Several reviews have been performed to evaluate interventions aimed at reducing adolescent pregnancies, with widely different standards for searching and analyzing the evidence. As a result, they have drawn different conclusions regarding effectiveness. Kirby found that four types of intervention programs result in increased contraceptive

use in adolescents: sex and HIV education curricula which emphasize that abstinence is the best method to prevent pregnancy and
STDs, but that condoms and contraception are safer than unprotected
sex; one-on-one clinician–patient protocols; service learning programs
involving voluntary community work; and an intensive youth development program [40]. DiCenso et al. concluded that primary prevention
strategies do not improve the use of contraception among young
women and found five studies (four involving abstinence-only programs) which showed evidence that the intervention might increase
pregnancies in partners of male participants [41]. The most promising results have come from intensive, multi-component, long-term,
youth development programs which target at-risk adolescents [42].
The evidence currently is not strong enough to support the conclusion
that one-time clinic consultations decrease unintended pregnancies
[43]. Nevertheless, multiple factors should be included (but often are
omitted) in clinicians' contraceptive counseling sessions with both
adolescents and adults (Table 7.2).

Contraceptive counseling of adolescents especially should take into
consideration factors such as risk-taking behaviors, fear of pelvic
exams, and inaccurate information obtained from peers or even school

Table 7.2 Important components of contraceptive counseling visits

- Evaluate the patient's cultural and religious background
- Explore the patient's reproductive goals
- Discuss how the methods work and their efficacy
- Discuss the most frequent side effects and transient nature of many of
  them
- Review non-contraceptive benefits of particular methods
- Dispel contraceptive myths such as: long-term use of hormonal methods
  can decrease future fertility; some methods can cause cancer or birth
  defects; the oral contraceptive pill causes weight gain
- Determine the best method for that individual patient
- Discuss and provide written instructions on proper use, what to do if doses
  are missed, and when a back-up method is needed. Encourage the patient
  to read accompanying manufacturer information
- Suggest practical measures such as establishing a regular pill-taking time
- Establish follow-up. Encourage and provide easy ways for patients to
  contact the office to have their questions answered
- Discuss the availability and use of emergency contraception and consider
  advance provision of prescriptions to women <18 years

sex education programs. Although adolescents may have concerns regarding confidentiality, if it is possible to integrate support from her parents, adherence to contraception may be improved. In one study, teenagers who chose more effective contraceptive methods reported more support from their mothers [44]. It is certainly appropriate to encourage adolescent patients to postpone sexual activity, but the declining teenage pregnancy rate in this country is primarily a result of improved contraceptive use and less so delayed sexual activity [37]. Counseling adolescents regarding sexuality must be a developmentally appropriate, non-judgmental, yet concrete discussion of effective contraception and ways to prevent STDs.

Longer term contraceptive methods that do not require daily adherence may be particularly appropriate for adolescents. DMPA is the third most popular method among adolescents after condoms and OCPs [37]. A recent study found that adolescents who chose DMPA for postpartum contraception were, at 1 year of follow-up, significantly more likely to be using any form of hormonal contraception and less likely to have had a repeat pregnancy [45]. Although DMPA has been found to have high discontinuation rates, the clinician can play a critical role in decreasing these rates by providing pre-administration counseling, particularly with regard to irregular bleeding and amenorrhea [46]. In one study, women using DMPA who had been educated regarding the possibility of amenorrhea and told to return to the clinic for side effects were found to be significantly more likely to continue use of the method [47]. RCTs performed in Mexico and China also found that women who received appropriate pretreatment counseling were significantly less likely to discontinue DMPA [13, 46]. On-line tools, such as that found on the Depo-Provera® Web site, which allow women to register to receive reminder e-mails regarding injections, may also be particularly helpful for younger women.

One concern many providers may have with regard to DMPA is the 2004 Food and Drug Administration's (FDA) "black-box" warning regarding DMPA and loss of bone mineral density. This warning recommends continued use beyond 2 years only if other contraceptive methods are inadequate and suggests dual x-ray absorptometry (DXA) monitoring after 2 years of use. However, the position of the American Congress of Obstetricians and Gynecologists (ACOG) is that DMPA has likely contributed to a decrease in adolescent pregnancies and that the "black-box" warning should not prevent practitioners from prescribing DMPA or limiting its use to two consecutive years since DMPA-associated bone density loss appears to be recovered with discontinuation of the method and is unlikely to place a woman at increased risk of fracture [48]. ACOG also does not recommend DXA monitoring solely in response to DMPA use.

Other long-acting forms of contraception that are quite appropriate for adolescent use include the subdermal single-rod etonogestrel contraceptive implant (Implanon®) and intrauterine devices (IUDs). Although not yet widely used by adolescents in this country, the etonogestrel subdermal implant is highly effective for up to 3 years and easy to insert. An IUD containing levonorgestrel (Mirena®) was FDA-approved in 2000, is associated with reduced menstrual bleeding or amenorrhea, and is another option in addition to the copper IUD (Paraguard®). Although IUDs have traditionally been thought of as a contraceptive method only for monogamous parous women with no history of STDs, thus limiting use in adolescents, the WHO gives IUDs a category 2 rating for women <20 years of age [49], indicating that the benefits generally outweigh the risks. ACOG supports the consideration of IUDs as first-line contraceptive methods for both nulliparous and parous adolescents [50]. It has been shown that with modern IUDs, the risk of pelvic inflammatory disease (PID) is primarily increased in the 3 weeks immediately following insertion [51]. Additionally, if there is no clinical evidence of infection, gonorrhea and chlamydia testing can be performed at the same time as IUD insertion rather than scheduling a follow-up visit for insertion. Studies show that that even if chlamydia testing returns positive, PID is unlikely to develop if treatment is initiated, even with the IUD retained [52, 53].

Adolescents with Chronic Medical Conditions

Increasing numbers of young women with conditions such as congenital heart disease and cystic fibrosis are surviving into adulthood. Adolescents with chronic medical conditions have been found to have the same sexual aspirations as those of their peers [54]. A 1996 study showed no difference between adolescents with and without chronic conditions with regard to ever having intercourse, age of first intercourse, or pregnancy [55]. However, many of these young women, despite encountering the health-care system on a frequent basis, do not receive appropriate counseling regarding their reproductive health. They may not be educated about the potentially significant risks to their health posed by pregnancy and therefore the importance of contraception. A recent study reported that only 51% of 116 women with congenital heart disease recalled receiving specific information from a nurse or doctor regarding contraception. Eighty of these women were felt to be at intermediate to high risk of cardiac complications during pregnancy, yet 34% of them did not recall having received this information [56]. A study of 55 young Australian women with cystic fibrosis found that although they were no less likely to be sexually active than their peers without cystic fibrosis, they were significantly less likely to use contraception [57]. For women with chronic conditions, it is not only important to communicate the potential risks to their health that pregnancy might confer, but also to help them find an appropriate and safe contraceptive. Some contraceptive types, typically estrogen-containing methods, are contraindicated in women with certain chronic conditions. But many chronically ill women are under the false assumption, or have been told in error by their health-care providers, that they are not candidates for certain types of highly effective contraception [58]. Not only do patients and clinicians need to be better educated, but there is also a need for improved collaboration between reproductive health-care providers and the providers who manage these women's chronic conditions.

Obesity

Obesity is an epidemic in the USA, with 33% of women aged 20 years or older classified as obese (body mass index [BMI] > 30 kg/m^2) [59]. Obesity significantly increases the risk of pregnancy complications including gestational hypertension, preeclampsia, gestational diabetes, cesarean delivery, and fetal macrosomia [60–63]. Because of these risks, the avoidance of unintended pregnancies in obese women is of particular importance. Several studies have examined whether obese women are less likely to use contraception or be adherent to a particular method. Kaneshiro et al. evaluated 6,690 women and found no differences in contraceptive use patterns or in the risk of unintended pregnancies between normal weight women and overweight or obese women [64]. Huber et al. enrolled 145 OCP users in a 5 week, diary-based study of adherence and found that obese women were no less likely to have adherence problems [65]. In contrast, Chuang et al. found an association between obesity and contraceptive nonuse in a sample of 7,943 women [66]. Similarly, Chin et al. found an association between a BMI $\geq$ 35 kg/m^2 and less use of the most effective contraceptive methods (OCPs, IUDs, and sterilization) at 12 months postpartum in a sample of 361 women [67].

If obese women are less likely to use contraception, the reasons behind this are not clear. A recent study found similar sexual activity levels among women of different BMI categories [68]. Fertility has been shown to be decreased among obese women [69] and it's possible that these women believe they are less likely to conceive. Although Kaneshiro et al. found no differences in perceived fertility between BMI categories [64], other studies have shown that women with diabetes, for example, perceive themselves to be less fertile [70, 71]. It is possible that chronic conditions, such as hypertension and diabetes, which often accompany obesity, might be determinants of less contraceptive use by obese women. This may be due to health-care providers being less likely to prescribe contraception because of safety concerns and patients less likely to accept it for similar reasons. Nevertheless, given the number of women of reproductive age in this country who are obese and develop associated health problems, finding effective, safe contraceptive methods for them is critically important and it is nearly always possible.

While it is well known that the contraceptive patch and first generation subdermal implants (Norplant$^{®}$) are less effective in obese women [72–74], studies regarding oral contraceptive efficacy in obese women have shown conflicting results [75–80]. No data currently exist to suggest that the single-rod etonogestrel implant is less effective in obese women. The use of DMPA, in either subcutaneous or intramuscular form, has not been associated with higher pregnancy rates in obese women [81]. Even if future studies confirm that OCPs have decreased effectiveness in the setting of obesity, this probably does not mean that this method should be avoided altogether in this population. One study estimated that the decreased effectiveness of OCPs in overweight or obese women translates into an additional two to four pregnancies per 100 woman years [75], meaning that the effectiveness still remains high. What is most important is to take into careful consideration the woman's weight, her co-morbid conditions, her ability to adhere to different contraceptive methods, and to weigh the risk of a particular method against the risk of pregnancy with less effective methods or no contraception at all. Pregnancy and childbirth among obese women are associated with more health risks than contraception [82].

With regard to reversible contraceptive methods, highly effective and longer term ones which do not contain estrogen, such as DMPA and IUDs, may be good options for obese women. It is important to keep in mind with regard to the woman's overall health, however, that DMPA has been associated with more weight gain in obese than non-obese women [83]. While both the levonorgestrel containing IUD and the copper IUD are associated with a decreased risk of endometrial cancer, the levonorgestrel-containing device may be particularly appropriate for obese women and can also effectively treat conditions such as menorrhagia and anemia [84].

Combined hormonal contraception and obesity represent independent risk factors for thromboembolism [85, 86]. One case–control study found a substantially higher risk of venous thromboembolism in obese women using combination OCPs than in normal weight OCP users [87]. However, the risk of thromboembolism from use of a combined method is still less than that posed by pregnancy [88]. Progesterone-only methods have not been shown to increase the risk of thromboembolism [89], so they may provide the best contraceptive options for some obese women.

Combination OCPs appear to cause a small increase in blood pressure [90, 91]. A WHO case–control study performed in European and developing countries found that combination OCPs in women with hypertension increase the risk of myocardial infarction [92]. A pooled analysis of two US case–control studies suggested that combination OCPs do not increase the risk of stroke in women with hypertension; however, the study was limited by too few women who were older than 35 years or had hypertension [93]. For women with well-controlled hypertension who are younger than 35 years, do not smoke, have no evidence of vascular disease, and are otherwise healthy, combined hormonal contraception may still be a reasonable option as the absolute risk of myocardial infarction or stroke remains low [94]. DMPA does not appear to increase blood pressure in normotensive or hypertensive women [95, 96]. Nor does DMPA appear to increase cardiovascular disease risk [89].

The authors of a 2006 Cochrane review of hormonal vs. non-hormonal contraceptives in women with diabetes type 1 or 2 concluded that there is insufficient evidence to determine whether progesterone-only or combination hormonal contraception alters diabetes control or the development of complications [97]. Due to theoretical concerns, the recommendations with regard to use of combination hormonal contraceptives by women with diabetes are similar to those for women with hypertension. Use should generally be limited to women younger than 35 years who have had diabetes for less than 20 years, are otherwise healthy, do not smoke, and have good glycemic control without evidence of vascular disease [49, 94].

The incidence of bariatric surgeries increased by 800% between 1998 and 2005, with 83% of surgeries in the 18- to 45-year-old age group being performed on women [98]. A recent systematic review performed by the Rand Corporation concluded that there is insufficient evidence regarding contraceptive efficacy in women who have undergone bariatric surgery, but concerns exist regarding potentially impaired absorption of OCPs [98]. The authors also stated that existing data suggest that bariatric surgery may have a beneficial effect on fertility with correction of the abnormal hormonal profiles seen in polycystic ovarian syndrome and an increased regularity of menses.

Policy Implications

Patient adherence is not only affected by individual behaviors, but also by complex policies and systems that create barriers to contraceptive knowledge, access, and use (Table 7.3).

For some women, problems with adherence stem from a basic inability to afford expensive brand name contraceptives. As described in a recent editorial, the practice of giving a woman several sample packs of a brand name contraceptive as well as a prescription which she subsequently cannot afford to fill may place her at risk for an unintended pregnancy once the free supply runs out [99]. Providers must discuss with patients their insurance status and ability

Table 7.3 Practices and policies which may impede contraceptive adherence

- Providing/prescribing expensive brand name contraceptives
- Inadequate funding of family planning services for low-income women
- Requiring a pelvic exam to initiate hormonal contraception
- Waiting to start hormonal contraception until the next menses
- Requiring teens to obtain a prescription for emergency contraception (EC).
- Lack of knowledge about EC among providers
- Abstinence-only sex education

to afford particular contraceptive types and suggest money-saving options. Many nationwide pharmacies now offer inexpensive generic OCPs and provide lists of these medications on their Web sites. Patients can sometimes also save money by using mail-out pharmacies to receive 3-month supplies.

Medicaid Title X was established by the Family Planning Services and Population Research Act of 1970 and is a vital source of funding for family planning clinics throughout the USA. These clinics primarily support young, low-income women who do not meet the narrow eligibility requirements of Medicaid. Services provided through Title X are on a sliding-scale based on income. Unfortunately, although family planning services may, from a societal perspective, save money in the long term by preventing unintended pregnancies and allowing women to improve their educational and economic status, funding for Title X has not kept up with inflation [100]. These funding limitations make it impossible for the program to achieve its stated goal of "making comprehensive voluntary family planning services readily available to all persons desiring such services [101]."

Many reproductive health-care providers argue that some of the current health-care practices related to contraceptive care impede access. ACOG, WHO, and the Planned Parenthood Federation of America support unbundling of services such that a pelvic exam is not required in order to initiate hormonal contraception [102]. Particularly for adolescents, the prospect of a pelvic exam can elicit fear and anxiety [103], which may result in avoidance to seek contraceptive services. In fact, for many young women their first family planning visit is to obtain a pregnancy test [104]. The California Office of Family Planning conducted an 18-month project in 1996–1997 where low-income women were offered hormonal contraceptives after a detailed medical history was elicited and blood pressure taken, but without the requirement of a pelvic exam [105]. Approximately 50% of the women were referred to an associated family planning clinic due to need for more extensive services and the majority of those women followed through with the referral within 6 weeks. Women in the project reported improved contraceptive patterns. Those who declined a pelvic exam were not found to be at higher risk of cervical neoplasia when compared with non-project participants [106]. Some women do have medical conditions such that they should not take hormonal contraception. However, for all such conditions as described by the WHO, a clinical breast or pelvic exam is unlikely to detect them and medical history and a blood pressure measurement are most useful [107]. Furthermore, some argue that requiring screening examinations to obtain contraception poses important ethical concerns in that women who are informed of the implications of a decision to defer screening should have the right to do so [107]. Certainly women should be educated regarding the importance of Pap smears and STD screening, but a woman's desire to defer a pelvic exam may not be enough reason to put her at risk for an unintended pregnancy.

The conventional practices of waiting to start hormonal contraception until the next menses and scheduling follow-up visits to have IUDs inserted, both of which aim to avoid contraceptive use during an undetected pregnancy, are not necessary. The WHO states that immediate start of contraception is acceptable if the woman has no signs or symptoms of pregnancy and meets any of the following criteria: she has not had intercourse since her last normal menses; she consistently and correctly uses a reliable contraceptive method; she is within 7 days of the start of a normal menses; she is less than 4 weeks postpartum and not breastfeeding; she is within 7 days of an abortion or miscarriage; or she is fully or nearly fully breastfeeding, amenorrheic, and less than 6 months postpartum [17]. The authors of a 2008 Cochrane review of five RCTs comparing immediate start to conventional start of various hormonal contraceptives concluded that there is limited evidence that immediate start reduces unintended pregnancies or increases method continuation [108]. However, one of the trials included in the review evaluated immediate injection of DMPA vs. a bridging contraceptive method and found fewer pregnancies during follow-up in the immediate start group and those women were also more satisfied with DMPA [109]. Guidelines for the use of back-up methods with immediate start of various contraceptives are listed in Table 7.4.

Table 7.4 Immediate start of contraception and the use of back-up methods

Combination OCPs[a]	DMPA[b]	IUDs[c]
If not initiating within 5 days of the start of menses, use a back-up method for 7 days	If not initiating within 7 days of the start of menses, use a back-up method for 7 days	– Copper T: No back-up method needed with immediate start – Levonorgestrel containing: If not inserting within 7 days of the start of menses, use a back-up method for 7 days

[a]OCPs Oral contraceptive pills
[b]Depot medroxyprogesterone acetate
[c]Intrauterine device
Source: [17]

Part of counseling patients regarding contraceptive adherence and avoiding unintended pregnancies involves the discussion of back-up methods. The FDA granted Plan B® emergency contraception (EC) nonprescription status for women aged 18 years and older in 2006. In 2009, the FDA approved Plan B One Step (a single, rather than two dose regimen) which is available over-the-counter to women 17 years and older. For women younger than 18 or 17 years, respectively, EC is available by prescription only. When used within 72 h of unprotected intercourse, EC has been estimated to prevent three out of four pregnancies that would otherwise occur [110]. The over-the-counter status was granted because EC meets FDA safety criteria in that it is nontoxic, nonaddictive, and has minimal side effects [111]. If a pregnant woman takes EC it will not harm the pregnancy [111]. Because EC does not contain estrogen and consists only of progesterone (levonorgestrel), it does not pose the risks of combination hormonal contraception and is safe for women with chronic medical conditions. Teenagers are no less able than older women to understand how to use EC properly [112, 113], and EC knowledge and access have not been found to adversely affect teen sexual behavior [114, 115]. Not only are there FDA restrictions on EC access for adolescents, but many clinicians are also not knowledgeable about EC and do not educate their patients, whether adolescents or adults, about its use and availability [116]. A 2007 systematic review found no convincing evidence that improved access to EC reduces unintended pregnancies [117]. One recent study indicated that this may be because some women with unrestricted access to EC may substitute it for their usual contraceptive method [118]. Another study, however, found that although advance provision of EC increased its use in a group of women aged 15–24 years, it did not increase sexually risky behavior or result in repeated use of EC in lieu of other contraceptive methods [119]. It should certainly be emphasized to women that EC is to be used as *back-up*, and is not a reliable first-line contraceptive method. But improved access and advance provision may be appropriate for some women and teenagers seeking to avoid an unintended pregnancy.

Until recently, the US federal government has promoted the abstinence-only-until marriage (AOUM) model as its primary sexual education method for teens. Programs which give information to teens regarding contraception or condoms (except to emphasize the methods' failure rates) have not been eligible for federal AOUM funding. This funding greatly expanded after 1996 with welfare reform and in 2001 the federal government started to directly fund community- and faith-based organizations to promote AOUM. Several studies have been conducted to evaluate the effects of AOUM curricula on the sexual behavior and reproductive outcomes of teenagers. An assessment of youth who took an abstinence pledge found that although they did delay the onset of intercourse for an average of 18 months as compared to non-pledgers, they were less likely than non-pledgers to use contraception when they did first have intercourse and 88% ultimately had intercourse prior to marriage [120]. Furthermore, after 6 years of follow-up, those who had taken an abstinence pledge did not have a decreased rate of STDs as compared to non-pledgers. In 2007, Mathematica Policy Research, an evaluation firm hired by the Department of Health and Human Services, published their results of an extensive evaluation of four AOUM programs [121]. The study found that there were no differences between intervention and control groups with regard to sexual initiation rates, age at first intercourse, condom use, number of sexual partners, pregnancy rates, or STD rates. Teenage pregnancy rates have been declining for nearly two decades. As mentioned previously, some of this decline is due to delayed sexual activity among teens, but the majority (75%) is due to more contraceptive use [37]. In addition, sexual experience rates for teens have not changed since 2001 despite increased federal funding for AOUM programs [122]. The benefits of abstinence should be emphasized to adolescents and they should be encouraged to delay sexual activity, but restricting their access to accurate reproductive health and contraceptive information as a policy is based on little evidence.

Summary

Most women spend decades of their lives trying to avoid pregnancy and using contraception. In light of the fact that nearly one-half of all women will have an unintended pregnancy during their lives [123], contraceptive adherence is clearly challenging and complex. Patient-specific factors, such as cultural or religious background, feelings about becoming pregnant, past experiences, partner and/or parental support, ability to establish a routine, and socioeconomic characteristics converge with health-care system and governmental practices and policies to determine a woman's ability to succeed at family planning. The clinician can play an important role in improving his or her patients' contraceptive care and adherence. Contraception is basic preventative care for women that should be an important part of all routine visits with primary care and reproductive health-care providers, even if only to confirm satisfaction with a current method. A patient-centered care model has been advocated as a good way to improve contraceptive care [101]. Patient-centered care means being respectful of and responsive to patients' preferences and needs, respectively, and ensuring that patients' values are what guide clinical decisions [124]. This approach has been shown to improve patient satisfaction and compliance in primary care [125–127]. It is by keeping the patient at the center of all interactions, decreasing barriers to access and use as much as possible, and providing accurate and up-to-date information that clinicians can be most effective in helping their individual patients achieve their reproductive goals.

References

1. Mosher WD, Martinez GM, Chandra A, et al. Use of contraception and use of family planning services in the United States: 1982–2002. *Adv Data*. 2004;350:1–36.

2. Trussell J. Contraceptive efficacy. In: Hatcher RA TJ, Nelson AL, Cates W, Stewart FH, Kowal D, eds. *Contraceptive technology. 19th Ed.* New York, NY: Ardent Media; 2007:747–826.

3. Finer LB, Henshaw SK. Disparities in rates of unintended pregnancy in the United States, 1994 and 2001. *Perspect Sex Reprod Health.* 2006;38(2): 90–96.

4. Rosenberg MJ, Waugh MS, Long S. Unintended pregnancies and use, misuse and discontinuation of oral contraceptives. *J Reprod Med.* 1995;40(5): 355–360.

5. Kost K, Landry DJ, Darroch JE. Predicting maternal behaviors during pregnancy: does intention status matter? *Fam Plann Perspect.* 1998;30(2):79–88.

6. Brown S, Eisenberg L. *The best intentions: Unintended pregnancy and the well-being of children and families.* Washington, DC: National Academy Press; 1995:50–90.

7. Trussell J. The cost of unintended pregnancy in the United States. *Contraception.* 2007;75(3):168–170.

8. Rosenberg MJ, Waugh MS, Burnhill MS. Compliance, counseling and satisfaction with oral contraceptives: a prospective evaluation. *Fam Plann Perspect.* 1998;30(2):89–92, 104.

9. Schwartz JL, Creinin MD, Pymar HC, et al. Predicting risk of ovulation in new start oral contraceptive users. *Obstet Gynecol.* 2002;99(2):177–182.

10. Murphy PA, Brixner D. Hormonal contraceptive discontinuation patterns according to formulation: investigation of associations in an administrative claims database. *Contraception.* 2008;77(4):257–263.

11. Nelson AL, Westhoff C, Schnare SM. Real-world patterns of prescription refills for branded hormonal contraceptives: a reflection of contraceptive discontinuation. *Obstet Gynecol.* 2008;112(4):782–787.

12. Rosenberg MJ, Waugh MS, Meehan TE. Use and misuse of oral contraceptives: risk indicators for poor pill taking and discontinuation. *Contraception.* 1995;51(5):283–288.

13. Lei ZW, Wu SC, Garceau RJ, et al. Effect of pretreatment counseling on discontinuation rates in Chinese women given depo-medroxyprogesterone acetate for contraception. *Contraception.* 1996;53(6):357–361.

14. Davie JE, Walling MR, Mansour DJ, et al. Impact of patient counseling on acceptance of the levonorgestrel implant contraceptive in the United Kingdom. *Clin Ther.* 1996;18(1):150–159.

15. Westhoff CL, Heartwell S, Edwards S, et al. Oral contraceptive discontinuation: do side effects matter? *Am J Obstet Gynecol.* 2007;196(4):412, e411–416; discussion 412, e416–417.

16. Blanc AK, Curtis SL, Croft TN. Monitoring contraceptive continuation: links to fertility outcomes and quality of care. *Stud Fam Plann.* 2002;33(2):127–140.

17. World Health Organization. *Selected practice recommendations for contraceptive use. 2nd Ed;* 2004. Available at: http://www.who.int/reproductive-health/publications/spr/spr.pdf. Accessed January 15, 2009.

18. Gaudet LM, Kives S, Hahn PM, et al. What women believe about oral contraceptives and the effect of counseling. *Contraception.* 2004;69(1):31–36.
19. Little P, Griffin S, Kelly J, et al. Effect of educational leaflets and questions on knowledge of contraception in women taking the combined contraceptive pill: randomised controlled trial. *Br Med J.* 1998;316(7149):1948–1952.
20. Melnick AL, Rdesinski RE, Creach ED, et al. The influence of nurse home visits, including provision of 3 months of contraceptives and contraceptive counseling, on perceived barriers to contraceptive use and contraceptive use self-efficacy. *Womens Health Issues.* 2008;18(6):471–481.
21. Petersen R, Albright J, Garrett JM, et al. Pregnancy and STD prevention counseling using an adaptation of motivational interviewing: a randomized controlled trial. *Perspect Sex Reprod Health.* 2007;39(1):21–28.
22. Peipert JF, Redding CA, Blume JD, et al. Tailored intervention to increase dual-contraceptive method use: a randomized trial to reduce unintended pregnancies and sexually transmitted infections. *Am J Obstet Gynecol.* 2008;198(6):630, e631–e638.
23. Matteson KA, Peipert JF, Allsworth J, et al. Unplanned pregnancy: does past experience influence the use of a contraceptive method? *Obstet Gynecol.* 2006;107(1):121–127.
24. Boyer CB, Shafer MA, Shaffer RA, et al. Evaluation of a cognitive-behavioral, group, randomized controlled intervention trial to prevent sexually transmitted infections and unintended pregnancies in young women. *Prev Med.* 2005;40(4):420–431.
25. Winikoff B, Mensch B. Rethinking postpartum family planning. *Stud Fam Plann.* 1991;22(5):294–307.
26. Hiller JE, Griffith E, Jenner F. Education for contraceptive use by women after childbirth. *Cochrane Database Syst Rev.* 2002;3:CD001863.
27. Gilliam M, Knight S, McCarthy M, Jr. Success with oral contraceptives: a pilot study. *Contraception.* 2004;69(5):413–418.
28. Halpern V, Grimes DA, Lopez L, et al. Strategies to improve adherence and acceptability of hormonal methods for contraception. *Cochrane Database Syst Rev.* 2006;1:CD004317.
29. Guttmacher Institute. U.S. Teenage Pregnancy Statistics: National and State Trends and Trends by Race and Ethnicity. Updated September; 2006. New York, NY: The Alan Guttmacher Institute. Available at: http://www.guttmacher.org/pubs/2006/09/12/USTPstats.pdf. Accessed January 15, 2009.
30. Ventura SJ, Abma JC, Mosher WD, et al. *Recent trends in teenage pregnancy in the United States, 1990–2002.* Health E-Stats. Hyattsville, MD: National Center for Health Statistics. Available at: http://www.cdc.gov/nchs/data/hestat/teenpreg1990–2002/teenpreg1990–2002.htm.
31. Hamilton BE, Martin JA, Ventura SJ. Births: preliminary data for 2005. *Natl Vital Stat Rep.* 2006;55(11):1–18.
32. Singh S, Darroch JE. Adolescent pregnancy and childbearing: levels and trends in developed countries. *Fam Plann Perspect.* 2000;32(1):14–23.

33. Abma JC, Martinez GM, Mosher WD, et al. Teenagers in the United States: sexual activity, contraceptive use, and childbearing, 2002. *Vital Health Stat.* 2004;23(24):1–48.

34. Darroch JE. Adolescent pregnancy trends and demographics. *Curr Womens Health Rep.* 2001;1(2):102–110.

35. Elfenbein DS, Felice ME. Adolescent pregnancy. *Pediatr Clin North Am.* 2003;50(4):781–800, viii.

36. Hoffman SD, Maynard RA. *Kids having kids: Economic costs and social consequences of teen pregnancy. 2nd Ed.* Washington, DC: Urban Institute; 2008.

37. Santelli JS, Lindberg LD, Finer LB, et al. Explaining recent declines in adolescent pregnancy in the United States: the contribution of abstinence and improved contraceptive use. *Am J Public Health.* 2007;97(1):150–156.

38. Zink TM, Shireman TI, Ho M, et al. High-risk teen compliance with prescription contraception: an analysis of Ohio Medicaid claims. *J Pediatr Adolesc Gynecol.* 2002;15(1):15–21.

39. O'Dell CM, Forke CM, Polaneczky MM, et al. Depot medroxyprogesterone acetate or oral contraception in postpartum adolescents. *Obstet Gynecol.* 1998;91(4):609–614.

40. Kirby D. Effective approaches to reducing adolescent unprotected sex, pregnancy, and childbearing. *J Sex Res.* 2002;39(1):51–57.

41. DiCenso A, Guyatt G, Willan A, et al. Interventions to reduce unintended pregnancies among adolescents: systematic review of randomised controlled trials. *Br Med J.* 2002;324(7351):1426.

42. Philliber S, Kaye JW, Herrling S, et al. Preventing pregnancy and improving health care access among teenagers: an evaluation of the Children's Aid Society-Carrera program. *Perspect Sex Reprod Health.* 2002;34(5):244–251.

43. Moos MK, Bartholomew NE, Lohr KN. Counseling in the clinical setting to prevent unintended pregnancy: an evidence-based research agenda. *Contraception.* 2003;67(2):115–132.

44. Harper C, Callegari L, Raine T, et al. Adolescent clinic visits for contraception: support from mothers, male partners and friends. *Perspect Sex Reprod Health.* 2004;36(1):20–26.

45. Thurman AR, Hammond N, Brown HE, et al. Preventing repeat teen pregnancy: postpartum depot medroxyprogesterone acetate, oral contraceptive pills, or the patch? *J Pediatr Adolesc Gynecol.* 2007;20(2):61–65.

46. Canto De Cetina TE, Canto P, Ordonez Luna M. Effect of counseling to improve compliance in Mexican women receiving depot-medroxyprogesterone acetate. *Contraception.* 2001;63(3):143–146.

47. Hubacher D, Goco N, Gonzalez B, et al. Factors affecting continuation rates of DMPA. *Contraception.* 1999;60(6):345–351.

48. Depot medroxyprogesterone acetate and bone effects. ACOG Committee Opinion No.415. American College of Obstetricians and Gynecologists. *Obstet Gynecol* 2008;112:727–730.

49. World Health Organization. *Medical eligibility criteria for contraceptive use. 3rd Ed*; 2004. Available at: http://www.who.int/reproductive-health/publications/mec/index.htm. Accessed December 31, 2008.
50. Intrauterine devices and adolescents. ACOG Committee Opinion No. 392. American College of Obstetricians and Gynecologists. *Obstet Gynecol* 2007;110:1493–1495.
51. Farley TM, Rosenberg MJ, Rowe PJ, et al. Intrauterine devices and pelvic inflammatory disease: an international perspective. *Lancet.* 1992;339(8796):785–788.
52. Faundes A, Telles E, Cristofoletti ML, et al. The risk of inadvertent intrauterine device insertion in women carriers of endocervical *Chlamydia trachomatis. Contraception.* 1998;58(2):105–109.
53. Skjeldestad FE, Halvorsen LE, Kahn H, et al. IUD users in Norway are at low risk for genital C. trachomatis infection. *Contraception.* 1996;54(4): 209–212.
54. Blum RW. Sexual health contraceptive needs of adolescents with chronic conditions. *Arch Pediatr Adolesc Med.* 1997;151(3):290–297.
55. Suris JC, Resnick MD, Cassuto N, et al. Sexual behavior of adolescents with chronic disease and disability. *J Adolesc Health.* 1996;19(2):124–131.
56. Kovacs AH, Harrison JL, Colman JM, et al. Pregnancy and contraception in congenital heart disease: what women are not told. *J Am CollCardiol.* 2008;52(7):577–578.
57. Sawyer SM, Phelan PD, Bowes G. Reproductive health in young women with cystic fibrosis: knowledge, behavior and attitudes. *J Adolesc Health.* 1995;17(1):46–50.
58. Rogers P, Mansour D, Mattinson A, et al. A collaborative clinic between contraception and sexual health services and an adult congenital heart disease clinic. *J Fam Plann Reprod Health Care.* 2007;33(1):17–21.
59. Ogden CL, Carroll MD, Curtin LR, et al. Prevalence of overweight and obesity in the United States, 1999–2004. *J Am Med Assoc.* 2006;295(13): 1549–1555.
60. Cedergren MI. Maternal morbid obesity and the risk of adverse pregnancy outcome. *Obstet Gynecol.* 2004;103(2):219–224.
61. Weiss JL, Malone FD, Emig D, et al. Obesity, obstetric complications and cesarean delivery rate – a population-based screening study. *Am J Obstet Gynecol.* 2004;190(4):1091–1097.
62. Sebire NJ, Jolly M, Harris JP, et al. Maternal obesity and pregnancy outcome: a study of 287,213 pregnancies in London. *Int J Obes Relat Metabol Disord.* 2001;25(8):1175–1182.
63. Young TK, Woodmansee B. Factors that are associated with cesarean delivery in a large private practice: the importance of prepregnancy body mass index and weight gain. *Am J Obstet Gynecol.* 2002;187(2):312–318; discussion 318–320.
64. Kaneshiro B, Edelman A, Carlson N, et al. The relationship between body mass index and unintended pregnancy: results from the 2002 National Survey of Family Growth. *Contraception.* 2008;77(4):234–238.

65. Huber LR, Hogue CJ, Stein AD, et al. Contraceptive use and discontinuation: findings from the contraceptive history, initiation, and choice study. *Am J Obstet Gynecol.* 2006;194(5):1290–1295.

66. Chuang CH, Chase GA, Bensyl DM, et al. Contraceptive use by diabetic and obese women. *Womens Health Issues.* 2005;15(4):167–173.

67. Chin JR, Swamy GK, Ostbye T, Bastian LA. Contraceptive use by obese women one year postpartum. *Contraception.* 2009;80(5):463–468.

68. Kaneshiro B, Jensen JT, Carlson NE, et al. Body mass index and sexual behavior. *Obstet Gynecol.* 2008;112(3):586–592.

69. Ramlau-Hansen CH, Thulstrup AM, Nohr EA, et al. Subfecundity in overweight and obese couples. *Hum Reprod.* 2007;22(6):1634–1637.

70. Holing EV, Beyer CS, Brown ZA, et al. Why don't women with diabetes plan their pregnancies? *Diab Care.* 1998;21(6):889–895.

71. St James PJ, Younger MD, Hamilton BD, et al. Unplanned pregnancies in young women with diabetes. An analysis of psychosocial factors. *Diab Care.* 1993;16(12):1572–1578.

72. Gu S, Sivin I, Du M, et al. Effectiveness of Norplant implants through seven years: a large-scale study in China. *Contraception.* 1995;52(2):99–103.

73. Grubb GS, Moore D, Anderson NG. Pre-introductory clinical trials of Norplant implants: a comparison of seventeen countries' experience. *Contraception.* 1995;52(5):287–296.

74. Zieman M, Guillebaud J, Weisberg E, et al. Contraceptive efficacy and cycle control with the Ortho Evra/Evra transdermal system: the analysis of pooled data. *Fertil Steril.* 2002;77(2 Suppl 2):S13–S18.

75. Holt VL, Scholes D, Wicklund KG, et al. Body mass index, weight, and oral contraceptive failure risk. *Obstet Gynecol.* 2005;105(1):46–52.

76. Holt VL, Cushing-Haugen KL, Daling JR. Body weight and risk of oral contraceptive failure. *Obstet Gynecol.* 2002;99(5 Pt 1):820–827.

77. Vessey M. Oral contraceptive failures and body weight: findings in a large cohort study. *J Fam Plann Reprod Health Care.* 2001;27(2):90–91.

78. Brunner Huber LR, Hogue CJ, Stein AD, et al. Body mass index and risk for oral contraceptive failure: a case-cohort study in South Carolina. *Ann Epidemiol.* 2006;16(8):637–643.

79. Brunner Huber LR, Hogue CJ. The association between body weight, unintended pregnancy resulting in a livebirth, and contraception at the time of conception. *Matern Child Health J.* 2005;9(4):413–420.

80. Brunner Huber LR, Toth JL. Obesity and oral contraceptive failure: findings from the 2002 National Survey of Family Growth. *Am J Epidemiol.* 2007;166(11):1306–1311.

81. Jain J, Dutton C, Nicosia A, et al. Pharmacokinetics, ovulation suppression and return to ovulation following a lower dose subcutaneous formulation of Depo-Provera. *Contraception.* 2004;70(1):11–18.

82. Grimes DA, Shields WC. Family planning for obese women: challenges and opportunities. *Contraception.* 2005;72(1):1–4.

83. Bonny AE, Ziegler J, Harvey R, et al. Weight gain in obese and nonobese adolescent girls initiating depot medroxyprogesterone, oral contraceptive

pills, or no hormonal contraceptive method. *Arch Pediatr Adolesc Med.* 2006;160(1):40–45.

84. Hubacher D, Grimes DA. Noncontraceptive health benefits of intrauterine devices: a systematic review. *Obstet Gynecol Surv.* 2002;57(2):120–128.

85. Samuelsson E, Hagg S. Incidence of venous thromboembolism in young Swedish women and possibly preventable cases among combined oral contraceptive users. *Acta Obstet Gynecol Scand.* 2004;83(7):674–681.

86. Samama MM. An epidemiologic study of risk factors for deep vein thrombosis in medical outpatients: the Sirius study. *Arch Intern Med.* 2000;160(22):3415–3420.

87. Nightingale AL, Lawrenson RA, Simpson EL, et al. The effects of age, body mass index, smoking and general health on the risk of venous thromboembolism in users of combined oral contraceptives. *Eur J Contracept Reprod Health Care.* 2000;5(4):265–274.

88. Mishell DR, Jr. Cardiovascular risks: perception versus reality. *Contraception.* 1999;59(1 Suppl):21S–24S.

89. Cardiovascular disease and steroid hormone contraception. Report of a WHO scientific group. *World Health Organ Tech Rep Ser.* 1998;877:i–vii, 1–89.

90. Narkiewicz K, Graniero GR, D'Este D, et al. Ambulatory blood pressure in mild hypertensive women taking oral contraceptives. A case-control study. *Am J Hypertens.* 1995;8(3):249–253.

91. Cardoso F, Polonia J, Santos A, et al. Low-dose oral contraceptives and 24-hour ambulatory blood pressure. *Int J Gynecol Obstet.* 1997;59(3):237–243.

92. Acute myocardial infarction and combined oral contraceptives: results of an international multicentre case-control study. WHO collaborative study of cardiovascular disease and steroid hormone contraception. *Lancet.* 1997;349(9060):1202–1209.

93. Schwartz SM, Petitti DB, Siscovick DS, et al. Stroke and use of low-dose oral contraceptives in young women: a pooled analysis of two US studies. *Stroke.* 1998;29(11):2277–2284.

94. Use of hormonal contraception in women with coexisting medical conditions. ACOG Practice Bulletin No. 73. American College of Obstetricians and Gynecologists. *Obstet Gynecol.* 2006;107:1453–1472.

95. Black HR, Leppert P, DeCherney A. The effect of medroxyprogesterone acetate on blood pressure. *Int J Gynecol Obstet.* 1978;17(1):83–87.

96. Taneepanichskul S, Reinprayoon D, Jaisamrarn U. Effects of DMPA on weight and blood pressure in long-term acceptors. *Contraception.* 1999;59(5):301–303.

97. Visser J, Snel M, Van Vliet HA. Hormonal versus non-hormonal contraceptives in women with diabetes mellitus type 1 and 2. *Cochrane Database Syst Rev.* 2006;4:CD003990.

98. Maggard MA, Yermilov I, Li Z, et al. Pregnancy and fertility following bariatric surgery: a systematic review. *J Am Med Assoc.* 2008;300(19):2286–2296.

99. Singh R, Frost J, Jordan B, et al. Beyond a prescription: strategies for improving contraceptive care. *Contraception.* 2009;79(1):1–4.

100. Stewart FH, Shields WC, Hwang AC. Title X: a sure-fire investment with at least a 300% return. *Contraception.* 2003;68(1):1.

101. Family Planning Services & Population Research Act. PLN 91-572. December 24; 1970.

102. Leeman L. Medical barriers to effective contraception. *Obstet Gynecol Clin North Am.* 2007;34(1):19–29, vii.

103. Larsen SB, Kragstrup J. Experiences of the first pelvic examination in a random samples of Danish teenagers. *Acta Obstet Gynecol Scand.* 1995;74(2):137–141.

104. Zabin LS, Emerson MR, Ringers PA, et al. Adolescents with negative pregnancy test results. An accessible at-risk group. *J Am Med Assoc.* 1996;275(2):113–117.

105. Harper C, Balistreri E, Boggess J, et al. Provision of hormonal contraceptives without a mandatory pelvic examination: the first stop demonstration project. *Fam Plann Perspect.* 2001;33(1):13–18.

106. Sawaya GF, Harper C, Balistreri E, et al. Cervical neoplasia risk in women provided hormonal contraception without a pap smear. *Contraception.* 2001;63(2):57–60.

107. Stewart FH, Harper CC, Ellertson CE, et al. Clinical breast and pelvic examination requirements for hormonal contraception: current practice vs evidence. *J Am Med Assoc.* 2001;285(17):2232–2239.

108. Lopez LM, Newmann SJ, Grimes DA, et al. Immediate start of hormonal contraceptives for contraception. *Cochrane Database Syst Rev.* 2008;2:CD006260.

109. Rickert VI, Tiezzi L, Lipshutz J, et al. Depo now: preventing unintended pregnancies among adolescents and young adults. *J Adolesc Health.* 2007;40(1):22–28.

110. Guttmacher Institute. Emergency contraception. Available at: www.guttmacher.org/media/supp/ec121702.html. Accessed January 15; 2009.

111. Harper CC, Weiss DC, Speidel JJ, et al. Over-the-counter access to emergency contraception for teens. *Contraception.* 2008;77(4):230–233.

112. Raymond EG, Dalebout SM, Camp SI. Comprehension of a prototype over-the-counter label for an emergency contraceptive pill product. *Obstet Gynecol.* 2002;100(2):342–349.

113. Raymond EG, Chen PL, Dalebout SM. "Actual use" study of emergency contraceptive pills provided in a simulated over-the-counter manner. *Obstet Gynecol.* 2003;102(1):17–23.

114. Graham A, Moore L, Sharp D, et al. Improving teenagers' knowledge of emergency contraception: cluster randomised controlled trial of a teacher led intervention. *Br Med J.* 2002;324(7347):1179.

115. Stewart HE, Gold MA, Parker AM. The impact of using emergency contraception on reproductive health outcomes: a retrospective review in an urban adolescent clinic. *J Pediatr Adolesc Gynecol.* 2003;16(5):313–318.

116. Golden NH, Seigel WM, Fisher M, et al. Emergency contraception: pediatricians' knowledge, attitudes, and opinions. *Pediatrics.* 2001;107(2):287–292.

117. Raymond EG, Trussell J, Polis CB. Population effect of increased access to emergency contraceptive pills: a systematic review. *Obstet Gynecol.* 2007;109(1):181–188.
118. Weaver MA, Raymond EG, Baecher L. Attitude and behavior effects in a randomized trial of increased access to emergency contraception. *Obstet Gynecol.* 2009;113(1):107–116.
119. Harper CC, Cheong M, Rocca CH, et al. The effect of increased access to emergency contraception among young adolescents. *Obstet Gynecol.* 2005;106(3):483–491.
120. Bearman P, Bruckner H. Promising the future: virginity pledges and the transition to first intercourse. *Am J Sociol.* 2001;106:859–912.
121. Trenholm C DB, Forston K, et al. Impacts of four Title V, Section 510 abstinence education programs. Princeton, NJ: Mathematica Research Group; 2007. Available at: http://aspe.hhs.gov/hsp/abstinence07/. Accessed December 31, 2008.
122. Eaton DK, Kann L, Kinchen S, et al. Youth risk behavior surveillance – United States, 2007. *Morb Mortal Wkly Rep, Surveil Summ.* 2008;57(4): 1–131.
123. Henshaw SK. Unintended pregnancy in the United States. *Fam Plann Perspect.* 1998;30(1):24–29, 46.
124. Institute of Medicine. *Crossing the quality chasm: A new health system for the 21st century.* Washington, DC: National Academy of Press; 2001.
125. Stewart M, Brown JB, Donner A, et al. The impact of patient-centered care on outcomes. *J Fam Pract.* 2000;49(9):796–804.
126. Kinnersley P, Stott N, Peters TJ, et al. The patient-centredness of consultations and outcome in primary care. *Br J Gen Pract.* 1999;49(446):711–716.
127. Cecil DW, Killeen I. Control, compliance, and satisfaction in the family practice encounter. *Fam Med.* 1997;29(9):653–657.
128. Rager KM, Omar HA. Hormonal contraception: noncontraceptive benefits and medical contraindications. *Adolesc Med Clin.* 2005;16(3):539–551.

Chapter 8
Chronic Pain and Adherence

Rebecca A. Shelby and Francis J. Keefe

Chronic pain of non-malignant etiology is a significant problem.
Chronic non-malignant pain is typically defined as pain that per-
sists for 3 months or longer and that is non-life threatening [1, 2].
Among the most common chronic pain conditions are chronic back
pain, migraine headaches, and tension headaches. Chronic pain is very
common. In the United States, 17% of patients seen in primary care
report chronic pain [3], and chronic pain accounts for almost 80% of
all physician visits [4]. A review of 15 epidemiologic studies found
that the prevalence of chronic pain ranges from 2 to 40% in the adult
population, with a median point prevalence of 15% [5]. The personal
and economic costs of chronic pain are substantial. A study of primary
care patients found that 13% of headache patients and 18% of back
pain patients were unable to maintain full-time work over a 3-year
period due to pain [6]. Chronic pain is often accompanied by substantial decreases in physical functioning, disruption of social and family
roles, and psychological distress [4].

A wide array of specialized treatments are available for chronic
pain. These include transcutaneous electrical nerve stimulation,
regional anesthesia, neuroaugmentation modalities (e.g., spinal col-
umn and deep brain stimulators), implantable drug delivery systems

R.A. Shelby (✉)
Medical Psychology, Duke University Medical Center, Durham, NC, USA
e-mail: shelb003@mc.duke.edu

H. Bosworth (ed.), *Improving Patient Treatment Adherence*,
DOI 10.1007/978-1-4419-5866-2_8,
© Springer Science+Business Media, LLC 2010

and neurodestructive surgical procedures. Despite the availability of these specialized treatment options, medications remain the mainstay of chronic pain treatment and by far are the most frequently used treatment for chronic pain [1]. Epidemiologic studies in the general population show that more than 60% of individuals with chronic pain use medications to treat their pain [7–9].

The goal of this chapter is to provide an overview of what is known about medication non-adherence in patients with chronic pain. The chapter is divided into four sections. In the first section, we examine types of medication non-adherence including medication underuse, overuse, and abuse in the context of chronic pain. For each type of non-adherence, we provide information about the scope of the problem, contributing factors, and consequences. In the second section, we describe and evaluate a variety of strategies for monitoring medication adherence in chronic pain. In the third section, we highlight approaches that can be used to enhance medication adherence in persons with chronic pain. In this section we highlight the potential utility of a number of approaches in preventing and modifying medication non-adherence in the context of chronic pain. In the final section, we identify a number of important clinical issues and future directions for research on medication adherence in persons suffering from chronic pain.

Adherence to Pain Medication

Clinicians often report that patients with chronic pain do not adhere to their medication as prescribed [10]. In chronic pain treatment, the term medication non-adherence encompasses three basic categories of behaviors: underuse of medication, overuse of medication, and abuse of medication. Table 8.1 summarizes key features of each of these types of non-adherence. For each type of non-adherence, we now discuss the scope of the problem, contributing factors, and consequences.

Underuse

In a recent review of medication adherence in patients with chronic pain [1], the percentage of patients using less medication than

Table 8.1 Medication non-adherence in patients with chronic pain

Type	Definition	Contributing factors	Consequences
Underuse	Taking less medication than prescribed or taking medications irregularly	• Poor communication with doctor • Mistrust in doctor • Side effect concerns • Psychological distress • Negative beliefs about pain medications	• Lose benefits of medication but still exposed to side effects • If unaware of underuse, doctor may discontinue medication, prescribe higher doses, or add medications
Overuse	Taking more medication than prescribed	• Greater perceived need for medication • History of substance abuse • Poor communication with doctor • Misinterpretation of medication instructions	• Toxicity • Severe adverse effects • Analgesic ceiling effect
Abuse	Maladaptive pattern of use manifested by significant and recurrent adverse consequences including a failure to fulfill major role obligations, repeated use when it is physically hazardous, legal problems, and social or interpersonal problems	• History of substance abuse • Strong belief that greater amounts of medication are needed to reduce pain • Current or past depression or anxiety disorders	• Toxicity • Severe adverse effects • Tolerance • Addiction • Withdrawal • Financial problems • Job loss • Legal problems • Social/interpersonal problems

prescribed averaged 29.9%. The fact that almost 30% of patients take less pain medication than prescribed means that many patients are on less than optimal medication regimens and may account for why these patients report that their medications are not very effective. Interestingly, although this rate of medication underuse may seem high, it is similar to rates of underuse of prescribed medication reported in studies of other chronic disease populations [11].

Several factors appear to contribute to the problem of pain medication underuse in persons suffering from chronic pain. Sewitch et al. [12] found that patients who reported problems communicating with their doctor were much more likely to underuse pain medications. Mistrust in one's doctor and concerns about side effects also have been linked to pain medication underuse [10]. A recent study [13] of 121 women with chronic pain found that those with higher levels of psychological distress were much more likely to skip doses or simply forget to take their medication. Paradoxically, this study found that women with lower affective pain ratings, a pattern usually linked to *low* levels of psychological distress, also were more likely to underuse their medication. Thus, these findings suggest that persons having either high levels of psychological distress *or* whose pain is not as affectively distressing may be at risk for underuse of pain medications [13].

There is growing evidence that negative beliefs and attitudes about taking pain medication are common in patients who underuse pain medication and represent a barrier to medication adherence [10, 14–16]. Recent qualitative studies [15–18] have identified several beliefs and attitudes linked to medication underuse in persons with chronic pain. First, many patients believe that, while one should adhere to most medications, it is appropriate to reduce or skip doses of pain medications. Many patients did not view underuse of pain medication as a problem mainly because they did not believe it would lead to negative health outcomes. Second, many patients believed that their ability to reduce or skip doses of pain medication was a sign of strength in that it showed that they were able to cope with pain and had a high pain tolerance. Third, older adults, in particular, reported that they did not want to waste the doctor's time or be seen as a nuisance so they did not ask questions about their pain medications. Many of these patients reported that not having their questions addressed contributed to their skipping or stopping use of their pain medications [17].

Finally, many patients were very concerned about the adverse effects of pain medications fearing that these drugs would lead to significant side effects (e.g., incapacitating constipation, nausea), internal organ damage, and addiction [17].

Cross-sectional studies indicate that the effectiveness of pain medication is reduced when patients underuse pain medications [19, 20]. Underuse is also associated with several important problems. When patients continually underuse pain medication they will most likely lose the benefits associated with taking the medication, but will continue to be exposed to the adverse effects associated with it. If unaware of medication underuse, doctors also may view a potentially effective medication as ineffective. In this case, doctors may discontinue the medication, prescribe higher doses of the medication, or prescribe additional medications to potentiate the effects of the originally prescribed medication, all of which could increase the risk of negative outcomes.

To our knowledge, there are no rigorous, prospective studies examining how pain medication underuse influences outcomes in persons suffering from chronic pain. Longitudinal studies clearly are needed and could provide important new insights into factors that predispose patients to underuse pain medication and could increase our understanding of the short- and long-term consequences of pain medication underuse.

Overuse

While there can be some overlap between pain medication overuse and abuse, there is growing recognition that these two types of behavior are distinct with each linked to its own specific risk factors and consequences. Medication overuse refers to taking more medication than prescribed or recommended. A recent review [1] found that the rates of medication overuse in persons with chronic pain ranged from 3.4 to 21%, with a weighted average of 13.7%.

A number of studies in patients with chronic pain have identified factors related to overuse of pain medication. McCracken et al. [10] found that patients who have a strong belief that they need pain medications in order to achieve any pain relief are much more likely to overuse medication. Interestingly, pain severity has not been consistently linked to overuse of pain medications [1]. McCracken and colleagues [10] found that, while pain severity was significantly and negatively associated with underuse, it was not significantly associated with overuse. However, in this study both pain severity and perceived need for medication were included in the model predicting overuse, which may have obscured the relationship between pain severity and pain medication overuse.

There is growing evidence that poor communication between patients and their health-care providers contributes to pain medication overuse [10, 21]. Robinson and colleagues [21] examined both patient and provider perspectives on treatment adherence in a chronic pain treatment program. Interestingly, there were many discrepancies between what health-care providers reported they recommended that patients do to manage their pain and what patients heard them recommend. Overall, health-care providers reported making many more treatment recommendations than patients recalled hearing. Particularly important for this chapter was the finding that discrepancies between patient and provider reports of treatment recommendations were highest for recommendations related to discontinuing old medications.

There is growing evidence that patients with chronic pain are prone to misinterpret or fail to understand the instructions they are given for use of their pain medications [15, 17]. For example, some pain medications are prescribed with the instructions "take as needed" or "as required." Sale et al. [15] found that some patients view these instructions as giving them permission to alter the amount or frequency of the recommended dose. There is a subgroup of patients with chronic pain who, when told to take pain medications as needed, may exceed the recommended dose (per 24 h) or take unsafe amounts of medication.

Converging lines of evidence suggest that patients with a history of substance abuse are not only more likely to abuse pain medications, but also prone to overuse pain medications [22, 23]. Patients with a history of drug or alcohol abuse, a family history of substance abuse, or a history of legal problems related to substance abuse are at increased risk for making unsanctioned escalations in the dose of their pain medication, unscheduled clinic or Emergency Department visits for more pain medication, and having toxicology screens positive for high doses of opioids [24].

Regularly overusing pain medications increases the likelihood of toxicity and severity of side effects. Although a wide array of medication is used to treat chronic pain, three classes of medications are used very often: nonopioid analgesics (acetaminophen and non-steroidal anti-inflammatory drugs), opioid analgesics, and adjuvant analgesics (e.g., antiepileptic drugs, tricyclic antidepressants). Table 8.2 summarizes the common side effects of these three classes of medications. Common side effects of acetaminophen and non-steroidal anti-inflammatory drugs (NSAIDs) include GI problems (e.g., dyspepsia, ulcers, perforation), liver dysfunction, kidney dysfunction, bleeding (i.e., antiplatelet effect), and central nervous system (CNS) effects [25]. Acute or chronic overuse of acetaminophen and some NSAIDs can cause liver or kidney toxicity. It is important to note that overuse of NSAIDs will not result in additional pain relief due to an analgesic ceiling effect, but dose escalations will contribute to increasing side effects and risk for toxicity. The side effects of opioids commonly used to treat chronic pain include sedation, mental clouding or confusion, mood changes, respiratory depression, changes in heart rate and blood pressure, nausea, vomiting, constipation, itching (i.e., pruritus), and urinary retention [25]. All opioids have the potential for addiction and this risk is increased with larger doses. Acute opioid toxicity is characterized by profound respiratory depression, apnea, deep sleep, stupor or coma, circulatory collapse, seizures, cardiopulmonary arrest, and death. Death related to opiod overdose is usually caused by respiratory arrest. Common side effects of antiepileptic drugs (AEDs) as a class include sedation, mental clouding, dizziness, nausea, and unsteadiness [26]. Older AEDs are associated with more serious adverse effects including hematologic abnormalities, liver dysfunction, hypersensitivity reactions, and rash. Finally, common side effects of tricyclic antidepressants (TCAs) include sedation, anticholinergic effects, and orthostatic hypertension [19]. While uncommon at dosages typically prescribed for chronic pain treatment, TCAs can have serious side effects including arrhythmias, MI, and stroke [19].

Several particularly problematic patterns of pain medication overuse have been identified. First, some patients engage in simultaneous overuse of several medications (e.g., a prescribed opioid, NSAID, along with over-the-counter pain medications). Simultaneous overuse of multiple medications dramatically increases the risk of serious adverse consequences, as the safe maximum dose for each medication will be limited when used in combination with other medications. Accidental overdose is much more likely to occur in patients taking a combination of pain medications. Second, a number of patients also show cyclic patterns of overuse and underuse. This

Table 8.2 Common side effects of nonopioid analgesics, opioid analgesics, and adjuvant analgesics

Medication	Side effects
Nonopioid analgesics	
Acetaminophen	• Liver damage with acute overdose
	• Liver toxicity, nephrotoxicity, and thrombocytopenia with chronic overdose
NSAIDs	• Gastrointestinal problems (e.g., ulcers, dyspepsia, bleeding)
	• Liver dysfunction
	• Kidney problems (e.g., renal insufficiency, acute renal failure)
	• Bleeding due to inhibited platelet aggregation
	• CNS effects (e.g., headache, dizziness, attention and memory deficits, drowsiness)
	• Hypersensitivity reactions
Opioid analgesics	• Sedation
	• Mental clouding and confusion
	• Nausea and vomiting
	• Constipation
	• Pruritus (itching)
	• Mood changes
	• Respiratory depression
	• Changes in heart rate and blood pressure
	• Urinary retention
Adjuvant analgesics	
Antiepileptic drugs	• Somnolence and fatigue
	• Sedation
	• Mental clouding
	• Nausea and vomiting
	• Dizziness and unsteadiness
	• Ataxia
Tricyclic antidepressants	• Sedation
	• Anticholinergic effects (e.g., dry mouth, blurred vision, constipation, urinary retention)
	• Orthostatic hypertension
	• Arrhythmias, MI, and stroke

pattern places patients at increased risk of inadequate analgesia, continuing or increased sensitivity to side effects, and toxicity [25, 26]. Third, entrenched patterns of pain medication overuse can motivate patients to search for other ways to get extra medication such as borrowing medication from relatives or friends, stealing medication, or purchasing medication without a prescription [27].

Abuse

For a subset of patients with chronic pain, overuse of pain medication may escalate into abuse [28]. The *Diagnostic and Statistical Manual of Mental Disorders, Fourth Edition* (DSM-IV) [29] defines substance abuse as a maladaptive pattern of substance use manifested by significant and recurrent adverse consequences including a failure to fulfill major role obligations, repeated medication use when it is physically hazardous, legal problems, and significant and recurrent social or interpersonal problems. Several studies of patients treated with opioids for chronic pain report that rates of opioid abuse are relatively high and range from 20 to 40% [30–32]. With the expanded use of opioid analgesics and increased reliance on high-dose extended-release opioid formulations for chronic pain management [33], there is growing concern about the problem of pain medication abuse [34, 35].

The most consistent predictor of medication abuse in persons with chronic pain is a prior history of substance abuse [23, 36–41]. In a prospective cohort study of 196 patients in a chronic pain management program, Ives and colleagues [23] found that past cocaine abuse, drug or DUI conviction, and past alcohol abuse were significant predictors of opioid abuse. Michna and colleagues [24] examined the association between substance abuse history and misuse of opioids in 145 patients treated in a hospital-based pain management program. Patients with a history of drug or alcohol abuse, a family history of substance abuse, or a history of legal problems related to substance abuse were at increased risk for having urine toxicology screens that were positive for illegal substances, nonprescribed opioid drugs, and high doses of opiate medication. Finally, Dunbar and Katz [42] examined outcomes of opioid treatment in patients with chronic pain who had substance abuse histories. Patients with a history of alcohol abuse alone were successfully managed on chronic opioid treatment. However, abuse of prescription opioids was common among patients with a history of polysubstance or oxycodone abuse suggesting that these patients were poor candidates for long-term opioid treatment.

Persons who have a strong belief that greater amounts of opioids are needed to reduce pain [37] are also at a much higher risk of pain medication abuse. Schieffer and colleagues [37] examined the relationship between pain medication beliefs and medication abuse in 288 patients with chronic pain. Patients who had abused medications were more likely to endorse beliefs that narcotic medications are effective for pain control, that medication use will improve mood, that they would be able to function better with free access to medication, and that they need higher amounts of narcotics to experience pain relief than other patients. These beliefs about medications mediated the relationship between substance abuse history and current pain medication misuse. Overall, these data suggest that the belief in a better quality of life associated with freer access and higher doses of medication may lead to medication abuse.

Recent evidence suggests that depression and anxiety disorders are linked to pain medication abuse. Several studies have found that a history of one or more major depressive episodes is associated with increased rates of opioid abuse in patients with chronic pain [27, 38, 43]. Kouyanou and colleagues [27] conducted a study of 125 patients with chronic pain. Patients who were abusing opioids had higher rates of depressive symptoms and were more likely to have had a depressive episode compared to patients who were not abusing their pain medications. Similar findings have emerged for anxiety disorders. Wilsey and colleagues [44] conducted a study of 113 patients with chronic pain who presented to Emergency Department and urgent care facilities for treatment. Patients with high levels of trait anxiety (i.e., STAI trait anxiety score >40), panic attacks, or posttraumatic stress disorder were significantly more likely to abuse their pain medication than other patients.

The relationship between psychiatric disorders and medication abuse may be due to a number of underlying causes. In a study examining the effects of opioids in patients with chronic pain and psychiatric morbidity, Wasan and colleagues [45] found that the effectiveness of opioids in reducing pain was diminished in patients with mood and anxiety disorders. Because patients with mood and anxiety disorders experience less pain control with opioid treatment, they may be more likely to increase doses of medication or seek additional medication to manage pain. Self-medication for depressive and anxious symptoms (i.e., chemical coping) also may contribute to pain medication abuse. Data from the National Survey on Drug Use and Health (2002 and

2003) found that adults who reported feeling depressed or anxious during the past year were two times more likely to initiate extra medical use (i.e., without a prescription or not as prescribed) of prescription pain relievers compared to individuals without these symptoms [46]. Of course, increased depression and anxiety may emerge secondary to the health and psychosocial consequences of medication abuse.

Abusing pain medications leads to a number of negative outcomes. Abuse dramatically increases the likelihood of severe adverse effects including liver or kidney toxicity, respiratory depression, heart rate and blood pressure changes, circulatory collapse, seizures, cardiopulmonary arrest, and death [26]. Patients who abuse pain medications are also at increased risk for tolerance and addiction. Further, pain medication abuse is often accompanied by legal, financial, and significant interpersonal problems. Patients who abuse pain medications must find ways to obtain medication without a prescription. Illegal activities such as prescription forgery, stealing drugs from others, and obtaining drugs from nonmedical sources can lead to significant legal problems [35]. Financial difficulties associated with abuse can result from deterioration in the ability to function at work, missing work, job loss, and the cost of obtaining drugs. Finally, abuse often results in an inability to fulfill family and social roles, relationship dysfunction, and social isolation [47, 48].

Monitoring Pain Medication Adherence

There is growing recognition that monitoring pain medication adherence is an important component of best practice in the management of chronic pain [49]. There is a particularly strong consensus about the need to carefully monitor medication adherence in those patients taking opioid medications. Table 8.3 summarizes several methods (self-report questionnaires, interview-based methods, toxicological screening, and formal Prescription Drug Monitoring Programs) used to monitor pain medication adherence. We describe and critically evaluate each of these monitoring methods in the following.

Self-Report Questionnaires

Several self-report questionnaires have been developed to assess risk for medication overuse and abuse [50]. The recently revised Screener

Table 8.3 Strategies for monitoring medication adherence in patients with chronic pain

Strategy	Description	Advantages	Limitations	Recommendation
Self-report questionnaires	Questionnaires that are completed by the patient: • Screener and Opioid Assessment for Patients with Pain • Opioid Risk Tool • Pain Medication Questionnaire • Current Opioid Misuse Measure • Morisky Medication Adherence Scale • Beliefs about Medicines Questionnaire	• Low cost • Easily administered • Time efficient	• Overestimate adherence • Vulnerable to social desirability • Difficult to complete for patients with low levels of literacy	• Useful for monitoring underuse, patients treated with over-the-counter medications, and patients at low risk for overuse and abuse. • Should be combined with other monitoring methods for patients treated with opioids and patients at increased risk for overuse or abuse.
Interview-based methods	Measures administered by the health-care provider: • Prescription Drug Use Questionnaire • Addiction Behaviors Checklist • Pain Assessment and Documentation Tool	• More objective than self-report • Assess substance abuse risk and problematic behaviors associated with abuse.	• Can be influenced by clinician's positive or negative biases • Vulnerable to social desirability • Limited by period of time spent interacting with patient	• Useful for assessing risk for abuse, and monitoring behaviors associated with abuse • Should be combined with other monitoring methods for patients treated with opioids and patients at increased risk for overuse and abuse

Table 8.3 (continued)

Strategy	Description	Advantages	Limitations	Recommendation
Toxicological screening	Urine testing to detect the presence of opioids or other substances	• Objective assessment of adherence • Fairly noninvasive • Easily administered • Good specificity and sensitivity	• Cannot identify all relevant agents and metabolites • Information limited to days preceding the appointment • Does not provide information about number of correct doses or time between doses	• Useful for monitoring adherence in patients treated with opioids and patients who are at increased risk for substance abuse
Prescription drug monitoring programs	Database of prescription information maintained and monitored by a state program	• Provides objective system for detecting prescribing aberrations or problems	• Does not monitor all types of pain medications • Prescribers may not have access to the database	• If available, useful for monitoring patients treated with opioids and those at high risk for substance abuse for prescription problems

and Opioid Assessment for Patients with Pain (SOAPP-R) is a 24-item self-administered questionnaire that is used to assess the risk potential for opioid abuse and the suitability of long-term opioid treatment for patients with chronic pain [51]. The SOAPP-R assesses risk factors in five areas: (1) history of substance abuse, (2) legal problems, (3) craving medication, (4) heavy smoking, and (5) mood swings. Items were developed based on input from an expert panel and a panel of patients treated with opioids. When completing the SOAPP-R, patients rate items on a 5-point scale (0=never to 5=very often) and items are summed to create a total risk score. A total score of 18 or higher is used to identify patients at high risk for opioid abuse, and this cutoff score has shown adequate sensitivity (0.81) and specificity (0.68) for predicting opioid misuse [51].

A second widely used self-report questionnaire that assesses risk for opioid misuse is the Opioid Risk Tool (ORT) [43]. The ORT includes five questions about family history of substance abuse, personal history of substance abuse, history of sexual abuse, psychiatric history, and age. Responses (yes vs. no) to items are weighted and summed to create a total risk score. Patients with scores of 0–3 are considered low risk for opioid abuse, scores of 4–7 are considered moderate risk, and scores of 8 or higher are considered to reflect high risk. The ORT has shown adequate sensitivity and specificity for identifying patients at risk for abuse of opioids [43]. The ORT takes approximately 5 min to complete.

The Pain Medication Questionnaire (PMQ) [52–54] is also a widely used self-report measure of risk for pain medication misuse or abuse. In contrast to other self-report screening tools, the PMQ items do not mention a specific type of pain medication (e.g., opioids) so that patients taking any form of pain medication can use this questionnaire. The PMQ includes 26 items that assess potentially problematic attitudes and behaviors surrounding pain medication use. The items were developed based on the literature addressing medication misuse in chronic pain treatment and extensive input from health-care providers (nurses, physicians, psychologists) working in pain clinics. Patients evaluate items on a 5-point response scale that uses verbal anchors and responses to items are summed to create a total risk score. This measure has demonstrated adequate long-term predictive validity for pain medication abuse and requests for early refills [53, 54]. Holmes and colleagues [53] administered the PMQ to 271 newly evaluated patients with chronic pain and followed patients for 6 months. Patients were divided into subgroups based on the lowest, middle, and highest third of PMQ scores. Patients with the highest PMQ scores were 2.6 times more likely to have a substance abuse problem and 3.2 times more likely to request early refills of prescription pain medication compared to patients with the lowest PMQ scores.

Another important use of self-report questionnaires is to monitor patients' pain medication adherence throughout the course of treatment. The Current Opioid Misuse Measure (COMM) [55] is a 17-item self-report questionnaire specifically designed to monitor medication overuse and abuse in chronic pain patients who have been taking opioids for an extended period of time. This measure was developed with extensive input from pain specialists, addiction experts, and primary care physicians. In a recent study of patients ($N=227$) taking opioids for chronic pain, the COMM demonstrated excellent internal consistency and test–retest reliability, as well as adequate sensitivity and specificity. The COMM can be used as a brief, self-report measure to assess problematic medication-taking behaviors in chronic pain patients that may indicate medication overuse or abuse.

Finally, monitoring underuse of pain medications is also important. The Morisky Medication Adherence Scale (MMAS) is probably the most widely used self-report measure of medication non-adherence [56]. This questionnaire focuses on medication underuse. The original four-item MMAS was recently expanded to include eight items [57, 58]. Each of the eight items assesses a medication-taking behavior related to underuse including forgetting to take medication, skipping doses, reducing or stopping medication when feeling better, and reducing or stopping medication when feeling worse. MMAS scores range from 0 to 8, and cutoffs have been developed for use in clinical practice: < 6 =low adherence, 6–7 =moderate adherence, and 8=high adherence. The MMAS has demonstrated excellent validity and reliability in patients with chronic diseases [57–60].

Because beliefs are linked to medication underuse, clinicians should consider systematically assessing patients' beliefs about their pain medications to identify those patients who may be at risk for medication underuse. The Beliefs about Medicines Questionnaire (BMQ) has been developed for use in patients with chronic diseases [61] and this questionnaire can be modified to refer to specific medications. The BMQ includes five items that assess the perceived necessity of medications (e.g., "My life would be impossible without my medicines," "My medicine protects me from becoming worse"), and five items that assess concerns about medications (e.g., "I sometimes worry about long-term effects of my medicines," "I sometimes worry about becoming too dependent on my medicines"). Patients rate their degree of agreement with each of the statements and individual item scores are summed to create a total necessity score and a total concerns score. The BMQ has been used to measure beliefs about a wide range of medications and has demonstrated excellent reliability and validity [62–65].

Comment: Self-report measures of medication non-adherence are easy to administer, low cost, and easily incorporated into a busy clinic setting. Self-report questionnaires offer several important advantages. First, self-report measures can provide detailed information about medication-taking behaviors that would be difficult to obtain during time-limited health-care provider–patient interactions. Second, the information obtained by self-report questionnaires can be used to guide conversations with patients and increase the likelihood that patients' primary concerns or problems are discussed. Finally, information from self-report questionnaires can be combined with other sources of information (e.g., interactions with the patient, toxicological screening) to thoroughly assess risk potential for medication abuse before starting treatment and to monitor medication-taking behaviors during treatment. Because patients may overestimate their own adherence [66], self-report questionnaires may be most useful when combined with information from interactions with patients and other methods of assessing pain medication adherence. Combining self-report with other adherence assessment methods is particularly important for clinicians who are prescribing opioids for chronic pain or working with patients who are at risk for overuse or abuse [49].

Interview-Based Methods

Most interview-based measures are designed to be used as part of an initial assessment that focuses on identifying ongoing substance abuse and assessing potential risk for future substance abuse. The majority of interview-based measures that assess substance abuse risk were not developed for use in patients with chronic pain and their utility for predicting pain medication abuse or misuse is unknown (e.g., the CAGE, Addiction Severity Index). We describe three widely used interview-based measures that were specifically developed for use in patients with chronic pain in the following.

The Prescription Drug Use Questionnaire (PDUQ) [50, 67] is one of the most widely used and well-validated interviews for assessing medication abuse in patients with chronic pain. The PDUQ is a 42-item interview-based instrument developed to help clinicians identify substance abuse in the context of chronic pain and opioid analgesic treatment. It takes approximately 20 min to administer and requires minimal training to administer. The PDUQ consists of a series of questions in which patients are asked about their pain condition, opioid use pattern, social and family factors, history of substance abuse, and psychiatric history. Items are marked as either present or absent (yes or no) and then items are summed to create a total risk score. The PDUQ items assessing psychiatric morbidity are not included in the total score. A total score of 15 or greater indicates that a patient is at high risk for medication abuse. The PDUQ has demonstrated adequate reliability, sensitivity, and specificity in patients with chronic pain [67].

A second interview-based instrument is the Addiction Behaviors Checklist (ABC) [68]. This 20-item instrument was designed to help clinicians monitor ongoing and current behaviors characteristic of prescription opioid medication addiction in patients with chronic pain. Items were based on the literature addressing medication abuse and addiction in chronic pain treatment. The ABC consists of a checklist completed by the clinician that focuses on observable behaviors noted both during and between clinic visits. For each item, the presence or absence (yes vs. no) of the behavior is indicated, and items are summed to create a total score (range 0–20). A score of 3 or greater is used to identify patients who are displaying inappropriate opioid use. The ABC has demonstrated adequate reliability, concurrent validity, and sensitivity and specificity [68].

The Pain Assessment and Documentation Tool (PADT) [69] is an interview-based measure that is completed using a two-sided chart note that can be included in the patient's medical record. This simple charting device takes approximately 5 min to complete and focuses on four key areas for managing patients with chronic pain who are treated with opioids: analgesia, activities of daily living, adverse events, and potential aberrant drug-related behaviors (e.g., requests frequent early refills, changes in route of administration). The PADT was developed based on the literature addressing medication misuse in chronic pain treatment, extensive input from physicians working in pain clinics, and field testing by clinicians who were treating patients on long-term opioid therapy for chronic pain. The PADT provides a consistent approach to assessing and documenting adherence and progress in pain management over the course of opioid treatment.

Comment: Interview-based measures have several advantages. First, because they are administered by the clinician, they reduce burden on the patient. Second, they can provide an independent and more objective assessment of adherence than is possible by self-report questionnaire alone. Finally, because these measures are standardized, they ensure that all important aspects of medication-taking behavior and risk factors for non-adherence are consistently assessed. Standardized interviews also enable clinicians to compare results obtained from a given patient across multiple clinic visits as well as compare the patient's results with others in a normative population or within one's own clinical setting. Interview-based measures also have limitations. While numerous interview-based measures have been developed to assess potential medication misuse or abuse, it may be challenging to incorporate some of these measures into busy clinic settings due to their length. If a brief interview-based measure is needed, it is important that the selected measure captures key high-risk behaviors for medication abuse [49]. Based on studies in patients with chronic pain, Chabal and colleagues [70] recommend consistently assessing and documenting the following high-risk behaviors: (1) an overwhelming and persisting focus on drug-related issues during pain clinic visits; (2) a pattern (three or more) of early refills or problems associated with their prescription; (3) multiple telephone calls or visits with requests for more medication; (4) reports of lost, spilled, or stolen medications; (5) obtaining opioids from multiple providers, emergency rooms, or illegal sources; and (6) escalating medication use in the absence of an acute change in the medical condition.

Toxicological Screening

Toxicological screenings provide objective information about medication intake, and there is evidence that their use may reduce medication abuse [49]. Urine testing for patients treated with opioids is often regarded as the gold standard for abuse/misuse screening because it is fairly noninvasive and has relatively good specificity, sensitivity, ease of administration, and cost [49]. In the treatment of chronic pain, urine testing is increasingly being used both to detect the presence of opioids or other substances at the start of treatment and to test for illicit drug use or medication abuse during treatment [71].

Toxicological screening tests have several important limitations. First, they cannot identify all relevant agents and metabolites so a negative screening test does not preclude misuse or abuse of all substances. Second, they only provide information about medication intake in the days preceding the appointment. Patients may misuse or abuse substances between appointments, but refrain from using substances in the days prior to a screening test in order to yield a negative screening result. It is also important to note that detection times for substances vary considerably depending on acute vs. chronic use, the particular drug used within a class, and individual characteristics of the patient (e.g., metabolism of medication) [49]. Finally, toxicological screening tests do not provide a measure of important medication-taking behaviors such as the correct number of daily doses taken and the time interval between doses [1]. Toxicological screening may not be able to identify long-term patterns of pain medication misuse such as simultaneous overuse of several medications in between appointments or cyclic patterns of medication overuse and underuse.

Despite their limitations, toxicological screenings are an essential component in the assessment and treatment of patients with chronic pain who are treated with opioids or who are at increased risk for medication abuse. The limitations of this type of screening can be mitigated by combining it with other methods of assessment such as self-report questionnaires that can provide information about daily medication-taking behaviors and interview-based screening that can provide a more objective assessment of potential risk for medication abuse and problematic medication-related behaviors.

Prescription Drug Monitoring Programs

Clinicians who treat chronic pain face the challenge of reducing prescription drug abuse while still assuring that patients can have

access to adequate pain treatment [49]. When prescribing opioids for
patients with a history of substance abuse, major concerns include
prescription forgery, medication diversion, and patients with multiple opioid prescriptions from multiple providers. Formal Prescription
Drug Monitoring Programs (PDMPs) have been introduced in some
states in response to concerns about prescription drug misuse/abuse.
These programs aim to educate practitioners and the public about
drug misuse/abuse, facilitate early identification and intervention in
cases of drug misuse or abuse, and aid in the investigation of drug
misuse or abuse. For the majority of PDMPs, pharmacies submit prescription information electronically, and the prescription information
in the PDMP database is monitored for prescribing aberrations or
problems (e.g., a patient with multiple opioid prescriptions from multiple providers). The manner in which PDMPs are implemented varies
across states. Some PDMPs notify providers when problems are identified while other programs allow prescribers to access the database. As
of 2008, 38 states had signed laws to authorize the creation of PDMPs,
32 had active programs, and 6 had implemented their programs [72].
The number of active PDMPs is expected to increase due to the pass-
ing of the National All Schedules Prescription Electronic Reporting
(NASPER) Act in 2005, which supports states in developing PDMPs.

Comment: While PDMPs might reduce the prevalence of prescription opioid abuse, their utility for monitoring patients in the clinical
setting and their impact on opioid abuse in persons with chronic pain
remains to be determined.

Strategies for Improving Medication Adherence

Non-adherence to pain medications is a complex problem influenced
by a variety of biological, psychological, and social factors. Non-
adherence is influenced by, and in turn influences, the health-care environment, patient–provider relationships, the availability of resources
such as social support, and characteristics of the patient [73]. For
some patients with chronic pain, medication non-adherence is mainly
related to a single or small number of factors (e.g., poor communication with health-care providers and fear of medication side effects) and
thus can be improved with brief, educational or information-focused

interventions. For other patients, the determinants of pain medication non-adherence are multiple, complex, and interacting. In such cases a treatment package that combines education/information with a number of other strategies is needed to improve adherence [49].

Table 8.4 summarizes several strategies for improving adherence and the contexts in which these strategies may be beneficial. In Fig. 8.1, we provide examples of monitoring and adherence enhancement programs for patients who underuse pain medication and for patients at high risk for medication abuse. We discuss each of the intervention strategies for improving adherence including pain medication instructions, collaborative treatment planning, pain education programs, patient–provider communication skills training, medication contracts, and substance abuse management in the following.

Pain Medication Instructions

Providing patients with detailed written instructions for taking pain medications is a low cost and easily administered strategy that may reduce underuse and overuse of medications. Studies testing the efficacy of medication instruction formats have found that the comprehension and recall of medication information are significantly improved when written drug-taking instructions are explicitly provided, instructions are organized in lists rather than paragraphs, and when pictorial icons are used to supplement written instructions [74–77]. Written instructions provide an important reference for patients regarding medication dosages, the timing of medications (e.g., take at bedtime), special instructions (e.g., take with food), and safety precautions. Specific and clear written instructions for taking pain medications are an essential component of adequate care and should be provided to all patients [78].

Collaborative Treatment Planning

In a collaborative treatment planning model, health-care providers partner with patients to develop a treatment plan for managing pain, and the patient is encouraged to participate in making treatment

Table 8.4 Strategies for enhancing medication adherence in patients with chronic pain

Intervention	Description	Advantages	Limitations	Recommendation
Medication instructions	Detailed written instructions for taking pain medications accompanied by pictorial icons	• Low cost • Easily administered • Easily incorporated into clinic setting	• May be less effective for patients with a low level of literacy	• Medication instructions should be given to all patients as part of adequate chronic pain care
Collaborative treatment planning	Involving the patient in treatment planning and giving patients an opportunity to articulate concerns and barriers	• Low cost • Increases treatment plan acceptability • Identifies patient concerns prior to starting treatment	• Not all patients desire collaborative treatment planning • Could be difficult to incorporate in some clinic settings due to time constraints	• Collaborative treatment planning should be offered to all patients as part of adequate chronic pain care
Pain education	Program that educates patients about pain and how medications fit into pain management	• Educates patients about chronic pain and treatments for chronic pain • Provides patients with skills for enhancing adherence and pain management	• Requires trained clinicians to provide pain education • Involves multiple sessions	• Used to improve adherence among patients who repeatedly underuse or overuse pain medications even after receiving written instructions and feedback from providers

Table 8.4 (continued)

Intervention	Description	Advantages	Limitations	Recommendation
Communication skills training	Intervention that teaches patients skills for communicating with health-care providers	• Improves patient–provider communication • Provides patients with strategies for conveying and remembering information	• Requires trained clinicians to provide program • Involves multiple sessions	• Useful for patients who repeatedly underuse or overuse pain medications • Can be used as a stand-alone intervention or as part of a pain education program
Medication contracts	Written contract that defines patient and physician responsibilities, expectations, and consequences for not meeting obligations	• Clearly explicates the benefits, burdens, risks, and consequences of pain medications	• Does not provide strategies or skills training to enhance adherence or help patients uphold medication contract	• Used for patients treated with opioids and for patients who are at high risk for substance abuse
Substance abuse management	Referral and appropriate drug treatment for patients suffering from substance abuse or dependence.			• Required for adequate management of chronic pain patients with substance abuse or dependence problems

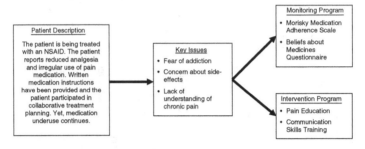

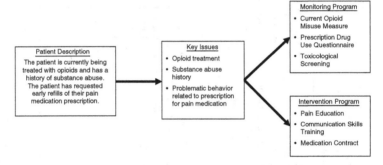

Fig. 8.1 Sample monitoring and adherence enhancement programs

decisions. This model utilizes the patient's knowledge of their pain, support network, resources, living and working conditions, value system, beliefs about using medication to treat pain, and willingness to take pain medications to develop a treatment plan and set treatment goals for managing pain. Collaborative treatment planning involves open discussion of all aspects of the treatment plan, including the potential benefits and risks of pain medications, and jointly agreed upon treatment goals. This process encourages patients to take an active part in planning treatment and making treatment decisions.

There are a number of advantages of this collaborative approach for the treatment of chronic pain. Involving patients in formulating their treatment plan can result in a treatment plan that is more realistic for the patient's particular circumstances, more consistent with the patient's beliefs about using medication to treat pain, and more acceptable to the patient (e.g., takes concerns about side effects into account). Collaborating with patients to develop their treatment plan also provides patients with an opportunity to articulate concerns and potential barriers to pain medication adherence so these issues can be addressed in advance. Further, patients may be more invested in treatment plans that are developed in collaboration with their provider rather than plans that are dictated by the provider [78]. Increasing patients' investment in their treatment plan and improving the patient-treatment plan match may result in improved pain medication adherence [78].

Pain Education Programs

Some patients may require a more intensive strategy to address multiple factors that contribute to pain medication non-adherence. A growing body of evidence suggests that programs that educate patients about pain and how medications fit into an overall program for managing pain yield higher rates of medication adherence [78, 79]. Traditional pain education programs usually include three central components. First, a pain education segment teaches patients about the complex nature of chronic pain using concepts such as the biopsychosocial model of pain. The biopsychosocial model of pain emphasizes that chronic pain is influenced not only by the biological factors highlighted in the biomedical model, but also by psychological factors and social factors [80]. Second, educational information about pharmacologic pain management is used to teach patients about the role of medication in treating chronic pain, how to appropriately take their pain medication, potential medication side effects, and tolerance and addiction. Third, patients are provided with an overview of non-pharmacologic strategies for managing pain (e.g., relaxation, heat, cold, massage) and their role as an adjunct to pain medication.

Pain education programs have been successful in improving medication adherence, changing patients' attitudes about using medications to treat pain, and reducing concerns about addiction, tolerance, and side effects [2, 78, 81–84]. There is evidence that pain education programs are most effective when delivered in small segments over a series of sessions [78]. Providing large blocks of information to patients at one time is less likely to yield benefits, especially for patients with low literacy levels, difficulty comprehending medical information, or whose cognitive status may be compromised by excessive or inconsistent pain medication use [78].

Communication Skills Training

Improving patient–health-care provider communication is important for increasing medication adherence in patients with chronic pain [21]. Communication skills training protocols teach patients strategies that are designed to improve patient–provider communication. In these protocols, patients learn to use pain-rating scales to communicate about pain and terminology for talking to their medical providers about pain. Patients also learn how to monitor and record symptoms and medication side effects, use effective verbal and non-verbal communication skills when talking with health-care providers, and use techniques to remember information communicated during medical appointments (e.g., taking notes, bringing someone with you, recording the conversation). Communication skills training can be delivered as a stand-alone intervention or as part of a larger pain education program. Communication skills training interventions have been successful not only in improving adherence to pain medications, but also in improving patient–provider communication and increasing patient satisfaction [85–87].

Medication Contracts

When medication overuse or abuse is the primary concern, medication contracts (or controlled substance agreements) are commonly used [49]. Medication contracts clarify the parameters of treatment, clearly define patient and physician responsibility, inform patients of expectations and roles, and outline the potential consequences for not meeting obligations and responsibilities. The most common features of medication contracts include explicit statements regarding the terms of treatment, prohibited behaviors, and reasons for terminating treatment [88]. Many medication contracts also include educational information about medications, emergency issues, and legal considerations. A 1999 study by Fishman et al. revealed that a requirement to submit to random urine drug testing was also a common feature of pain clinic opioid contracts [88]. Recently, the American Academy of Pain Medicine released a sample patient–physician medication agreement form for long-term opioid treatment for chronic pain (www.painmed.org/productpub/statement/sample.html).

Several studies have found that medication contracts reduce overuse and abuse of pain medications [89–91]. Further, many clinicians use medication contracts to help explicate the benefits, burdens, risks, and consequences of the medications used for chronic pain management [49]. A recent study [91] of medical residents found that the majority (90%) found medication contracts useful for discussing potential problems related to opioid treatment. This study also found that medication contracts were helpful for reducing patients' use of multiple prescribers, reducing requests for early refills or additional drugs, and identifying patients who were abusing pain medications [91].

Substance Abuse Management

There is growing agreement that chronic pain cannot be adequately managed and may worsen in the context of current substance abuse [28, 48, 49, 92]. If a person with chronic pain is found to be currently suffering from substance abuse or dependence, the health-care provider must initiate and support drug addiction treatment interventions. Principles of addiction treatment for patients with chronic pain include referral to and involvement with formal drug treatment, the use of medication contracts for pain medication use, intensive medication monitoring, and aggressively managing pain with nonopioid and non-pharmacologic interventions [47, 92]. If possible, patients should be treated by a drug treatment program experienced in the care of patients with chronic pain.

During treatment for substance abuse, it is important that health-care providers continue to provide ongoing pain management and ensure that the pain management needs of the patient are being adequately addressed. While patients who have abused pain medications are not necessarily precluded from future opioid treatment for chronic pain, careful monitoring of medication use and support by appropriate health-care providers must be consistently provided [28, 49].

Case Examples

A variety of monitoring and intervention strategies are available for enhancing medication adherence in patients with chronic pain. When creating a plan to monitor and address non-adherence in the clinic setting, several key factors should be considered: (1) type of medication being used (e.g., NSAIDs vs. opioids); (2) type of non-adherence behaviors being exhibited by the patient (e.g., underuse vs. overuse vs. abuse); and (3) individual characteristics of the patient (e.g., past history of substance abuse). Figure 8.1 illustrates adherence monitoring and intervention plans for two exemplar patients. The top panel of Fig. 8.1 presents a plan for a patient who continues to underuse pain medication after receiving written medication instructions and participating in collaborative treatment planning. For this patient, self-report questionnaires are chosen to monitor underuse because the patient is being treated with an NSAID and the risk of overuse or abuse is low. Because prior written instructions and collaborative treatment planning did not improve adherence, a more intensive intervention approach (i.e., pain education and communication skills training) is selected to address the patient's concerns about pain medications, educate the patient about chronic pain management, and improve the patient's ability to communicate with health-care providers.

The bottom panel of Fig. 8.1 presents an adherence monitoring and intervention plan for a patient who is at high risk for pain medication abuse. This particular patient is being treated with an opioid medication, has a substance abuse history, and has requested early prescription refills. An intensive monitoring approach that combines multiple methods of assessment is used for this patient. In this patient, combining self-report and interview-based monitoring with toxicological screening will allow us to triangulate information from different sources and will increase our ability to identify problematic medication-taking behaviors [49]. It is important to note that the use of self-report questionnaires alone or an interview alone would not be advised in this context [49]. The intervention plan for this patient is also intensive as it combines pain education and communication skills training with a medication contract. Medication contracts are commonly used for patients treated with opioids, but they do not provide strategies or skills training to enhance adherence. Medication contracts may be most beneficial for high-risk patients when combined with interventions that help patients develop skills for adhering to their medication and upholding their medication contract.

Summary and Future Directions

Pain medication non-adherence is a significant problem in the treatment of chronic pain [1, 49] and monitoring adherence is an essential component of adequate care for patients with chronic pain [49]. While it is often overlooked or not assessed, pain medication underuse is a common problem that contributes to inadequate analgesia for a substantial proportion of patients [1]. Routine monitoring for underuse can help to identify patients who are experiencing reduced analgesia, do not understand the role of medication in managing chronic pain, or do not fully understand the instructions for taking their pain medication. Regular monitoring for medication overuse and abuse is also critical, especially for patients taking opioid medications. Clinicians who are prescribing opioids for chronic pain or working with patients who are at risk for medication abuse should use multiple strategies to monitor medication adherence including self-report questionnaires, interview methods, and toxicological screening [49].

Basic strategies for enhancing adherence such as written medication instructions and collaborative treatment planning should be incorporated into the care of all patients with chronic pain. These strategies are low cost, easy to administer, and can be incorporated into most clinic settings [76]. There is also growing recognition that pain education programs are important for enhancing adherence as well as improving overall pain management and patient outcomes [2, 78, 81–84]. Increasingly, these programs are being viewed as an integral part of chronic pain management rather than a nice extra [93]. It is unclear how often written medication instructions, collaborative treatment planning, and pain education strategies are currently employed in clinics that treat patients with chronic pain [94]. Routinely incorporating these strategies into patient care and increasing patients' access to these resources are important for improving adherence to pain medication and patient outcomes.

The use of technology for enhancing adherence is rapidly expanding. Medication reminder systems and cueing devices (e.g., day-of-the-week pillboxes, mechanical or electronic medication diaries) are widely available [78]. Increasingly, these types of tools are using technology to remind patients to take their medication, alert patients when medications are taken outside of the regular dosing schedule, and notify providers when extra medication prescriptions are requested or filled. Technologies that are currently being used include cell phones, personal digital assistants (e.g., Palm Pilots), the Internet, and Interactive Voice Response (IVR) systems [87, 95–97]. As various technologies advance and become more accessible to patients, the options for providing individualized, cost-effective, and easily administered interventions will continue to expand.

Finally, the goal of this chapter was to provide an overview of what is known about medication non-adherence in patients with chronic pain. While medications continue to be the most frequently used treatment for chronic pain [1], the availability of specialized treatment options (e.g., transcutaneous electrical nerve stimulation, regional anesthesia, implantable drug delivery systems) is increasing [94]. Each specialized treatment is associated with unique benefits and challenges for adherence. Understanding the adherence issues associated with specific treatment modalities as well as intervention strategies that might enhance adherence to these treatments is increasingly important as more patients have access to specialized treatments.

References

1. Broekmans S, Dobbels F, Milisen K, Morlion B, Vanderschueren S. Medication adherence in patients with chronic non-malignant pain: is there a problem? *Eur J Pain*. 2009;13(2):115–123.
2. Jackman RP, Purvis JM, Mallett BS. Chronic nonmalignant pain in primary care. *Am Fam Physician*. 2008;78(10):1155–1162.
3. Gureje O. Persistent pain and well-being: a world health organization study in primary care. *JAMA*. 1998;280:147–151.
4. Gatchel RJ, Peng YB, Peters ML, Fuchs PN, Turk DC. The biopsychosocial approach to chronic pain: scientific advances and future directions. *Psychol Bull*. 2007;133(4):581–624.
5. Verhaak PF, Kerssens JJ, Dekker J, Sorbi MJ, Bensing JM. Prevalence of chronic benign pain disorder among adults: a review of the literature. *Pain*. 1998;77(3):231–239.
6. Stang P, Von Korff M, Galer BS. Reduced labor force participation among primary care patients with headache. *J Gen Intern Med*. 1998;13:296–302.

7. Andersson HI, Ejlertsson G, Leden I, Schersten B. Impact of chronic pain on health care seeking, self care, and medication. Results from a population-based Swedish study. *J Epidemiol Comm Health.* 1999;53(8):503–509.

8. Catala E, Reig E, Artes M, Aliaga L, Lopez JS, Segu JL. Prevalence of pain in the Spanish population: telephone survey in 5000 homes. *Eur J Pain.* 2002;6(2):133–140.

9. Vallerand AH, Fouladbakhsh J, Templin T. Patients' choices for the self-treatment of pain. *Appl Nurs Res.* 2005;18(2):90–96.

10. McCracken LM, Hoskins J, Eccleston C. Concerns about medication and medication use in chronic pain. *J Pain.* 2006;7(10):726–734.

11. DiMatteo MR. Variations in patients' adherence to medical recommendations: a quantitative review of 50 years of research. *Med Care.* 2004;42(3): 200–209.

12. Sewitch MJ, Dobkin PL, Bernatsky S, et al. Medication non-adherence in women with fibromyalgia. *Rheumatology (Oxford).* 2004;43(5):648–654.

13. Dobkin PL, Sita A, Sewitch MJ. Predictors of adherence to treatment in women with fibromyalgia. *Clin J Pain.* 2006;22(3):286–294.

14. Monsivais D, McNeill J. Multicultural influences on pain medication attitudes and beliefs in patients with nonmalignant chronic pain syndromes. *Pain Manag Nur.* 2007;8(2):64–71.

15. Sale JE, Gignac M, Hawker G. How "bad" does the pain have to be? A qualitative study examining adherence to pain medication in older adults with osteoarthritis. *Arthritis Rheum.* 2006;55(2):272–278.

16. Peters M, Huijer Abu-Saad H, Vydelingum V, Dowson A, Murphy M. The patients' perceptions of migraine and chronic daily headache: a qualitative study. *J Headache Pain.* 2005;6(1):40–47.

17. Lansbury G. Chronic pain management: a qualitative study of elderly people's preferred coping strategies and barriers to management. *Disabil Rehabil.* 2000;22(1–2):2–14.

18. Liddle SD, Baxter GD, Gracey JH. Chronic low back pain: patients' experiences, opinions and expectations for clinical management. *Disabil Rehabil.* 2007;29(24):1899–1909.

19. Institute for Clinical Systems Improvement (ICSI) Work Group. *Adult low back pain.* ICSI Health Care Guideline. Bloomington, MN: ICSI; 1999.

20. Institute for Clinical Systems Improvement (ICSI). *Adult low back pain.* Bloomington, MN: Institute for Clinical Systems Improvement; 2004.

21. Robinson ME, Bulcourf B, Atchison JW, et al. Compliance in pain rehabilitation: patient and provider perspectives. *Pain Med.* 2004;5(1):66–80.

22. Berndt S, Maier C, Schütz H-W. Polymedication and medication compliance in patients with chronic non-malignant pain. *Pain.* 1993;52(3):331–339.

23. Ives TJ, Chelminski PR, Hammett-Stabler CA, et al. Predictors of opioid misuse in patients with chronic pain: a prospective cohort study. *BMC Health Serv Res.* 2006;6:46.

24. Michna E, Ross EL, Hynes WL, et al. Predicting aberrant drug behavior in patients treated for chronic pain: importance of abuse history. *J Pain Symptom Manage.* 2004;28(3):250–258.

25. Max MB, Payne R, Edwards WT. *Principles of analgesic use in the treatment of acute pain and cancer pain. 4th Ed.* Glenview, IL: American Pain Society; 1999.
26. Portenoy RK, McCaffery M. Adjuvant analgesics. In: McCaffery M, Pasero C., ed. *Pain clinical manual. 2nd Ed.* St. Louis, MO: Mosby, Inc.; 1999: 300–361.
27. Kouyanou K, Pither CE, Wessely S. Medication misuse, abuse and dependence in chronic pain patients. *J Psychosom Res.* 1997;43(5):497–504.
28. Manchikanti L. Prescription drug abuse: what is being done to address this new drug epidemic? Testimony before the Subcommittee on Criminal Justice, Drug Policy and Human Resources. *Pain Physician.* 2006;9(4):287–321.
29. American Psychiatric Association. *Diagnostic and statistical manual of mental disorders. 4th Ed.* Washington, DC: American Psychiatric Association; 1994.
30. Katz N, Fanciullo GJ. Role of urine toxicology testing in the management of chronic opioid therapy. *Clin J Pain.* 2002;18(4 Suppl):S76–S82.
31. Reid MC, Engles-Horton LL, Weber MB, Kerns RD, Rogers EL, O'Connor PG. Use of opioid medications for chronic noncancer pain syndromes in primary care. *J Gen Intern Med.* 2002;17(3):173–179.
32. Fishbain DA, Rosomoff HL, Rosomoff RS. Drug abuse, dependence, and addiction in chronic pain patients. *Clin J Pain.* 1992;8(2):77–85.
33. Jamison RN, Anderson KO, Peeters-Asdourian C, Ferrante FM. Survey of opioid use in chronic nonmalignant pain patients. *Reg Anesth.* 1994;19(4): 225–230.
34. Manchikanti L. National drug control policy and prescription drug abuse: facts and fallacies. *Pain Physician.* 2007;10(3):399–424.
35. Manchikanti L, Singh A. Therapeutic opioids: a ten-year perspective on the complexities and complications of the escalating use, abuse, and nonmedical use of opioids. *Pain Physician.* 2008;11(2 Suppl):S63–S88.
36. Portenoy RK. Opioid therapy for chronic nonmalignant pain: a review of the critical issues. *J Pain Symptom Manage.* 1996;11(4):203–217.
37. Schieffer BM, Pham Q, Labus J, et al. Pain medication beliefs and medication misuse in chronic pain. *J Pain.* 2005;6(9):620–629.
38. Manchikanti L, Cash KA, Damron KS, Manchukonda R, Pampati V, McManus CD. Controlled substance abuse and illicit drug use in chronic pain patients: an evaluation of multiple variables. *Pain Physician.* 2006;9(3): 215–225.
39. Manchikanti L, Pampati V, Damron KS, Fellows B, Barnhill RC, Beyer CD. Prevalence of opioid abuse in interventional pain medicine practice settings: a randomized clinical evaluation. *Pain Physician.* 2001;4(4):358–365.
40. Manchikanti L, Pampati V, Damron KS, Beyer CD, Barnhill RC. Prevalence of illicit drug use in patients without controlled substance abuse in interventional pain management. *Pain Physician.* 2003;6(2):173–178.
41. Manchikanti L, Damron KS, Beyer CD, Pampati V. A comparative evaluation of illicit drug use in patients with or without controlled substance abuse in interventional pain management. *Pain Physician.* 2003;6(3):281–285.

42. Dunbar SA, Katz NP. Chronic opioid therapy for nonmalignant pain in patients with a history of substance abuse: report of 20 cases. *J Pain Symptom Manage*. 1996;11:163–171.

43. Webster LR, Webster RM. Predicting aberrant behaviors in opioid-treated patients: preliminary validation of the Opioid Risk Tool. *Pain Med*. 2005;6(6):432–442.

44. Wilsey BL, Fishman SM, Tsodikov A, Ogden C, Symreng I, Ernst A. Psychological comorbidities predicting prescription opioid abuse among patients in chronic pain presenting to the emergency department. *Pain Med*. 2008;9(8):1107–1117.

45. Wasan AD, Davar G, Jamison R. The association between negative affect and opioid analgesia in patients with discogenic low back pain. *Pain*. 2005;117(3):450–461.

46. Dowling K, Storr CL, Chilcoat HD. Potential influences on initiation and persistence of extramedical prescription pain reliever use in the US population. *Clin J Pain*. 2006;22(9):776–783.

47. Savage SR, Kirsh KL, Passik SD. Challenges in using opioids to treat pain in persons with substance use disorders. *Addict Sci Clin Pract*. 2008;4(2):4–25.

48. Savage SR. Long-term opioid therapy: assessment of consequences and risks. *J Pain Symptom Manage*. 1996;11(5):274–286.

49. Manchikanti L, Atluri S, Trescot AM, Giordano J. Monitoring opioid adherence in chronic pain patients: tools, techniques, and utility. *Pain Physician*. 2008;11(2 Suppl):S155–S180.

50. Turk DC, Swanson KS, Gatchel RJ. Predicting opioid misuse by chronic pain patients: a systematic review and literature synthesis. *Clin J Pain*. 2008;24(6):497–508.

51. Butler SF, Fernandez K, Benoit C, Budman SH, Jamison RN. Validation of the revised Screener and Opioid Assessment for Patients with Pain (SOAPP-R). *J Pain*. 2008;9(4):360–372.

52. Dowling LS, Gatchel RJ, Adams LL, Stowell AW, Bernstein D. An evaluation of the predictive validity of the Pain Medication Questionnaire with a heterogeneous group of patients with chronic pain. *J Opioid Manag*. 2007;3(5):257–266.

53. Holmes CP, Gatchel RJ, Adams LL, et al. An opioid screening instrument: long-term evaluation of the utility of the pain medication questionnaire. *Pain Pract*. 2006;6(2):74–88.

54. Adams LL, Gatchel RJ, Robinson RC, et al. Development of a self-report screening instrument for assessing potential opioid medication misuse in chronic pain patients. *J Pain Symptom Manage*. 2004;27(5):440–459.

55. Butler SF, Budman SH, Fernandez KC, et al. Development and validation of the current opioid misuse measure. *Pain*. 2007;130(1–2):144–156.

56. Morisky DE, Green LW, Levine DM. Concurrent and predictive validity of a self-reported measure of medication adherence. *Med Care*. 1986;24(1):67–74.

57. Krousel-Wood M, Islam T, Webber LS, Re RN, Morisky DE, Muntner P. New medication adherence scale versus pharmacy fill rates in seniors with hypertension. *Am J Manag Care*. 2009;15(1):59–66.

58. Morisky DE, Ang A, Krousel-Wood M, Ward HJ. Predictive validity of a medication adherence measure in an outpatient setting. *J Clin Hypertens* (Greenwich). 2008;10(5):348–354.

59. Babamoto KS, Sey KA, Camilleri AJ, Karlan VJ, Catalasan J, Morisky DE. Improving diabetes care and health measures among hispanics using community health workers: results from a randomized controlled trial. *Health Educ Behav*. 2009;36(1):113–126.

60. Islam T, Muntner P, Webber LS, Morisky DE, Krousel-Wood MA. Cohort study of medication adherence in older adults (CoSMO): extended effects of Hurricane Katrina on medication adherence among older adults. *Am J Med Sci*. 2008;336(2):105–110.

61. Horne R, Weinman J, Hankins M. The beliefs about medicines questionnaire: the development and evaluation of a new method for assessing the cognitive representation of medication. *Psychol Health*. 1999;14:1–24.

62. Kumar K, Gordon C, Toescu V, et al. Beliefs about medicines in patients with rheumatoid arthritis and systemic lupus erythematosus: a comparison between patients of South Asian and White British origin. *Rheumatology (Oxford)*. 2008;47(5):690–697.

63. Menckeberg TT, Bouvy ML, Bracke M, et al. Beliefs about medicines predict refill adherence to inhaled corticosteroids. *J Psychosom Res*. 2008;64(1): 47–54.

64. Clifford S, Barber N, Horne R. Understanding different beliefs held by adherers, unintentional nonadherers, and intentional nonadherers: application of the necessity-concerns framework. *J Psychosom Res*. 2008;64(1):41–46.

65. Horne R, Weinman J. Patients' beliefs about prescribed medicines and their role in adherence to treatment in chronic physical illness. *J Psychosom Res*. 1999;47(6):555–567.

66. Osterberg L, Blaschke T. Adherence to medication. *N Engl J Med*. 2005;353(5):487–497.

67. Compton P, Darakjian J, Miotto K. Screening for addiction in patients with chronic pain and "problematic" substance use: evaluation of a pilot assessment tool. *J Pain Symptom Manage*. 1998;16(6):355–363.

68. Wu SM, Compton P, Bolus R, et al. The addiction behaviors checklist: validation of a new clinician-based measure of inappropriate opioid use in chronic pain. *J Pain Symptom Manage*. 2006;32(4):342–351.

69. Passik SD, Kirsh KL, Whitcomb L, Portenoy RK, Katz NP, Kleiman L, Dodd SL, Schein JR. A new tool to assess and document pain outcomes in chronic pain patients receiving opioid therarpy. *Clin Ther*. 2004;26:552–561.

70. Chabal C, Erjavec MK, Jacobsen L, Mariano A, Chaney E. Prescription opiate abuse in chronic pain patients: clinical criteria, incidence, and predictors. *Clin J Pain*. 1997;13:150–155.

71. Hammett-Stabler CA, Pesce AJ, Cannon DJ. Urine drug screening in the medical setting. *Clin Chim Acta*. 2002;315(1–2):125–135.

72. Drug enforcement administration. Questions and answers: state prescription drug monitoring programs. http://www.deadiversion.usdoj.gov/faq/rx_monitor.htm. Accessed January 5, 2009.

73. Turk DC, Rudy TE. Neglected topics in the treatment of chronic pain patients – Relapse, noncompliance, and adherence enhancement. *Pain*. 1991; 44(1):5–28.
74. Morrow DG, Hier CM, Menard WE, Leirer VO. Icons improve older and younger adults' comprehension of medication information. *J Gerontol B Psychol Sci Soc Sci*. 1998;53(4):P240–P254.
75. Morrow DG, Leirer VO, Andrassy JM, Hier CM, Menard WE. The influence of list format and category headers on age differences in understanding medication instructions. *Exp Aging Res*. 1998;24(3):231–256.
76. Morrow DG, Weiner M, Steinley D, Young J, Murray MD. Patients' health literacy and experience with instructions: influence preferences for heart failure medication instructions. *J Aging Health*. 2007;19(4):575–593.
77. Morrow DG, Weiner M, Young J, Steinley D, Deer M, Murray MD. Improving medication knowledge among older adults with heart failure: a patient-centered approach to instruction design. *Gerontologist*. 2005;45(4):545–552.
78. Rains JC, Penzien DB, Lipchik GL. Behavioral facilitation of medical treatment for headache – Part II: theoretical models and behavioral strategies for improving adherence. *Headache*. 2006;46(9):1395–1403.
79. Banbury P, Feenan K, Allcock N. Experiences of analgesic use in patients with low back pain. *Br J Nurs*. 2008;17(19):1215–1218.
80. Waters SJ, McKee DC, Keefe FJ. Cognitive behavioral approaches to the treatment of pain. *Chronic Comorbidity in CNS Med* 2004;1:45–51.
81. Edworthy SM, Devins GM. Improving medication adherence through patient education distinguishing between appropriate and inappropriate utilization. Patient Education Study Group. *J Rheumatol*. 1999;26(8):1793–1801.
82. Fahey KF, Rao SM, Douglas MK, Thomas ML, Elliott JE, Miaskowski C. Nurse coaching to explore and modify patient attitudinal barriers interfering with effective cancer pain management. *Oncol Nurs Forum*. 2008;35(2): 233–240.
83. Hill J, Bird H, Johnson S. Effect of patient education on adherence to drug treatment for rheumatoid arthritis: a randomised controlled trial. *Ann Rheum Dis*. 2001;60(9):869–875.
84. Schlenk EA, Dunbar-Jacob J, Engberg S. Medication non-adherence among older adults: a review of strategies and interventions for improvement. *J Gerontol Nurs*. 2004;30(7):33–43.
85. Bieber C, Muller KG, Blumenstiel K, et al. A shared decision-making communication training program for physicians treating fibromyalgia patients: effects of a randomized controlled trial. *J Psychosom Res*. 2008;64(1):13–20.
86. Leveille SG, Huang A, Tsai SB, Allen M, Weingart SN, Iezzoni LI. Health coaching via an internet portal for primary care patients with chronic conditions: a randomized controlled trial. *Med Care*. 2009;47(1):41–47.
87. Lorig KR, Ritter PL, Laurent DD, Plant K. The internet-based arthritis self-management program: a one-year randomized trial for patients with arthritis or fibromyalgia. *Arthritis Rheum*. 2008;59(7):1009–1017.
88. Fishman SM, Bandman TB, Edwards A, Borsook D. The opioid contract in the management of chronic pain. *J Pain Symptom Manage*. 1999;18(1):27–37.

89. Manchikanti L, Manchukonda R, Damron KS, Brandon D, McManus CD, Cash K. Does adherence monitoring reduce controlled substance abuse in chronic pain patients? *Pain Physician.* 2006;9(1):57–60.
90. Manchikanti L, Manchukonda R, Pampati V, et al. Does random urine drug testing reduce illicit drug use in chronic pain patients receiving opioids? *Pain Physician.* 2006;9(2):123–129.
91. Fagan MJ, Chen JT, Diaz JA, Reinert SE, Stein MD. Do internal medicine residents find pain medication agreements useful? *Clin J Pain.* 2008;24(1): 35–38.
92. Savage SR. Addiction in the treatment of pain: significance, recognition, and management. *J Pain Symptom Manage.* 1993;8(5):265–278.
93. Lorig K. Self-management education: more than a nice extra. *Med Care.* 2003;41(6):699–701.
94. Turk DC. Clinical effectiveness and cost-effectiveness of treatments for patients with chronic pain. *Clin J Pain.* 2002;18(6):355–365.
95. Naylor MR, Keefe FJ, Brigidi B, Naud S, Helzer JE. Therapeutic Interactive Voice Response for chronic pain reduction and relapse prevention. *Pain.* 2008;134(3):335–345.
96. Naylor MR, Helzer JE, Naud S, Keefe FJ. Automated telephone as an adjunct for the treatment of chronic pain: a pilot study. *J Pain.* 2002;3(6):429–438.
97. Lorig K, Ritter PL, Villa F, Piette JD. Spanish diabetes self-management with and without automated telephone reinforcement: two randomized trials. *Diab Care.* 2008;31(3):408–414.

Chapter 9
Adherence and Psychotherapy

Jennifer L. Strauss, Vito S. Guerra, Christine E. Marx, A. Meade Eggleston, and Patrick S. Calhoun

Psychotherapists target a wide range of clinical disorders, adopt diverse theoretical approaches, and operate within multiple treatment settings. As such, a unifying definition of *adherence* in the field of psychotherapy is not yet tenable. We therefore limit the scope of this chapter to an examination of adherence in the context of individual outpatient psychotherapy delivered to adult populations, with particular attention paid to evidence-based, cognitive-behavioral treatments. In this context, issues of adherence may be broadly summarized into two categories. The first, *premature termination,* has relevance across the full range of theoretical approaches. The second, failure to complete *between-session tasks and exercises*, is more specific to cognitive-behavioral interventions.

Premature Termination

> Eighty percent of success is just showing up. (Woody Allen)

We use the term *premature termination* to refer only to cases in which the patient unilaterally decides to end treatment (i.e., patient

J.L. Strauss (✉)
Department of Psychiatry and Behavioral Sciences, Duke University Medical Center; Investigator, Mid-Atlantic Research Educational and Clinical Center Health Scientist, Durham VAMC Center for Health Services Research in Primary Care, Durham, NC, USA
e-mail: jennifer.strauss@duke.edu

H. Bosworth (ed.), *Improving Patient Treatment Adherence*,   215
DOI 10.1007/978-1-4419-5866-2_9,
© Springer Science+Business Media, LLC 2010

"dropout"), against the therapist's recommendation and contrary to any existing agreement of treatment length. Premature termination is most likely to occur early in therapy, before the patient has experienced significant improvement, and thus is arguably the most significant obstacle to effective mental health service delivery [1]. That said, premature termination and treatment failure are not synonymous terms. Certainly, many patients who terminate therapy earlier than planned have made significant strides and, regardless of the clinician's perspective, may feel sufficiently helped and satisfied with the outcome. Hence, treatment may have been successful or partially successful, despite suboptimal adherence.

Prevalence of Premature Termination

Estimates of the prevalence of premature termination vary considerably, ranging from 30 to 60%, in part because researchers have operationalized it in different ways [2]. In their seminal meta-analysis, Wierzbicki and Pekarik found that the prevalence of premature termination averaged 48% (SD = 24%) across studies that examined therapist ratings of unilateral patient dropout [2]. Data suggest that approximately two-thirds of patients attend fewer than 10 sessions, that the majority attend less than 8 sessions, and that 14–44% attend only 1–2 sessions [3–5].

Lower rates of premature termination have been reported in clinical research settings than in non-research settings. For example, average premature termination rates reported in the National Institute of Mental Health Treatment of Depression Collaborative Research Program (TDCRP) for two manualized therapies were 32% (cognitive-behavioral therapy) and 23% (interpersonal therapy) [6], respectively, as compared to a 50% premature termination rate in private practice delivery of cognitive therapy for depression [7]. This likely reflects multiple factors. In research settings, for example, patient selection criteria may exclude more complex patients (e.g., those with comorbid substance abuse or significant Axis II pathology), therapists may provide increased pretherapy education about the schedule and processes involved in treatment (informed consent), and patients may develop a sense of commitment to the research. The pretherapy orientation to treatment length/course that occurs during the informed consent process may be particularly important, as lower dropout rates have been reported when prespecified time limits to therapy are established at treatment outset (32 versus 67%) [8].

Predictors of Premature Termination

Several comprehensive reviews of research on premature termination have been published within the past three decades [2, 9, 10]. Summarized below, reviews have examined patient demographic and clinical variables, therapist variables, and patients' expectations of treatment. Given the ubiquity of examinations of the patient–therapist relationship in the therapy outcome literature, we also briefly review associations between strength of the treatment alliance and premature termination.

Patient Characteristics

Patients who discontinue therapy prematurely are more likely to be female [9], unmarried [2], of younger age [2, 11–13], less educated (≤high school degree) [2, 3, 10, 14, 15], of minority race [2, 10, 12, 14], and of lower socioeconomic status (SES) [2, 9–12]. With respect to the latter, there exist multiple logistical barriers to completing therapy that are strongly associated with low SES, including work constraints, lack of child care, transportation problems, and lack of mental health insurance coverage [11, 16, 17]. Those who terminate treatment prematurely also tend to be high users of mental health services [1] and to have limited social support [9, 18].

Clinical diagnoses and characteristics associated with higher rates of dropout include history of an eating disorder [3], comorbid depressive- and anxiety-spectrum disorders [12], substance use disorders [9, 14], personality disorders [7, 14, 19, 20], psychotic symptoms and/or suspiciousness [14], hostility [14, 21], suicidality [14], and *psychological reactance* (i.e., emotional response that motivates one to restore threatened or reduced behavioral freedoms) [22]. Several investigations have demonstrated a link between patients' level of *psychological mindedness* (i.e., the ability to recognize psychological problems, use psychological terminology, and acknowledge possible psychological causes to problems) and treatment continuation [23]. Conversely, patient characteristics associated with poor psychological mindedness, such as low frustration tolerance, poor motivation, and impulsivity, have been associated with dropout [16].

However, associations between premature termination and patient demographic and clinical variables have not been consistently replicated. For example, though personality disorders tend to be predictive of higher dropout rates, at least one study found symptoms of borderline personality disorder to be associated with higher rates of session attendance [19]. Even where the data are more robust, effect sizes tend to be of small-to-moderate magnitude [10, 16]. For these reasons, researchers interested in premature termination have underscored the importance of looking beyond the sociodemographic characteristics and symptom profiles of patients [2].

Therapist Characteristics

Higher rates of premature termination have been associated with lower levels of therapist experience [9] and education [3], although type of training (e.g., social work, clinical psychology) has not [16]. Patients' perceptions of therapists' professional and personal qualities also may play a role: Patients are less likely to drop out of treatment if their therapists are perceived to be expert, trustworthy, and physically attractive [11, 24].

Patient Expectations, Beliefs, and Satisfaction

Ideally, patient and therapist agree on the goals and course of therapy at the outset of treatment, at least in broad strokes. Therapist and patient may commit to a prespecified number of sessions or agree to an approximate length of treatment that is subject to revision as therapy unfolds, depending on progress toward goals and the complexity of the case. Likewise, ideally the timing of treatment termination is mutually agreed upon and discussed well in advance of actual termination.

In reality, expectations regarding the length and course of treatment often go unaddressed. This is unfortunate, as patients' expectations of treatment duration consistently predict actual number of sessions attended across clinical settings, with correlations ranging from 0.28 to 0.38. Therapists, on the other hand, appear to underestimate the likelihood of early termination and overestimate treatment length [4, 5, 15].

Patients' expectations of treatment duration are, in fact, a better predictor of treatment length than problem severity, patient demographic variables, and therapist characteristics [3–5]. Additionally, it may be that some patient-level variables function as proxies for the degree of alignment between patients' and therapists' expectations for therapy [10, 16]. For example, several investigations have found that the association between lower socioeconomic status and premature termination can be statistically accounted for by patients' expectations of treatment length [2, 4, 5].

Patients' perceptions, attitudes and assumptions about mental illness (e.g., that problems are a sign of weakness), and psychotherapy (e.g., that seeking help will reflect poorly on one's family) may also influence willingness to engage and remain in therapy [11, 16]. Although relatively little extant research has examined associations between socialization practices and the emergence of beliefs regarding mental illness and psychotherapy, there is interest in further elucidating these relations and developing culturally sensitivity interventions to improve treatment adherence and engagement [16].

Finally, patients who discontinue treatment prematurely are more likely than treatment completers to report dissatisfaction with treatment and, paradoxically, are also more likely to report symptom improvement or problem abatement [3]. In other words, patients leave therapy when the perceived benefits do not justify the ongoing investment of time and energy, either because the patient believes that therapy or the therapist is ineffective, because presenting problems have dissipated and the patient no longer perceives a "need" for therapy, or both.

Treatment Alliance

The treatment alliance refers to the collaborative and personal bond between a patient and a therapist, as well as to the extent of patient–therapist agreement on the tasks and goals of therapy. Empirical reviews [25, 26] and meta-analytic studies [27, 28] have concluded that, regardless of patient diagnosis or therapist orientation, the alliance is a reliable and strong predictor of treatment outcomes. Indeed, several studies have demonstrated an inverse association between the strength of the alliance early in therapy, generally measured between sessions 1 and 5, and premature termination

[12, 29–36]. Although these studies do not explicate the bases for a weak treatment alliance, such findings are consistent with the idea that patients sometimes leave treatment because they distrust, dislike, or simply do not "connect" with their therapists and underscore the importance of establishing a collaborative, trusting alliance early in the course of therapy. Interestingly, limited evidence also suggests that *very* strong early alliances, perhaps representing unrealistic initial expectations, may also be related to poor outcomes and premature termination [37].

Forging a strong alliance may be particularly important when providing treatment to patient with pronounced interpersonal difficulties, such as those with personality disorders. For example, among patients enrolled in a trial of cognitive therapy for avoidant and obsessive-compulsive personality disorders, Strauss and colleagues found that those with more severe symptoms at baseline formed weaker treatment alliances, suggesting the need for extra attention to developing a treatment relationship with such patients. Higher early alliance scores were positively associated with session attendance [34].

Therapist–Patient In-Session Interactions

Several studies have examined associations between specific in-session interactions and premature termination. Such therapy process studies generally rely on review and coding of audiotaped sessions. Given the time intensity and potential intrusiveness of such designs, relatively few of these studies have been conducted. A common theme, however, has been the examination of therapists' contributions to premature termination and poor outcomes.

Several studies have examined in-session interactions in psychodynamic therapies. Using data from the Vanderbilt II study, Najavits and Strupp compared effective and ineffective psychodynamic therapists (relative "effectiveness" was defined on the basis of patient outcomes and length of treatment). As compared to those deemed less effective, more effective therapists demonstrated more positive relationship-oriented behaviors, such as warmth, and more self-criticism [38]. Piper and colleagues evaluated predictors of premature termination among patients enrolled in a trial of time-limited, interpretive individual therapy. Therapy process variables that distinguished early dropouts from matched completers included less early engagement in *dynamic work* (defined as the degree to which the patient identified, elaborated, and causally linked dynamic factors, such as wishes, fears, and defenses, related to his or her problems), less patient exploration of his or her problems, greater patient and therapist focus on transference, and weaker treatment alliances both early in treatment and at the session prior to dropout [39]. Review of the session prior to dropout revealed a common pattern in which "Patient and therapist seemed to be caught up in an unproductive power struggle that increased the frustration of both. Persistent use of transference interpretations on the therapist's part was not successful in resolving the impasse" (p. 121).

This pattern is consistent with that observed by the same investigators in an earlier study in which high use of transference interpretations was associated with weaker alliance and less favorable outcomes [40]. In both cases, treatment was delivered by highly experienced therapists, suggesting that this pattern is not simply attributable to "rookie error." Relatedly, several investigators have observed therapy interfering behaviors among even experienced therapists when in-session flexibility is compromised in favor of technical adherence to manualized psychodynamic [41, 42] and cognitive therapy [43]. Of note, these observations have occurred in the context of research studies, in which therapists' adherence to the treatment model is closely monitored, and may not generalize to other settings. In contrast, in analyses that excluded patients who left treatment prematurely, Loeb and colleagues reported a positive association between therapists' adherence to two manualized therapies for bulimia nervosa and strength of the alliance among treatment completers; the association between protocol adherence and treatment outcome was not significant [44] (Table 9.1).

Significance of Premature Termination

There are significant consequences of premature termination including, most prominently, reduced treatment efficacy. As noted above, the majority of patients entering psychotherapy attend fewer than eight sessions. Yet recent data suggest that a minimum of 11–13 sessions of evidence-based psychotherapy are needed for 50–60% of clients to recover [16]. Thus, a significant proportion of patients may not receive an adequate "dose" of therapy.

Table 9.1 Factors that predict premature termination

Patient demographic characteristics

1. Female gender
2. Younger age
3. Unmarried
4. Minority race/ethnicity
5. Less education (≤high school degree)
6. Low socioeconomic status

Patient health-related and clinical characteristics

1. Overutilization of health-care services
2. Low "psychological mindedness"
3. Low frustration tolerance
4. High impulsivity
5. Poor motivation
6. Hostility
7. Suicidality
8. Psychosis
9. Reactance
10. History of an eating disorder
11. Substance use disorder
12. Comorbid depressive- and anxiety-spectrum disorders
13. Personality disorder

Therapist characteristics

1. Less experience
2. Less education
3. Less warm
4. Perceived as less expert, less trustworthy, or physically unattractive

Treatment characteristics

1. Misaligned therapist–patient expectations regarding treatment length
2. Weak treatment alliance
3. Patient dissatisfaction or perceived abatement of problems

Decreased cost-effectiveness is another significant consequence of premature termination [2, 10]. Unused clinic time can result in lost revenues and, particularly in community clinic settings, inefficient resource allocation and reduced ability to meet the high demand for mental health services [1, 16]. To the extent that dropouts may be perceived to reflect patients' dissatisfaction with services, premature termination also may lower the credibility of the therapist, the clinic, and, more broadly, the field of psychotherapy within the community [45].

In addition to not receiving the full benefit of treatment, patients who terminate prematurely often experience a sense of dissatisfaction, failure, self-blame, wasted effort, and/or hopelessness, which may exacerbate symptoms, increase distress, and – importantly – lead to demoralization and a decreased likelihood of treatment seeking in the future [1, 3, 39]. Finally, premature terminations can bruise a therapist's morale and confidence, particularly early career therapists and trainees, and may contribute to the high rate of burnout among mental health professionals [1, 10, 39, 45].

Between-Session Tasks and Exercises

Just showing up doesn't get the job done. (John Wayne in Rio Bravo)

Between-session tasks and exercises are designed to encourage patients to practice and master new skills and strategies, facilitate generalization of these skills and strategies to novel settings, enhance self-efficacy, and reduce vulnerability to relapse [46]. Most contemporary psychologists employ between-session tasks and exercises ("homework") in their practices [47], and they are an integral component of cognitive-behavioral, manualized treatments for a broad range of clinical conditions [48]. Completion of homework is considered a specific "active ingredient" of cognitive-behavioral therapy (CBT) that is distinct from the nonspecific effects of most helping relationships [49]. Current research on the role of homework in psychotherapy is largely limited by reliance on retrospective reports, correlational designs, and secondary analyses with inadequate statistical power. However, there is a growing movement in the field to redress these shortcomings, particularly with respect to the role of homework in CBT for depression [49].

Prevalence and Moderators of Homework Adherence

At present there is no consensus on the prevalence of homework nonadherence, although most agree it is pervasive [46]. Likewise, definitive studies are lacking to explain why some patients complete assignments and others do not [49, 50].

Patient Characteristics

Homework completion has not been associated with baseline symptom severity [46, 51], personality disorders [46], or coping skills [51, 52]. However, clinical observation suggests that perfectionism, fear of failure, and fear of displeasing the therapist may negatively influence adherence rates [49, 53]. Of note, such obstacles also may reflect traits that brought the patient to therapy in the first place. One study of patients receiving cognitive therapy for depression showed a negative association between number of previous depressive episodes and adherence [51]. An interpretation of this finding offered by the investigators is that patients who have experienced more prior depressive episodes may feel more resigned to their depression and thus less motivated to complete between-session tasks. Patients' attributions about their illness may also influence homework adherence [54]. Consistent with the literature on session adherence, reviewed above, most research on homework adherence has focused on the role of patient characteristics, despite limited evidence of a strong predictive association [46].

Patient Expectancies

Establishing patients' expectations about the essential role of between-session tasks in therapy is central to much of what has been written on this topic. A therapist who assigns homework makes the implicit assumption that treatment efficacy is somewhat contingent upon the extent to which the patient actively works on therapy-related issues outside of the therapist's office. Likewise, patients who enter therapy expecting to be passive recipients of treatment and to be "fixed" by the therapist may not anticipate or appreciate the provider's perspective regarding the importance of between-session tasks. As such, it is paramount that the therapist stress the critical nature of homework completion and instill in the patient confidence that he or she can complete the tasks assigned. To this end, Burns and Auerbach delineate three common therapist errors: (1) failure to effectively explain the rationale for homework; (2) failure to create homework assignments that are relevant to the client; and (3) failure to develop meaningful therapeutic goals [55]. Although an association between these tasks and homework adherence rates was not supported in one small study of patients receiving cognitive therapy for depression, results did indicate that therapists' in-session review of the previous week's assignment predicted stronger adherence to subsequent assignments [51].

Therapist Characteristics

In their thoughtful review of the role of homework in cognitive therapy for depression, Thase and Callan underscore the clinical skill involved in persuading patients to complete between-session tasks, balancing use of homework with the usual flow of in-session contact, reinforcing successive approximations, addressing nonadherence, and matching assignments to patients' needs, abilities, and readiness [49]. Although the focus is on treatment of depression, these observations are applicable to a wide range of treatment modalities and clinical populations. Likewise, Waddington notes the import of patient–therapist rapport in encouraging patients to attempt aversive tasks, both within and between sessions [56]. However, ratings of therapist empathy, an independent predictor of outcome, were not associated with homework adherence in one large study of CBT for depression [57], suggesting that rapport alone may not influence patients' willingness to complete assignments. Not surprisingly, therapists who regularly assign homework elicit greater adherence [51]. Perhaps therapists, like their patients, are more likely to master skills and techniques with repeated practice! (Table 9.2)

Chicken Versus Egg

Does homework matter? Do patients get better *because* they complete homework assignments, or are those who get better simply more likely to complete between-session tasks? Or does a third variable, such as motivation, mediate both symptom improvement and homework adherence? Although predominantly correlational, the emergent literature, consistent with theory, suggests that completion of between-session tasks does improve clinical outcomes [49, 50].

Table 9.2 Factors that predict homework nonadherence

Patient health-related and clinical characteristics

1. Perfectionism
2. Fear of failure
3. Fear of displeasing therapist
4. History of multiple major depressive episodes

Therapist characteristics

1. Failure to clearly convey rationale for homework
2. Failure to match assignments to specific needs/readiness of patient
3. Failure to reinforce homework completion (e.g., by reviewing in session)

Treatment characteristics

1. Misaligned therapist–patient expectations regarding homework
2. Weak treatment alliance

One meta-analysis of 27 CBT studies (1,702 total participants) conducted between 1980 and 1998 reported a weighted average association of $r = 0.36$ between the assignment of homework and therapy outcomes, with larger effects obtained when assignments were varied during the course of treatment rather than limited to one specific type of task (e.g., relaxation skills training) [48]. With regard to homework adherence, the weighted average correlation between homework completion and outcomes was $r = 0.22$ [48].

Several studies suggest that treatment benefits associated with homework completion are stronger for more symptomatic patients. In one such study, 70 patients seeking treatment for depression were provided CBT in a private practice setting [7]. Among patients with more severe baseline symptoms (Beck Depression Inventory (BDI) [58] scores >19), homework completers experienced an average symptom reduction of 81%, whereas homework non-completers experienced an average symptom reduction of only 0.60%. Among patients with less severe baseline BDI scores, the corresponding between-group discrepancy was less pronounced, as homework completers and non-completers experienced average symptom reductions of 64 and 45%, respectively. Research by Neimeyer and Feixas [59] likewise points to the possibility that treatment benefits of homework adherence are most salient among highly symptomatic patients. In that study, which provided for randomized assignment of homework in the context of group cognitive therapy for depression, a significant association between homework completion and treatment outcome was found only among patients with more severe depression symptoms. Not all available data comport with this pattern of findings, however. Burns and colleagues [60], for example, studied the delivery of outpatient CBT for depression among 521 patients being seen in an independent specialty clinic. Although homework completion was significantly associated with posttreatment symptom reduction, the data did not suggest that effects associated with homework adherence were moderated by baseline severity of depressive symptoms. Taken together, current evidence suggests that completion of between-session tasks likely contributes to positive outcomes in general and that homework completion may be of particular import to the successful treatment of patients with severe symptomatology.

Interventions

> Consider the postage stamp; its usefulness consists in the ability to stick to one thing till it gets there. (Josh Billings)

Numerous interventions and techniques to enhance adherence have been proposed by clinicians and researchers. What follows is an overview of commonly proposed approaches, with an emphasis on those for which there is strong consensus and/or empirical support. We first summarize general orientation techniques that may function to reduce both premature termination and homework noncompliance, followed by a discussion of more targeted strategies.

Orientation Strategies to Enhance Adherence

Pretherapy Preparation

Several interventionists have developed orientation processes, ranging from intensive and highly structured to cursory, to introduce patients to the therapy process; to establish expectations for treatment length, structure, content, roles and outcomes; and to enhance patients' treatment motivation and willingness to actively participate in therapy. A review of 16 empirical studies supports the effectiveness of such techniques [61]. For example, a 12-min pretherapy preparation videotape resulted in significantly fewer treatment dropouts among 125 patients who sought outpatient treatment at an HMO clinic [23]. In a second study, a comparison of a verbal interview versus written orientation strategy yielded comparable advantages for both delivery methods [62].

In addition to educating the patient about the therapy process, such strategies may identify and address apprehensions and misconceptions about therapy, reduce incongruence between patients' and therapists' treatment expectations, enhance patients' motivation and readiness for change, and encourage the foundation of a strong treatment alliance [1]. Pretherapy orientation techniques may be particularly appropriate for patients who are "therapy naïve" [61]. Given potentially vast differences between individual therapists and theoretical orientations, even those with previous therapy experience may benefit from an introductory discussion to establish, for example, expectations regarding the amount of specific direction and advice the therapist will provide and the amount of between-session work to be expected.

Motivational Enhancement

As opposed to focusing on education, a related orientation approach focuses on enhancing patients' treatment motivation. Such strategies draw heavily from motivational interviewing, a technique initially developed to enhance motivation and readiness for change among patients engaged in substance abuse treatment [63]. Motivational interviewing techniques are designed to elicit behavior change by helping patients explore and resolve ambivalent feelings about addressing their problems. Following an initial assessment of a patient's readiness for change, the therapist employs nondirective interviewing techniques to guide the patient through the process of initially contemplating change, preparing to engage in the change process, and taking action. Patients are encouraged to express their concerns and consider the pros and cons of making changes [16].

A recent example of an application of this approach is the VA's REACH (Reaching out to Educate and Assist Caring, Healthy Families) intervention, which incorporates motivational interviewing procedures to review the advantages and disadvantages of engaging a veteran's family in a 9-month group therapy, including a focus on the patient's individual treatment goals and logistical issues [64].

Motivational interviewing techniques have repeatedly been shown to enhance substance abuse treatment engagement and retention. However, applications to other patient populations are described with less frequency and, to date, empirical support for such applications has not been consistent.

Planned Termination

Particularly in the context of brief, time-limited therapy (e.g., when insurance coverage is limited or when the patient is preparing for a scheduled event, such as an upcoming marriage or the birth of a child), therapists may consider preparing patients for termination at the beginning of therapy [65]. Assuming that therapists approach such discussions sensitively, in a manner likely to minimize the chance that the patient will feel rejected or abandoned (particularly those for whom issues of separation and loss are important), potential benefits of planned termination may include improved patient buy-in to the treatment rationale, goals and format and, thus, potentially improved treatment adherence. For some, such discussions may also raise important interpersonal issues that may be the subject of treatment [65]. When time is limited, it is particularly important to focus on what can be accomplished and to establish positive (but realistic) expectations. On the other hand, encouraging patient autonomy and self-confidence is particularly important in long-term cases in which overdependency on the therapist is a risk. Knowing that therapy will be time limited may motivate some patients to persevere through difficult patches [1]. Relevant strategies, in addition to an initial discussion of treatment length and structure, may include tapering the frequency of sessions, having the patient take greater control of the therapeutic agenda, and having the patient devise his or her own homework assignments [65].

Additional Considerations

Despite our best efforts, a significant proportion of patients may be expected to terminate treatment prematurely, some quite early in the process. With this reality in mind, therapists may consider devoting a portion of initial sessions to addressing patients' immediate concerns, thereby ensuring provision of some assistance to the large proportion of patients who may be expected to attend only a handful of sessions

[45]. Finally, regardless of specific technique, orientation processes should be tailored to match the individual patient's beliefs about their illness and perceptions of well-being [50]. Despite therapists' best intentions and efforts, adherence is ultimately the patient's decision. As such, attempts to modify adherence rates or, frankly, any other aspect of a patient's behavior should acknowledge and respect that it is the patient's choice to make.

Strategies to Reduce Premature Termination

The vast majority of the literature on intervention strategies to reduce premature termination is based on clinical theory and lore; a recent review identified a mere 15 empirical studies published between 1970 and 2004 [1]. In their review of predictors of premature termination, the authors suggest that the problem is generally multifactorial and, as such, that multiple strategies may be needed to improve session adherence across patients and treatment settings.

Initial Session Attendance and Prompts

Several strategies have been proposed to improve rates of initial session attendance, including mailing videotapes, written brochures and letters, scheduling preparatory interviews, and initiating telephone contacts and reminders in advance of an initial appointment. Likewise, brief prompts, such as reminder calls, may increase regular session attendance [45]. Providing flexible hours and brief wait time for appointments may also improve retention. Some suggest establishing a written contract with patients to formalize a commitment to attend a prespecified number of sessions [45]. Such contracts may be revisited and revised regularly in accordance with treatment gains.

Case Management

Case management may be introduced as an adjunct to therapy to assist patients, particularly those with limited resources, to manage difficult life circumstances or events. More traditionally a component of care for patients with severe mental illness, a recent study demonstrated that the addition of telephone-based case management resulted in a near 50% reduction in premature termination among ethnically diverse, economically impoverished, primary care patients enrolled in group CBT for depression [66].

Foster Open Dialogue

To the extent that premature termination may occur when patients are dissatisfied with therapy or their therapist, encouraging an open dialogue about such issues early in the therapy process may help to avert drop out. To this end, therapists should endeavor to create a safe atmosphere in which patients feel free to ask questions and express doubts or dissatisfaction [1]. One caveat to this suggestion is that its proper execution will require clinical finesse to avoid an overemphasis, and potentially destructive focus, on negative affect, the treatment relationship, or the therapy process at the expense of addressing the patient's clinical concerns.

Strategies to Enhance Homework Adherence

Framing Homework Assignments

Burns and Auerbach posit that the "art" of therapy entails both fostering a shared appreciation for the essential role of between-session tasks to the therapeutic process and matching the focus and difficulty level of tasks to the individual patient [55]. Application of such strategies underscores the importance of orienting patients to the therapy process early in treatment. Patients' difficulty completing a between-session task may indicate that the therapist has failed to clearly describe the exercise, has selected a task that is too demanding or advanced, did not clearly link the task to material addressed in-session, or has misperceived the patient's endorsement of the relevance and importance of completing the assignment [49, 50]. One technique used to identify possible obstacles to task completion is to ask the patient to visualize going through the steps of completing a proposed assignment while in-session [50]. This brief exercise may enhance homework adherence by helping patient and therapist to identify and address skills or resource deficits in advance.

Thase and Callan note that the therapist tacitly conveys the importance of between-session tasks by regularly devoting session time to reviewing progress and explicitly linking the patient's independent work into session content [49]. Through the example of their own actions, therapists may also instill the importance of devoting between-session time to the case. For example, therapists may assign themselves parallel homework assignments (e.g., locating a copy of a relevant magazine article for the patient) or express thoughts about the patient that occurred between sessions (e.g., "I've been thinking about what you said last week"; "A thought occurred to me after our last session") [65]. Such actions model for patients the importance of working on therapy daily, rather than just within the formal therapy session.

In cases of nonadherence, it may be necessary to devote session time to troubleshooting obstacles [46, 50]. Burns, Adams, and Anastopoulos [67] have devised a list of common reasons for homework nonadherence that may be used to guide troubleshooting efforts (see Table 9.3). Because a homework "failure" may diminish patient confidence, subsequent to planning the next between-session task clinicians may want to briefly check in by asking patients to rate their confidence in their ability to complete the assignment and consider revising the plan and/or bolstering patients' support when confidence is weak [50].

Several clinical theorists suggest incorporating role playing and role reversals to change beliefs and enhance the motivation of ambivalent patients [68, 69]. For example, the patient may be asked to play the role of therapist and engage the "patient" (therapist) in a discussion about the importance of completing between-session tasks. Methods

Table 9.3 Common reasons for homework nonadherence

1. All or no thinking
2. Fear of disapproval
3. Hopelessness
4. Unexpressed anger
5. Coercion sensitivity
6. Depressive realism
7. Conceptual mismatch
8. Entitlement
9. Fear of shame
10. Shame

Adapted from Burns et al. [67]

to enhance motivation to complete other behavioral tasks, such as exercise, may also be applied to enhance homework adherence. For example, greater enjoyment of the task may be achieved when patients set specific goals, perceive that they have choice and control over the tasks, incorporate family and friends into activities if appropriate and feasible, have flexibility in assignment completion, and are assigned tasks that are both challenging and personally rewarding [70]. In the context of substance abuse treatment, Miller has long espoused-related strategies to enhance motivation and perceived control, including providing choices among various homework alternatives and discussing the pros and cons of completing homework assignments [71].

Therapists may also discuss the importance of self-reinforcement, particularly when social support is lacking or when negative feedback following behavior change may be predicted (e.g., increased self-assertion with a domineering spouse) [50]. The process of learning to develop and implement a self-reinforcement plan can be presented as a possible treatment goal and an important life skill in its own right. Patients should also be encouraged to enlist the support of existing social networks.

An interesting literature exists within the field of health behavior change on "message framing" which suggests that people are more receptive to a behavior change that is framed in terms of its associated benefits versus costs. Thus, at least in theory, patients should be more likely to complete between session tasks when told that doing so will help them to feel better as opposed to being told that not completing a task may compromise treatment progress [72]. Finally, it is arguably unfortunate that the term "homework" has persisted in the literature. To the extent that the term holds negative and paternalistic connotations for many, therapists may consider using alternate descriptors (e.g., "practice sessions" or "self-help exercises") that convey a sense of autonomy and independence.

Structuring Assignments

Several authors suggest using preprinted homework forms, handouts, and other prepared materials to help patients to structure and monitor completion of between-session assignments [50, 73]. Consistent with findings in the medical adherence literature, providing written versus verbal assignments may improve adherence rates by reducing ambiguity, improving recall, and increasing the perceived importance of task completion [74]. Therapists may consider assigning relatively simple tasks initially, reinforcing small gains and successive approximations of task completion, and gradually building up to more demanding and complex assignments [75]. It may be fruitful to devote a portion of the session to helping the patient develop a specific schedule and plan for task completion and to conveying very specific details about task completion including how, when, for how long, and in what circumstances the assigned behavior is to be carried out [75]. Briefly checking with the patient – via telephone, email, or text message – can enhance accountability and allow for some troubleshooting if the patient feels stymied or stuck. Enlisting the support of a significant other, as appropriate, may also be beneficial.

Summary

In this chapter we discuss the role of adherence in outpatient psychotherapy with adult populations. We specifically focus on two types of treatment adherence: premature termination, which is broadly applicable to a range of treatment approaches, and failure to complete between session tasks and exercises, which is more specific to cognitive-behavioral therapies. Both adherence problems are highly prevalent and both pose significant obstacles to effective and efficient delivery of mental health care. We summarize patient, therapist, and treatment characteristics associated with treatment nonadherence, as well as intervention strategies to enhance adherence. Our overarching goal, of course, is to provide clinically relevant information and guidance. The following broad recommendations summarize the more detailed content presented above.

General Strategies to Enhance Adherence

- Establish realistic expectations about the focus, content, and length of treatment, including the role of the patient and therapist. Consensus on these components early in the therapy process sets the stage for all that follows. Such discussions may be iterative and, importantly, may provide opportunities to identify and address patient concerns, misconceptions, and ambivalence about therapy and to enhance patient motivation and readiness for change.

- Balance early discussions about the process of therapy, described above, with session time devoted to addressing the patient's immediate concerns. This will increase the likelihood that even patients who leave therapy prematurely receive at least some assistance, and early gains may enhance treatment motivation and retention.

- Recognize and respect that adherence is ultimately the patient's responsibility and choice to make.

Strategies to Enhance Session Attendance

- Use prompts and reminders, such as introductory letters and reminder calls, to enhance session attendance.

- Case management may be an appropriate adjunct to help some patients, particularly those with limited resources, manage difficult life circumstances and events.

- Encourage open dialogue about the patient's experience in and satisfaction with therapy and the therapist. Strive to create an atmosphere in which patients feel safe to ask questions and express concerns.

Strategies to Enhance Homework Adherence

- Individualize assignments. Match the focus, difficulty, and nature of between-session tasks to the patient.

- Orient the patient to the importance of between-session tasks, assess and address patient's ambivalence about the tasks, and clearly link assignments to session material and the patient's treatment goals. Frame tasks in terms of associated benefits to the patient (e.g., greater/more efficient treatment gains) versus associated costs (e.g., less/slower treatment progress). Before finalizing an assignment, ensure that the patient understands the tasks; believes that completion of assigned tasks is personal, relevant, and important; and feels confident in his or her ability to complete the assignments.

- Because the term "homework" holds negative connations for some, consider alternate terms, such as "practice sessions" or "self-help exercises," that convey autonomy and independence.
- Enlist the patient's existing support network and bolster self-reinforcement skills, as necessary, to assist with task completion.
- Provide clear instructions and confirm that the patient understands the task before ending the session.
- Written instructions and printed materials may help patients structure and monitor task completion.
- Consider devoting a portion of session time to developing a schedule and detailed plan for task completion.
- Consider briefly checking in with the patient between sessions to enhance accountability and briefly troubleshoot adherence obstacles.
- Given the importance of between-session tasks, it is appropriate to devote a portion of session time to troubleshoot obstacles that interfere with homework adherence.

References

1. Ogrodniczuk JS, Joyce AS, Piper WE. Strategies for reducing patient-initiated premature termination of psychotherapy. *Harv Rev Psychiatry.* 2005;13(2):57–70.
2. Wierzbicki M, Pekarik G. A meta-analysis of psychotherapy dropout. *Profess Psychol Res Prac.* 1993;24:190–195.
3. Mueller M, Pekarik G. Treatment duration prediction: client accuracy and its relationship to dropout, outcome, and satisfaction. *Psychotherapy.* 2000;37(2):117–123.
4. Pekarik G. Relationship of expected and actual treatment duration for child and adult clients. *J Clin Child Psychol.* 1991;20:121–125.
5. Pekarik G, Wierzbicki M. The relationship between clients' expected and actual treatment duration. *Psychotherapy.* 1986;23(4):532–534.
6. Elkin I, Shea MT, Watkins JT, et al. National Institute of Mental Health Treatment of Depression Collaborative Research Program. General effectiveness of treatments. *Arch Gen Psychiatry.* 1989;46(11):971–982; discussion 983.
7. Persons JB, Burns DD, Perloff JM. Predictors of dropout and outcome in cognitive therapy for depression in a private practice setting. *Cogn Ther Res.* 1988;12:557–575.
8. Sledge WH, Moras K, Hartley D, Levine M. Effect of time-limited psychotherapy on patient dropout rates. *Am J Psychiatry.* 1990;147(10):1341–1347.

9. Baekeland F, Lundwall L. Dropping out of treatment: a critical review. *Psychol Bull.* 1975;82(5):738–783.
10. Garfield SL. Research on client variables in psychotherapy. In: Berger AE, Garfield SL, eds. *Handbook of psychotherapy and behavior change. 4th Ed.* New York, NY: Wiley; 1994.
11. Edlund MJ, Wang PS, Berglund PA, Katz SJ, Lin E, Kessler RC. Dropping out of mental health treatment: patterns and predictors among epidemiological survey respondents in the United States and Ontario. *Am J Psychiatry.* 2002;159(5):845–851.
12. Arnow BA, Blasey C, Manber R, et al. Dropouts versus completers among chronically depressed outpatients. *J Affect Disord.* 2007;97(1–3):197–202.
13. Foulks EF, Persons JB, Merkel RL. The effect of patients' beliefs about their illnesses on compliance in psychotherapy. *Am J Psychiatry.* 1986;143(3):340–344.
14. Richmond R. Discriminating variables among psychotherapy dropouts from a psychological training clinic. *Profes Psychol Res Pract.* 1992;23:123–130.
15. Rabinowitz J, Renert N. Clinicians' predictions of length of psychotherapy. *Psychiatr Serv.* 1997;48(1):97–99.
16. Barrett MS, Chua WJ, Crits-Christoph P, Gobbons MB, Thompson D. Early withdrawal from mental health treatment: implications for psychotherapy practice. *Psychother Theor, Res, Pract, Train.* 2008;45(2):247–267.
17. Mukherjee S, Sullivan G, Perry D, et al. Adherence to treatment among economically disadvantaged patients with panic disorder. *Psychiatr Serv.* 2006;57(12):1745–1750.
18. Hilsenroth MJ, Handler L, Toman KM, Padawer JR. Rorschach and MMPI-2 indices of early psychotherapy termination. *J Consult Clin Psychol.* 1995;63(6):956–965.
19. Hilsenroth MJ, Castlebury FD, Holdwick DJ, Jr., Blais MA. The effects of DSM-IV Cluster B personality disorder symptoms on the termination and continuation of psychotherapy. *Psychotherapy.* 1998;35:163–176.
20. Barber JP, Morse JQ, Krakauer ID, Chittams J, Crits-Christoph P. Change in obsessive-compulsive and avoidant personality disorders following time-limited supportive-expressive therapy. *Psychotherapy.* 1997;24:133–143.
21. Smith TE, Koenigsberg HW, Yeomans FE, Clarkin JF, Selzer MA. Predictors of dropout in psychodynamic psychotherapy. *J Psychother Pract Res.* 1995;4:205–213.
22. Seibel CA, Dowd ET. Reactance and therapeutic noncompliance. *Cogn Ther Res.* 1999;23:373–379.
23. Reis BF, Brown LG. Preventing therapy dropout in the real world: the clinical utility of videotape preparation and client estimate of treatment duration. *Profes Psychol Res Pract.* 2006;37:311–316.
24. McNeil B, May R, Lee V. Perceptions of counselor source characteristics by premature and successful terminators. *J Counsel Psychol.* 1987;34:86–89.
25. Horvath AO, Bedi RP. The alliance. In: Norcross JC, ed. *Psychotherapy relationships that work: Therapist contributions and responsiveness to patients.* New York, NY: Oxford University Press; 2002:37–69.

26. Orlinsky DE, Grawe K, Parks BK. Process and outcome in psychother- apy – noch einmal. In: Garfield AEBSL, ed. *Handbook of psychotherapy and behavior change. Vol. 4.* New York, NY: Wiley; 1994:270–376.

27. Horvath AO, Symonds BD. Relation between working alliance and outcome in psychotherapy: a meta-analysis. *J Counsel Psychol.* 1991;38:139–149.

28. Martin DJ, Garske JP, Davis MK. Relation of the therapeutic alliance with outcome and other variables: a meta-analytic review. *J Consult Clin Psychol.* Jun 2000;68(3):438–450.

29. Mohl PC, Martinez D, Ticknor C, Huang M, Cordell L. Early dropouts from psychotherapy. *J Nerv Ment Dis.* Aug 1991;179(8):478–481.

30. Tryon GS, Kane AS. The helping alliance and premature termination. *Counsel Psychol Quarter.* 1990;3:223–238.

31. Tryon GS, Kane AS. Relationship of working alliance to mutual and unilateral termination. *J Counsel Psychol.* 1993;40:33–36.

32. Tryon GS, Kane AS. Client involvement, working alliance, and type of therapy termination. *Psychother Res.* 1995;5:189–198.

33. Yeomans FE, Gutfreund J, Selzer MA, Clarkin J, Hull JW, Smith TE. Factors related to drop-outs by borderline patients: treatment contract and therapeutic alliance. *J Psychothera Pract Res.* 1994;3:16–24.

34. Strauss JL, Hayes AM, Johnson SL, et al. Early alliance, alliance ruptures, and symptom change in a nonrandomized trial of cognitive therapy for avoidant and obsessive-compulsive personality disorders. *J Consult Clin Psychol.* Apr 2006;74(2):337–345.

35. Beckham EE. Predicting patient dropout in psychotherapy. *Psychotherapy.* 1992;27:177–182.

36. Samstag LW, Batchelder ST, Muran JC, Safran JD, Winston A. Early iden- tification of treatment failures in short-term psychotherapy. An assessment of therapeutic alliance and interpersonal behavior. *J Psychother Pract Res.* 1998;7(2):126–143.

37. Joyce AS, Piper WE. Expectancy, the therapeutic alliance, and treatment outcome in short-term individual psychotherapy. *J Psychother Pract Res.* 1998;7(3):236–248.

38. Najavits LM, Strupp HH. Differences in the effectiveness of psychodynamic therapists: a process-outcome study. *Psychotherapy.* 1994;31:114–123.

39. Piper WE, Ogrodniczuk JS, Joyce AS, McCallum M, Rosie JS, O'Kelly JG. Prediction of dropping out in time-limited, interpretive individual psychother- apy. *Psychotherapy.* 1999;36(2):114–122.

40. Piper WE, Azim HFA, Joyce AS, McCallum M. Transference interpretations, therapeutic alliance and outcome in short-term individual psychotherapy. *Arch Gen Psychiat.* 1991;48:946–953.

41. Henry WP, Schacht TE, Strupp HH, Butler SF, Binder JL. Effects of training in time-limited dynamic psychotherapy: mediators of therapists' responses to training. *J Consult Clin Psychol.* 1993;61:441–447.

42. Henry WP, Strupp HH, Butler SF, Schacht TE, Binder JL. Effects of training in time-limited dynamic psychotherapy: changes in therapist behavior. *J Consul Clin Psychol.* 1993;61(434–440).

43. Castonguay LG, Goldfried MR, Wiser S, Raue PJ, Hayes AM. Predicting the effect of cognitive therapy for depression: a study of unique and common factors. *J Consult Clin Psychol.* 1996;64(3):497–504.

44. Loeb KL, Wilson GT, Labouvie E, et al. Therapeutic alliance and treatment adherence in two interventions for bulimia nervosa: a study of process and outcome. *J Consult Clin Psychol.* 2005;73(6):1097–1107.

45. Pekarik G. Coping with dropouts. *Profess Psychol: Res Pract.* 1985;16:114–123.

46. Detweiler JB, Whisman MA. The role of homework assignments in cognitive therapy for depression: potential methods for enhancing adherence. *Clin Psychol: Sci Pract.* 1999;6(3):267–282.

47. Kazantzis N, Deane FP. Psychologists' use of homework assignments in clinical practice. *Profess Psychol: Sci Pract.* 1999;30:581–585.

48. Kazantzis N, Deane FP, Ronan KR. Homework assignments in cognitive and behavioral therapy: a meta-analysis. *Clin Psychol: Sci Pract.* 2000;7(2):189–202.

49. Thase ME, Callan JA. The role of homework in cognitive behavior therapy for depression. *J Psychothera Integr.* 2006;16(2):162–177.

50. Robinson P. Putting it on the street: homework in cognitive behavioral therapy. In: O'Donohue WT, Fisher JE, eds. *General principles and empirically supported techniques of cognitive behavior therapy.* New York, NY: Wiley; 2009:358–369.

51. Bryant MJ, Simons AD, Thase ME. Therapist skill and patient variables in homework compliance: controlling an uncontrolled variable in cognitive therapy outcome research. *Cogn Ther Res.* 1999;23:381–399.

52. Burns DD, Nolen-Hoeksema S. Coping styles, homework compliance, and the effectiveness of cognitive-behavioral therapy. *J Consult Clin Psychol.* 1991;59(2):305–311.

53. Persons JB. *Cognitive therapy in practice: A case formulation approach.* New York, NY: Norton and Company; 1989.

54. Addis ME, Jacobson NS. Reasons for depression and the process and outcome of cognitive-behavioral psychotherapies. *J Consult Clin Psychol.* 1996;64(6):1417–1424.

55. Burns DD, Auerbach AH. Does homework compliance enhance recovery from depression? *Psychia Ann.* 1992;22:464–469.

56. Waddington L. The therapy relationship in cognitive therapy: a review. *Behavi Cogn Psychother.* 2002;30:179–191.

57. Burns DD, Nolen-Hoeksema S. Therapeutic empathy and recovery from depression in cognitive-behavioral therapy: a structural equation model. *J Consult Clin Psychol.* 1992;60(3):441–449.

58. Beck AT. *Depression: causes and treatment.* Philadelphia, PA: University of Pennsylvania Press; 1972.

59. Neimeyer RA, Feixas G. The role of homework and skill acquisition in the outcome of group cognitive therapy for depression. *Behav Ther.* 1990;21:281–292.

60. Burns DD, Spangler DL. Does psychotherapy homework lead to improve-
    ments in depression in cognitive behavioral therapy: a structural equation
    model. *J Consul Clin Psychol*. 2000;68:46–56.
61. Walitzer KS, Dermen KH, Connors GJ. Strategies for preparing clients for
    treatment: a review. *Behav Modification*. 1999;23:129–151.
62. Garrison JE. Written vs. verbal preparation of patients for group psychother-
    apy. *Psychotherapy*. 1978;15:130–134.
63. Miller WR, Rollnick S. *Motivational interviewing: Preparing people to
    change addictive behaviors*. New York, NY: Guilford Press; 1991.
64. Sherman MD, Fischer E, Bowling UB, Dixon L, Ridener L, Harrison D. A
    new engagement strategy in a VA-based family psychoeducation program.
    Psychiat Service. 2009;60:254–257.
65. Newman CF. The therapeutic alliance in short-term cognitive therapy. In:
    Safran JD, Muran JC, eds. *The therapeutic alliance in brief psychotherapy*.
    Washington, DC: American Psychological Association; 1998:95–122.
66. Miranda J, Azocar F, Organista KC, Dwyer E, Areane P. Treatment of depres-
    sion among impoverished primary care patients from ethnic minority groups.
    Psychiat Service. 2003;54:219–225.
67. Burns DD, Adams RL, Anastopoulos AD. The role of self-help assignments in
    the treatment of depression. In: Leber EEBWR, ed. *Handbook of depression:
    treatment, assessment, and research*. Homewood: IL: Dorsey; 1985:634–668.
68. DiMatteo MR, DiNicola DD. *Achieving patient compliance: The psychology
    of the medical practitioner's role*. New York, NY: Pergamon; 1982.
69. Turk DC, Salovey P. Cognitive-behavior treatment of illness behavior. In:
    Smith PMNTW, ed. *Managing chronic illness: A biopsychological perspec-
    tive*. Washington, DC: American Psychological Association; 1995:245–284.
70. Wankel LM. The importance of enjoyment to adherence and psychological
    benefits from physical activity. *Int J Sports Psychol*. 1993;24:151–169.
71. Miller WR. Motivation for treatment: a review with special emphasis on
    alcoholism. *Psycholo Bull*. 1985;98:84–107.
72. Rothman AJ, Salovey P. Shaping perceptions to motivate healthy behavior: the
    role of message framing. *Psychol Bull*. 1997;121:3–19.
73. Broder MS. Making optimal use of homework to enhance your therapeutic
    effectiveness. *J Rational-Emotive Cognitive-Behavioral Ther*. 2000;18:3–18.
74. Cox DJ, Tisdelle DA, Culbert JP. Increasing adherence to behavioral home-
    work assignments. *J Behav Med*. 1988;11:519–522.
75. Shelton JL, Levy RL. *Behavioral assignments and treatment compliance: A
    handbook of clinical strategies*. Champaign, IL: Research Press; 1981.

Chapter 10
Adherence to Treatment for Depression

Carol D. Saur and David C. Steffens

Major depressive disorder (MDD) is often a chronic, recurrent, and debilitating health problem with a lifetime prevalence of 16.2% and a 12-month prevalence of 6.6% in the USA [1]. Left untreated, depression can have a significant negative impact on a person's social, physical, and mental well-being and place an enormous burden on society. Patients with depression experience a higher incidence of premature death related to cardiovascular disease [2, 3] and are 4.5 times more likely to suffer a myocardial infarction than those without depression [3]. Depression in patients with diabetes is associated with increasing rates of vascular complications and increased mortality [4]. In terms of economic burden, the total cost of depression in the USA was estimated at $83.1 billion in 2000 [5]. Major contributors to depression-related cost were lost productivity and direct medical expenses, which accounted for $30–$50 billion each year [6]. Compared with nondepressed patients, health service costs for depressed patients are 50–100% greater, mainly due to higher overall medical utilization [7, 8].

MDD frequently presents in the primary care setting, with a reported prevalence range of 5–13% among medical outpatients [9]. Other primary care patients with treated depression may continue to experience residual symptoms of generalized and somatic anxiety,

C.D. Saur (✉)
Department of Medicine, Duke University Medical Center, Durham, NC, USA
e-mail: carol.saur@duke.edu

H. Bosworth (ed.), *Improving Patient Treatment Adherence*,
DOI 10.1007/978-1-4419-5866-2_10,
© Springer Science+Business Media, LLC 2010

irritability, and persistent social dysfunction despite having few remaining depressive symptoms [10]. It is more prevalent in patients with common chronic medical conditions, such as obstructive pulmonary disease, hypertension, diabetes, stroke, coronary artery disease, asthma, and chronic pain [1]. In addition to its association with medical morbidity and mortality, depression has a negative impact on self-care behaviors, including medication adherence in patients with chronic medical illnesses, and on health-related behaviors such as exercise, smoking, and weight control [11–13]. As a result, comorbid MDD is a major barrier to effective care of chronic medical illnesses.

Despite the burdens that it imposes, detection and diagnosis of depression remains problematic in primary care; many medical patients have depression that is undiagnosed and/or untreated [14, 15]. Less than one third of adults with depression obtain appropriate professional treatment [16]. Several studies have demonstrated that early recognition and treatment of depression in the primary care setting can improve social function, increase productivity, and decrease absenteeism in the workplace [17, 18].

Adherence to treatment is another issue facing clinicians and depressed patients. Non-adherence during the acute phase of antidepressant treatment is high, with rates of premature discontinuation ranging from 20 to 60% during the first 3 months of care [19–22]. One recent study reported that among adults in the USA who initiate treatment with an antidepressant, 42.4% discontinued their medication during the first 30 days of treatment and 72.4% discontinued medication during the first 90 days [23]. About 25% of depressed patients do not inform their physicians when discontinuing treatment [20, 24]. In the primary care setting, non-adherence by depressed patients is a problem not only for depression treatment but also for treatment prescribed for comorbid chronic medical illnesses [1]. A meta-analytic review of 12 studies showed that depressed patients were three times more likely than nondepressed patients to be non-adherent to treatment recommendations for medical disorders [25]. Some have speculated that non-adherence to depression treatment may contribute to increased morbidity and mortality among depressed patients who have diabetes or heart disease [26].

Greater antidepressant adherence is associated with better acute and long-term mood outcomes among depressed samples [27], while non-adherence has been linked to less improvement of depressive symptoms [19, 28] and greater relapse and recurrence of depression [29, 30]. Enhancing adherence to depression treatment has been identified as an important research challenge for primary care [31].

Limited research exists on a variety of social, psychological, and clinical factors related to adherence to antidepressant treatment. There have also been few studies on interventions to improve adherence. In this chapter, we will review this literature and provide illustrative case examples based on clinical experience providing depression treatment in primary care, with a focus on improving antidepressant medication adherence.

Factors Related to Adherence to Antidepressant Treatment

Several studies have examined factors related to adherence to antidepressant medication use in the primary care setting. These include demographic factors, psychological/attitudinal factors, and clinical factors.

Demographic Factors

One group obtained data from the Medical Expenditure Panel Survey for 1996–2001 and found that among 829 adults who initiated antidepressant treatment for depression, antidepressant discontinuation during the first 30 days of treatment was highest among Hispanics, patients with less than 12 years of education, and patients with low family incomes [23]. Cooper et al. found that African Americans and Hispanic Americans had lower odds than Caucasians of finding antidepressant medications acceptable [32]. In this study, African Americans were slightly less likely than Caucasians to find counseling acceptable, whereas Hispanic Americans were slightly more likely to find counseling acceptable than Caucasians. Others have noted lower adherence rates generally for ethnic minorities, suggesting that part of the issue may be locus of control: African Americans and Hispanic Americans feel more strongly than Caucasians that they have less control over their own health status [33].

Psychological/Attitudinal Factors

In the Vantaa Depression Study, 198 psychiatric clinic patients with an initial episode of major depression were provided treatment and followed for 18 months [34]. The investigators assessed adherence to and attitudes toward both antidepressants and psychotherapeutic support/psychotherapy. Most (about 88%) depressed patients received antidepressants in the early acute phase, but 49% terminated treatment prematurely and tended to have poor depression outcomes. Premature termination was associated with negative attitudes, specifically fear of dependence on or side effects from antidepressants. As for non-pharmacological treatments, nearly all patients (98%) received some form of acute-phase psychosocial treatment and 16% had weekly psychotherapy during the follow-up. About a quarter of patients admitted non-adherence to ongoing treatments.

More recently, Russell and Kazantzis examined attitudes about medication and adherence in a general medical practice [35]. After a primary care visit, patients completed questionnaires that measured beliefs about antidepressant medication, self-reported adherence to antidepressant treatment, and depression severity. Interestingly, the authors failed to find a significant relationship between beliefs in the necessity of antidepressants and adherence. Patient concerns with medications were positively associated with non-adherence. They observed greater reported adherence in cases where beliefs about the necessity of antidepressants outweighed concerns about taking the medication. Finally, fewer depressive symptoms were also associated with greater adherence. The authors concluded that since adherence to depression care appeared to be most related to continuity of treatment, finding ways to improve ongoing treatment is a crucial step in maximizing outcomes of patients with MDD. Denial of illness and fear of social stigma are two primary barriers to proper identification and treatment of depression [36].

Clinical Factors

The nature of depression itself may play a role in non-adherence. Some have suggested that depression might contribute to non-adherence because of hopelessness and a lack of positive beliefs and expectations regarding the efficacy of treatment, social isolation limiting opportunities for social support, impairment in memory or cognition, or the motivation necessary for following treatment recommendations related to medication adherence [25].

Adverse reactions and response to antidepressant treatment may also play a role in non-adherence. Results of efficacy trials suggest that perceived side effects are the most common reason for antidepressant discontinuation, but naturalistic studies provide evidence that favorable response to treatment may be a reason, such that patients may perceive they no longer need treatment [1]. Perceived lack of efficacy and reported adverse events may contribute more to early discontinuation of treatment, while patient misperceptions may explain later discontinuation of treatment [20].

In summary, multiple factors (demographic, psychological/attitudinal, and clinical) contribute to antidepressant medication non-adherence. In the following sections, we will provide case reports to illustrate the role of the primary care clinician in patients' decisions about taking an antidepressant medication and identify strategies to improve adherence.

Case Report: Non-adherence

Ms. M. is a 65-year-old patient followed by her primary care physician (PCP) for multiple medical problems including type 2 diabetes mellitus, hypertension, hypercholesterolemia, obesity, and left radiculopathy. During a clinic visit, the PCP observed that the patient appeared discouraged. When questioned, the patient reported that she was unable to follow her recommended diabetic diet, checked finger sticks only intermittently, was not exercising regularly, and was not losing weight. Aware of recent news reports and published studies linking depression and diabetes [37–39], the PCP inquired about changes in sleep, energy level, and concentration, which the patient endorsed. The PCP suggested the patient was experiencing symptoms of depression and recommended treatment. The patient attributed her low mood to the burden of having multiple medical problems, but reluctantly agreed to a trial of sertraline 50 mg daily and to return in 1 month. She returned in 3 months for follow-up. The patient reported she tried sertraline for 1 week before discontinuing it since she saw no benefit. In addition, her husband expressed concern about her becoming dependent on "drugs." There was no improvement in the patient's self-care management. The PCP explained to the patient that it would take at least 2–3 weeks to notice benefit and encouraged her to trial another SSRI. The patient expressed reluctance, stating she did not like taking medications and was already taking too many with costly co-payments. Her PCP prescribed fluoxetine 20 mg daily and strongly encouraged the patient to engage in a 4-week trial to determine benefit. The patient returned in 6 months for a post-hospitalization appointment, having suffered an acute myocardial infarction. She had never started the fluoxetine as recommended by her PCP.

This case example highlights the outcome (non-adherence) when patient concerns are not actively addressed and the decision-making process in non-collaborative. This patient did not meet the "Choice Triad" described by Shea (2006):

1. Patients start medications because they recognize something is wrong (depressive symptoms).
2. Patients feel motivated to try to get help with what is wrong through the use of a medication (relief from suffering, improved sense of health and well-being).
3. Patients decide the pros of taking a medication will, in the long run, outweigh the cons.

Clinician/Patient Communication

Communication between clinician and patient around length of treatment for depression may also play a role in adherence and early treatment discontinuation. One group conducted a telephone interview of 401 depressed patients being treated with a selective serotonin reuptake inhibitor (SSRI) in the setting of a health maintenance organization outpatient clinic [40]. In addition, 137 prescribing physicians completed written surveys regarding communication around antidepressant treatment. While 99 physicians (72%) reported that they usually ask patients to continue using antidepressants for at least 6 months, only 137 patients (34%) reported that their physicians asked them to continue using antidepressants for this duration, and 228 (56%) reported receiving no instructions. Patients who said they were told to take their medication for less than 6 months were three times more likely to discontinue therapy compared with patients who said they were told to continue therapy longer. Patients who discussed adverse effects with their physicians were less likely to discontinue therapy than patients who did not discuss them, and those who reported discussing adverse effects with their physicians were more likely to switch medications. The authors advocate that explicit instructions about expected duration of therapy and discussions about medication adverse effects throughout treatment may reduce discontinuation of SSRI use. With effective communication, an "active care partnership" between the clinician and the patient is established.

Therapeutic Alliance

The development of a collaborative alliance between the clinician and the patient is critical to improving patient health outcomes. As described by Peplau [41], characteristics include a significant, therapeutic, human interaction that is goal directed and deliberately planned to make illness a learning experience for the patient. Guadagnino [42] reported that patients receiving "patient-centered collaborative care" strongly agree they are receiving "exactly the care they want and need, exactly when and how they need it."

Interventions That Improve Adherence

Strategies That Focus on the Clinician–Patient Interaction

In one study, the investigators examined specific educational messages, side effects, and features of doctor–patient collaboration that influence adherence [43]. One hundred fifty-five patients enrolled in a health maintenance organization who were newly prescribed antidepressants for depression were interviewed 1 and 4 months after starting antidepressant medication. Approximately 28% of patients stopped taking antidepressants during the first month of therapy, and 44% had stopped taking them by the third month of therapy. Patients who received the following five specific educational messages – (1) take the medication daily; (2) antidepressants must be taken for 2–4 weeks for a noticeable effect; (3) continue to take medicine even if feeling better; (4) do not stop taking antidepressant without checking with the physician; and (5) specific instructions regarding what to do to resolve questions regarding antidepressants – were more likely to comply during the first month of antidepressant therapy. Asking about prior experience with antidepressants and discussions about scheduling pleasant activities also were related to early adherence. Interestingly, neuroticism, depression severity, and other patient characteristics did not predict adherence.

Models of Care

There have been several studies over the last decade that have examined the use of a "depression specialist," often an advanced practice nurse or a social worker, in the primary care setting, who receives supervision from a psychiatrist and actively collaborates with the primary care physician to provide depression care. One such model that has received particular attention in the care of older depressed adults has been the "Improving Mood: Promoting Access to Collaborative Treatment" (IMPACT) study [44]. IMPACT was a randomized controlled trial that included 1,801 patients 60 years or older from 18 primary care clinics from eight health-care organizations in five states. Patients had major depression, dysthymic disorder, or both, and were randomly assigned to the IMPACT intervention. Intervention patients had access for up to 12 months to a depression care manager (DCM), supervised by a psychiatrist and a primary care expert. The DCM provided psychoeducation, behavioral activation/pleasant event scheduling, and care management including tracking outcomes. The IMPACT treatment algorithm suggested an initial choice of either an antidepressant medication (prescribed by the patient's primary care physician) or a course of problem-solving treatment in primary care (PST-PC), a brief, structured psychotherapy for depression. Treatment was adjusted based on clinical outcomes according to the evidence-based algorithm (stepped care). After 1 year, compared with usual care patients, intervention patients not only had better depression outcomes, but experienced greater rates of depression treatment, expressed greater satisfaction with depression care, and reported less functional impairment and a significantly improved quality of life. The IMPACT model has also demonstrated that enhanced depression care improved not only symptoms of depression but also symptoms of pain in older patients with arthritis and depression [45].

There has also been research focusing on collaborative models of care that improve adherence after treatment of an acute episode of depression. One study in primary care examined a relapse prevention intervention to improve adherence to antidepressant medication and improve depression outcomes in 386 high-risk patients compared with usual care [46]. Patients with recurrent major depression or dysthymia who had largely recovered after 8 weeks of antidepressant treatment by their primary care physicians were randomized to a relapse prevention program or usual primary care. The intervention group received two primary care visits with a depression specialist and three telephone visits over a 1-year period aimed at enhancing adherence to antidepressant medication, recognition of prodromal symptoms, monitoring of symptoms, and development of a written relapse prevention plan. Those in the intervention group had significantly greater adherence to adequate dosage of antidepressant medication for 90 days or more within the first and second 6-month periods and were significantly more likely to refill medication prescriptions during the 12-month follow-up compared with usual care controls. Intervention patients had significantly fewer depressive symptoms, but not fewer episodes of relapse/recurrence over the 12-month follow-up period.

In a recent literature review, Katon and Seelig examined studies of models of depression care in primary care [47]. They identified 37 randomized trials of collaborative care that integrated mental health specialists into the primary care clinic to provide greater support for management of depressed patients by their primary care clinicians. Results showed that collaborative care, compared with usual primary care (the patient and the primary care provider), was associated with twofold increase in antidepressant adherence, improvements in depressive outcomes that last up to 2–5 years, increased patient satisfaction with depression care, and improved primary care satisfaction with treating depression.

Case Report: Adherence

Ms. B. is a 60-year-old patient followed by her PCP for multiple medical problems including coronary artery disease, hypercholesterolemia, hypertension, obesity, and osteoarthritis. During a clinic visit, her PCP observed the patient appeared discouraged and expressed his concern about her well-being. She reported that she was not feeling like herself and did not feel like doing things she used to enjoy. She noted she was eating more than usual and "sleeping too much." Her PCP raised the possibility that she may be experiencing symptoms of depression, emphasizing that it was "a treatable disorder." He recommended that she meet the clinic's mental health nurse who worked with him to further evaluate her symptoms and provide collaborative care if indicated. She expressed some concern about what people would think, but agreed to set up an appointment since the nurse was part of the clinic practice. The initial mental health appointment focused on actively engaging the patient in a therapeutic alliance, providing psychoeducation, and fostering an explicit expectation of improvement. The patient revealed recurrent episodes of major depression that were untreated and endorsed current symptoms of MDD on the PHQ-9 [48]. A hierarchy of treatment targets was developed with the patient, and she reluctantly agreed to initiate a trial of citalopram 10 mg and to engage in behavioral activation (pleasant events, exercise). A 4-week follow-up appointment was scheduled and she was provided with the nurse's contact information if she had any questions or concerns before her next appointment. She returned for the appointment at week 4 and endorsed some improvement in mood/affect and behavior (function). The benefit of combined treatment (antidepressant medication and behavioral activation) was reviewed, and further upward titration of the citalopram to 20 mg was discussed. The patient revealed that her partner had expressed concern about her becoming dependent on "drugs." Simple psychoeducation was provided about how we understand antidepressant medications to work (increasing brain "neurotransmitters"), resulting in symptom reduction/relief. She was encouraged to assertively review this information with her partner and also to invite her partner to her next appointment if helpful. She agreed with the plan and expressed appreciation. Upward titration of citalopram was reviewed with the consulting psychiatrist, and a recommendation was forwarded to the patient's primary care clinician, who then authorized the increase. At week 8, the patient identified significant and persistent back and knee pain (7 out of 10) that interfered with physical function, along with cognitive distortions ("I should be able to handle it") and nonassertive communication ("I don't want to bother my doctor"), each of which contributed to persistent depressive symptoms. Psychotherapy focused on challenging cognitive distortions, developing realistic reappraisals, and practicing how to effectively communicate her needs and concerns. Her assigned homework was to make an appointment with her PCP and assertively address her pain experience. At that appointment, pain medication was prescribed and adequate pain control was achieved (2 out of 10). She was able to increase her physical activity and resumed bike-riding, which she greatly enjoyed. At week 12, she reported "I'm really enjoying my life and feel so much better that sometimes it's scary." In addition to an improved sense of well-being, she reported improved satisfaction with personal relationships. She was focused on maintaining wellness and managing her hypertension and chronic pain. She assertively expressed appreciation for collaborative care and comfort in receiving mental health care in her PCP's clinic.

Psychoeducation

One study examined 386 patients at high risk for depression recurrence or relapse following successful acute phase treatment were randomly assigned to receive a low intensity 12-month intervention or continued usual care [49]. The intervention combined education about depression, shared decision making regarding use of maintenance pharmacotherapy, and cognitive-behavioral strategies to promote self-management. The investigators found that intervention patients had significantly greater self-efficacy for managing depression and were more likely to keep track of depressive symptoms, monitor early warning signs, and plan for dealing with high-risk situations at all four quarterly assessments compared with usual care patients. In terms of outcomes, self-efficacy for managing depression, keeping track of depressive symptoms, monitoring for early warning signs, engaging in pleasant activities, and engaging in social activities were each associated with improvement in depression.

Practice Guidelines

Use of practice guidelines may improve depression outcomes. In one study, among 45 primary care practices, greater adherence to depression practice guidelines among care providers significantly predicted fewer depressive symptoms at 12, 18, and 24 months after initiation of treatment [50]. In 2002, the US Preventive Services Task Force (USPSTF) recommended screening adults for depression in clinical practices that have systems in place to assure accurate diagnosis, effective treatment, and follow-up. At that time, the USPSTF concluded that the evidence was insufficient to recommend for or against routine screening of children or adolescents for depression. This latter conclusion was reversed in March 2009, when the following statement was released: The USPSTF recommends screening of adolescents (12–18 years of age) for major depressive disorder (MDD) when systems are in place to ensure accurate diagnosis, psychotherapy (cognitive-behavioral or interpersonal), and follow-up. Finally, guidelines have been developed to monitor progress and track outcomes [51, 52]. The Patient Health Questionnaire [53] has been used to measure change in depression symptoms in the primary care setting [54, 55].

Use of the Internet

Use of the Internet in medicine has gained increasing attention from health services researchers. In a recent randomized trial, primary care patients with one of three chronic conditions, including depression, chronic pain, and impaired mobility, were studied using a nurse coach intervention conducted entirely through a patient Internet portal [56]. The results were mixed. More intervention than control patients reported their PCP gave them specific advice about their health (94 vs. 84%; $P = 0.03$) and referred them to a specialist (51 vs. 28%; $P = 0.002$). However, they found no differences in detection or management of screened conditions, symptom ratings, and quality of life between groups. Interestingly, control patients reported more medication changes than intervention patients (29 vs. 15%, respectively; $P = 0.03$). Future studies will need to examine the effects of Internet coaching on adherence to treatment.

Summary

Adherence to depression management in primary care is important not only to improve mood but also to enhance outcomes of comorbid medical illnesses and overall functional status. At an individual patient level, several approaches may improve depression care adherence, including establishing an "active care partnership" between clinician and patient (see Table 10.1). In this model, the clinician provides psychoeducation about depression and its treatment, helps the patient generate pros and cons of antidepressant treatment, and engages the patient in shared decision-making. At the level of clinic management, patient adherence to recommended depression treatment will be facilitated if clinicians use standard tools for tracking clinical outcomes.

Table 10.1 Strategies to improve antidepressant medication adherence in primary care

1. Develop a strong therapeutic alliance and active care partnership with the patient ("I can't do it without you!")
2. Avoid asking or telling the patient he/she is depressed. Rather, wonder about depression as a contributing factor
3. Assess with a screening tool (PHQ-2 or PHQ-9), identify patient's symptom profile, and provide education about depression as a treatable disorder
4. Provide antidepressant medication education and explain anticipated outcomes of treatment; actively instill hopefulness
5. Discuss antidepressant treatment pros and cons, elicit any stigma, social, and financial issues, and address fear of dependence and side-effect concerns.
6. If patient agrees, provide close follow-up: Schedule a 4-week return visit, ask the patient to contact you with any questions or concerns that may occur between appointments
7. If patient expresses reservation about initiating antidepressant treatment, provide close follow-up (same as above), express your concern about the patient's health and well-being, and encourage further discussion at the 4-week return visit.
8. At the beginning of the return visit, screen for non-adherence, readminister the tracking tool (PHQ-9) to evaluate response to treatment, review goal of symptom remission, and facilitate treatment planning and informed decision-making by the patient
9. Focus on short-term goal (symptom remission), address continuation treatment when depressive symptoms are in remission

Finally, at an overall systems level, adherence will improve if mental health care is integrated into the primary care setting.

References

1. Trivedi MH, Lin EH, Katon WJ. Adherence with antidepressant therapy and successful patient self-management. *CNS Spectr*. 2007;12(8 Suppl 13):1–27.
2. Musselman DL, Evans DL, Nemeroff CB. The relationship of depression to cardiovascular disease: epidemiology, biology, and treatment. *Arch Gen Psychiatry*. 1998;55:558, 580–592.
3. Pratt LA, Ford DE, Crum RM, et al. Depression, psychotropic medication, and risk of myocardial infarction. Prospective data from the Baltimore ECA follow-up. *Circulation*. 1996;94:3123–3129.
4. Black SA, Markides KS, Ray LA. Depression predicts increased incidence of adverse health outcomes in older Mexican Americans with type 2 diabetes. *Diab Care*. 2003;26:2822–2828.
5. Greenberg PE, Kessler RC, Birnbaum HG, et al. The economic burden of depression in the United States: how did it change between 1990 and 2000? *J Clin Psychiatry*. 2003;64:1465–1475.
6. Rice DP, Miller LS. Health economics and cost implications of anxiety and other mental disorders in the United States. *Br J Psychiatry Suppl*. 1998;172(suppl 34):4–9.
7. Simon GE, VonKorff M. Recognition, management, and outcomes of depression in primary care. *ArchFam Med*. 1995;4:99–105.
8. Henk HJ, Katzelnick DJ, Kobak KA, et al. Medical costs attributed to depression among patients with a history of high medical expenses in a health maintenance organization. *Arch Gen Psychiatry*. 1996;53:899–904.
9. Coyne JC, Fechner-Bates S, Schwenk TL. Prevalence, nature, and comorbidity of depressive disorders in primary care. *Gen Hospital Psychiatry*. 1994;16:267–276.
10. Alexander JL, Richardson G, Grypma L, et al. Collaborative depression care, screening, diagnosis and specificity of depression treatments in the primary care setting. *Expert Rev Neurother*. 2007;7:S59–80.
11. Katon W, Sullivan M, Walker E. Medical symptoms without identified pathology: relationship to psychiatric disorders, childhood and adult trauma, and personality traits. *Ann Intern Med*. 2001;134:917–925.
12. Lin EH, Katon W, Von Korff M, et al. Relationship of depression and diabetes self-care, medication adherence, and preventive care. *Diab Care*. 2004;27:2154–2160.
13. Ciechanowski PS, Katon WJ, Russo JE, et al. The relationship of depressive symptoms to symptom reporting, self-care and glucose control in diabetes. *Gen Hosp Psychiatry*. 2003;25:246–252.
14. Goldman LS, Nielsen NH, Champion HC. Awareness, diagnosis, and treatment of depression. *J Gen Intern Med*. 1999;14:569–580.

15. Hirschfeld RM, Keller MB, Panico S, et al. The National Depressive and Manic-Depressive Association consensus statement on the undertreatment of depression. *J Am Med Assoc.* 1997;277:333–340.

16. Judd LL, Paulus MP, Wells KB, et al. Socioeconomic burden of subsyndromal depressive symptoms and major depression in a sample of the general population. *Am J Psychiatry.* 1996;153:1411–1417.

17. Coulehan JL, Schulberg HC, Block MR, et al. Treating depressed primary care patients improves their physical, mental, and social functioning. *Arch Intern Med.* 1997;157:1113–1120.

18. Rost K, Smith JL, Dickinson M. The effect of improving primary care depression management on employee absenteeism and productivity. A randomized trial. *Med Care.* 2004;42:1202–1210.

19. Demyttenaere K, Mesters P, Boulanger B, et al. Adherence to treatment regimen in depressed patients treated with amitriptyline or fluoxetine. *J Affect Disord.* 2001;65:243–252.

20. Demyttenaere K, Enzlin P, Dewe W, et al. Compliance with antidepressants in a primary care setting, 1: beyond lack of efficacy and adverse events. *J Clin Psychiatry.* 2001;62(Suppl 22):30–33.

21. Thompson C, Peveler RC, Stephenson D, et al. Adherence with antidepressant medication in the treatment of major depressive disorder in primary care: a randomized comparison of fluoxetine and a tricyclic antidepressant. *Am J Psychiatry.* 2000;157:338–343.

22. Warden D, Trivedi MH, Wisniewski SR, et al. Predictors of attrition during initial (citalopram) treatment for depression: a STAR*D report. *Am J Psychiatry.* 2007;164:1189–1197.

23. Olfson M, Marcus SC, Tedeschi M, et al. Continuity of antidepressant treatment for adults with depression in the United States. *Am J Psychiatry.* 2006;163:101–108.

24. Kobak KA, Taylor L, Katzelnick DJ, et al. Antidepressant medication management and Health Plan Employer Data Information Set (HEDIS) criteria: reasons for nonadherence. *J Clin Psychiatry.* 2002;63:727–732.

25. DiMatteo MR, Lepper HS, Croghan TW. Depression is a risk factor for noncompliance with medical treatment: meta-analysis of the effects of anxiety and depression on patient adherence. *Arch Intern Med.* 2000;160:2101–2107.

26. Katon WJ, Rutter C, Simon G, et al. The association of comorbid depression with mortality in patients with type 2 diabetes. *Diab Care.* 2005;28: 2668–2672.

27. Akerblad A, Bengtsson F, von Knorring L, et al. Response, remission and relapse in relation to adherence in primary care treatment of depression: A 2-year outcome study. *Int Clin Psychopharmacol Bull.* 2006;21:117–124.

28. Peveler R, George C, Kinmonth AL, et al. Effect of antidepressant drug counselling and information leaflets on adherence to drug treatment in primary care: randomised controlled trial. *Br Med J.* 1999;319:612–615.

29. Melfi CA, Chawla AJ, Croghan TW, et al. The effects of adherence to antidepressant treatment guidelines on relapse and recurrence of depression. *Arch Gen Psychiatry.* 1998;55:1128–1132.

30. Thase ME, Nierenberg AA, Keller MB, et al. Efficacy of mirtazapine for prevention of depressive relapse: a placebocontrolled double-blind trial of recently remitted high-risk patients. *J Clin Psychiatry.* 2001;62:782–788.
31. Lester H, Howe A. Depression in primary care: three key challenges. *Postgrad Med J.* 2008;84:545–548.
32. Cooper LA, Gonzales JJ, Gallo JJ, et al. The acceptability of treatment for depression among African-American, Hispanic, and white primary care patients. *Med Care.* 2003;41:479–489.
33. Schraufnagel TJ, Wagner AW, Miranda J, et al. Treating minority patients with depression and anxiety: what does the evidence tell us? *Gen Hosp Psychiatry.* 2006;28:27–36.
34. Melartin TK, Rytsala HJ, Leskela US, et al. Continuity is the main challenge in treating major depressive disorder in psychiatric care. *J Clin Psychiatry.* 2005;66:220–227.
35. Russell J, Kazantzis N. Medication beliefs and adherence to antidepressants in primary care. *New Zeal Med J* 2008;121:14–20.
36. Halfin A. Depression: the benefits of early and appropriate treatment. *Am J Manage Care.* 2007;13 (4 Suppl):S92–S97.
37. Bogner HR, Morales KH, Post EP, et al. Diabetes, depression, and death: a randomized controlled trial of a depression treatment program for older adults based in primary care (PROSPECT). *Diab Care.* 2007;30:3005–3010.
38. Carnethon MR, Biggs ML, Barzilay JI, et al. Longitudinal association between depressive symptoms and incident type 2 diabetes mellitus in older adults: the cardiovascular health study. *Arch Intern Med.* 2007;167:802–807.
39. Katon W, Fan MY, Unutzer J, et al. Depression and diabetes: a potentially lethal combination. *J Gen Intern Med.* 2008;23:1571–1575.
40. Bull SA, Hu XH, Hunkeler EM, et al. Discontinuation of use and switching of antidepressants: influence of patient-physician communication. *JAMA.* 2002;288:1403–1409.
41. Peplau H. *Interpersonal relations in nursing.* New York, NY: Putnam; 1952.
42. Guadagnino C. Practicing patient-centered collaborative care (Physician News website), 2006.
43. Lin EH, Von Korff M, Katon W, et al. The role of the primary care physician in patients' adherence to antidepressant therapy. *Med Care.* 1995;33:67–74.
44. Unutzer J, Katon W, Callahan CM, et al. Collaborative care management of late-life depression in the primary care setting: a randomized controlled trial. *JAMA.* 2002;288:2836–2845.
45. Lin EH, Katon W, Von Korff M, et al. Effect of improving depression care on pain and functional outcomes among older adults with arthritis: a randomized controlled trial. *JAMA.* 2003;290:2428–2429.
46. Katon W, Rutter C, Ludman EJ, et al. A randomized trial of relapse prevention of depression in primary care. *Arch Gen Psychiatry.* 2001;58:241–247.
47. Katon WJ, Seelig M. Population-based care of depression: team care approaches to improving outcomes. *J Occup Environ Med.* 2008;50:459–467.
48. Kroenke K, Spitzer RL, Williams JB. The PHQ-9: validity of a brief depression severity measure. *J Gen Intern Med.* 2001;16:606–613.

49. Ludman E, Katon W, Bush T, et al. Behavioural factors associated with symptom outcomes in a primary care-based depression prevention intervention trial. *Psycholog Med.* 2003;33:1061–1070.

50. Hepner KA, Rowe M, Rost K, et al. The effect of adherence to practice guidelines on depression outcomes. *Ann Intern Med.* 2007;147:320–329.

51. Cheung AH, Zuckerbrot RA, Jensen PS, et al. Guidelines for Adolescent Depression in Primary Care (GLAD-PC): II. Treatment and ongoing management. *Pediatrics.* 2007;120:e1313–e1326.

52. Schulberg HC, Katon W, Simon GE, et al. Treating major depression in primary care practice: an update of the Agency for Health Care Policy and Research Practice Guidelines. *Arch Gen Psychiatry.* 1998;55:1121–1127.

53. Spitzer RL, Kroenke K, Williams JBW, et al. Validation and utility of a self-report version of PRIME-MD: The PHQ Primary Care Study. *JAMA.* 1999;282:1737–1744.

54. Dobscha SK, Gerrity MS, Corson K, et al. Measuring adherence to depression treatment guidelines in a VA primary care clinic. *Gen Hosp Psychiatry.* 2003;25:230–237.

55. Nease DE, Jr., Nutting PA, Dickinson WP, et al. Inducing sustainable improvement in depression care in primary care practices. *Joint Commission J Q Patient Saf.* 2008;34:247–255.

56. Leveille SG, Huang A, Tsai SB, et al. Health coaching via an internet portal for primary care patients with chronic conditions: a randomized controlled trial. *Med. Care.* 2009;47:41–47.

Chapter 11
Adherence in the Treatment of HIV and Other Infectious Diseases

Karen Moore Goldstein

Over the last decade, survival in patients with human immunodeficiency virus (HIV) has lengthened dramatically due to improvements in the robust options for antiretroviral therapy (ART) [1]. Clinicians caring for HIV-positive patients now face many of the same challenges encountered by those with other chronic conditions (e.g., cardiovascular disease, complications from diabetes, aging) [2]. One particular issue that plagues all clinicians caring for patients with chronic diseases is how to promote optimal adherence to prescribed treatment over time. Adherence to treatment for HIV has some unique features that make its assessment and measurement challenging. In this chapter, we will review the ways in which this disease differs from and is similar to other chronic diseases. Lastly, we will identify methods and techniques that clinicians may use to enhance adherence among individuals with HIV. Of note, we will be specifically focusing on issues pertaining to the treatment of HIV in the USA.

HIV-positive patients who do not take their antiretroviral therapy (ART) as prescribed run the risk of poor clinical outcomes. The connection between non-adherence and poor virologic outcome is clear. Current Department of Health and Human Services (DHHS)

K.M. Goldstein (✉)
Department of General Internal Medicine, University of Pennsylvania,
Philadelphia, PA, USA
e-mail: karen.goldstein@uphs.upenn.edu

H. Bosworth (ed.), *Improving Patient Treatment Adherence*,
DOI 10.1007/978-1-4419-5866-2_11,
© Springer Science+Business Media, LLC 2010

guidelines recommend virologic suppression to maximal levels for an indefinite time period [3]. Patients who demonstrate measurable viral loads have lower levels of adherence [4] and those patients who exhibit non-adherence are at greater risk of virologic failure [5]. Conversely, those who report 100% adherence are more likely to achieve virologic suppression [6]. In the long term, non-adherence is also related to immunologic outcome; however, the response in CD4 count measurements often takes longer to manifest [7].

One major difference with HIV from other non-infectious chronic diseases is that non-adherence jeopardizes more than the patient's health during the period of non-adherence; it can also decrease treatment options for the future. While the pattern of adherence that leads to a lack of viral suppression may have differences from that which leads to viral resistance [4], it is clear that adherence levels are related to both. At one end of the spectrum, a fully adherent patient will be able to suppress viral replication and decrease the risk of viral mutation and subsequent resistance development. Similarly, a patient who is completely non-adherent is less likely to develop resistance due to the lack of drug-induced selection pressure, which allows for the predominance of a wild-type virus of generally superior replication capacity. It is the patients who are partially adherent (i.e., those who take their medications intermittently) who are at greatest risk for developing resistance as they have enough drug present to select for resistant virus, but not enough to suppress replication [8] (see Fig. 11.1). Vrijens (2005) describes this as the "critical concentration zone" when drug levels are low enough to allow for viral replication but high enough to exert selection pressure [9]. The added danger is that non-adherence to one ART regimen can send patients into a self-destructive spiral; missed dosages lead to resistance that in turn can force a patient to move onto a more complicated and costly regimen with increased barriers to adherence and lead to subsequent further failures down the road [10].

Poor adherence jeopardizes not only the individual patient's future treatment options, but, potentially, also the options for others in the community. Because virologic resistance is transmissible as long as it does not compromise viral fitness [11], one person's resistance to certain antiretroviral therapy can be transferred to another through infection and thus limit the newly infected patient's options for initial and subsequent treatment. This risk has been confirmed by the increase

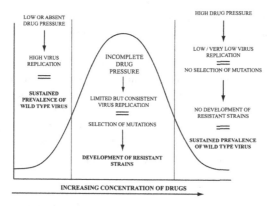

Fig. 11.1 Relationship between adherence and the development of resistance. Reproduced with permission from [8].

of newly infected patients in the USA exhibiting ART resistance at baseline testing [12, 13]. So, the development of virologic resistance is both an individual-level and population-level danger.

Gaps in adherence can also lead to poor clinical outcomes in HIV-positive individuals. Hogg et al. found that patients with less than 75% adherence in the first year of therapy had higher morality rates [14]. Evidence borne from treatment interruption trials revealed that patients who stopped their ART at specified immunologic cutoffs were more likely to experience disease progression and mortality [15, 16]. So, even though patients who stop their medication altogether may not develop viral resistance due to their non-adherence, their overall clinical course is likely still to suffer. Further evidence exists from patient-initiated "drug holidays" of greater than 48 h which have been shown to correlate with the development of major mutations conferring interclass cross-resistance [17]. At this point, planned treatment interruptions or "drug holidays" are not recommended [3].

One important variable of the impact of adherence on ART is the strength and ability of a particular regimen to prevent resistance development, known as the forgiveness of a regimen. Forgiveness is governed by the interplay between the genetic barrier, the pharmacokinetics, and pharmacodynamics of the different drugs. In general, higher and more consistent adherence to ART leads to better virologic suppression and CD4 response [6, 18, 19]; however, some

ART medications are recognized to have higher genetic barriers to the development of resistance and thus subsequent virologic failure [20]. The reverse is also true; older generation non-nucleoside reverse transcriptase inhibitors (NNRTIs) (i.e., efavirenz, nevirapine) are susceptible to complete resistance with the development of one mutation and thus have a low genetic barrier [8]. To make this more complicated, NNRTIs have longer half-lives such that discontinuation of combination regimens containing NNRTIs and a nucleoside reverse transcriptase inhibitor (NRTI) backbone, which have shorter half-lives, can lead to inadvertent NNRTI monotherapy and subsequent viral resistance [10]. However, ritonavir-based boosting of protease inhibitors enhance their genetic barrier to resistance (e.g., darunavir/norvir, atazanavir/norvir); thus, multiple genetic mutations are required to confer resistance to boosted PI-based regimens, and patients may get away with a lower level of adherence without the development of resistance [4, 21].

Thus, the consequences of suboptimal adherence in the treatment of HIV with ART are potentially dire and always complicated. It is imperative that HIV providers develop an understanding of adherence, from barriers to adequate adherence, to methods of assessment, to adherence promotion interventions among their patients.

Prevalence of Non-adherence to ART Medication

Average prevalence of adherence to ART in HIV-positive populations has been described in observational studies and clinical trials as ranging from 63 to 86.7% [5, 21–27] with approximately half of patients taking all their medication appropriately and on-time [19]. Others have measured adherence by the frequency of missed doses noting that up to one third of patients report missing at least one dose in the previous 5 days [28]. Some have noted that this level of adherence is higher than what is generally seen in other chronic conditions [23]. Regardless of how it is defined, evidence supports the fact that adherence to ART is not perfect.

Given this imperfect and wide range of ART adherence, one needs to know if the healthcare system is doing "enough". In general, the conclusion is that evidence indicates that the majority of patients have suboptimal adherence [22]. Most adherence studies use a reference cut-off of 95% or greater adherence as the level which is necessary for viral suppression [24]. Of note, these data were derived from HIV-infected patients many of whom experienced NNRTIs, receiving a non-boosted PI-based regimen, primarily nelfinavir. Others suggest that patients with undetectable viral loads (defined as <400 or <50 depending on the study) tend to have adherence ranging from 82 to 93% [4, 23]. Differences in noted levels of adherence required may be due to differences in study design, patient population, ART used, and study duration [7]. As noted previously, others have suggested that lower levels of adherence may be sufficient for virologic suppression when using newer, more potent regimens [4, 21]. While in general it seems that higher levels of adherence are best, it does appear that incremental increases in adherence below the highest cut-off of 95% are still associated with improved virologic control [27]. So, the ideal level of adherence for various regimens of ART remains undetermined and is information which is desperately needed [9].

As with therapies for other chronic conditions, adherence or non-adherence is not a dichotomous condition [9]. Adherence to ART has been described to be highest at initiation of therapy and deteriorates over time with treatment fatigue [4, 6]. Consequently, adherence support is required over the life of an HIV-positive patient and must be able to meet the changing needs of that patient overtime [29]. In order to provide that comprehensive care, it is important to understand the barriers that can compromise patient adherence.

Barriers to Adherence HIV Treatment

In considering adherence to ART, it is important to recognize common barriers to adherence in the HIV-positive population. Barriers can be thought of as being specific to the patient, the regimen, the provider, and the larger system in which ART is being prescribed and taken. Perhaps the easiest way to start to understand patient-specific barriers to ART adherence is through a review of patient reports on why they missed taking their medications.

Commonly cited reasons for missing medication include being busy or forgetting, being away from home, having a change in routine, stressful life events, confidentiality concerns, and running out of medications [4, 6, 22, 24, 28, 30]. Problems specific to particular regimens, for example having too many pills, confusing dosage instructions (i.e., dietary restrictions), and drug toxicity, tend to be less commonly cited reasons for missing medications [22, 28, 30]. Patients also report that lack of "readiness" to start taking medications on a regular basis at time of ART initiation can lead to poor adherence [31].

Other patient-specific factors found to be associated with non-adherence include non-white race [6, 23, 24], lower educational attainment [23, 32], psychiatric comorbidity [17, 24, 28], and active drug and/or alcohol use [22, 33, 34]. Conversely, increased adherence was associated with use of more adherence aids [23], and older age [24, 27, 35]. While various markers of socioeconomic status are found to have positive associations to adherence in some studies [23, 24, 30, 32], a recent systematic review was unable to find conclusive evidence establishing a relationship [36]. Finally, some data suggest that the particular patient-specific factors that determine an individual's adherence experience may change over time [6], such that pill burden might be important at the initiation of therapy while forgetting to take the evening dose of a medication may be more important in later years of treatment. Of note, gender and length of time since infection have not been found to be associated with adherence [30, 37].

Regimen-specific barriers to adherence have long been a concern in the treatment of HIV, specifically the complexity of the regimen and its side effects. Early in the era of ART, there were significant and often overwhelming pill burdens – up to 20 pills per day. Adherence studies conducted in the setting of these more complicated regimens often focused on complexity of the regimen, food restriction, pill burden, and dosing frequency as reasons for missing medications [30, 38]. Today, recommended first-line regimens range from 1 to 6 pills per day [3]. The advent of better tolerated drugs, fixed-dose combinations, and ritonavir-based boosting of proteases enables clinicians to design simple, well-tolerated, and compact regimens that facilitate adherence and enhance virologic success [39]. Likewise, side effects of earlier ART regimens included prohibitive amounts of diarrhea, nausea, neuropathy, and more serious complications such as lactic acidosis or hepatitis. Current regimens are much better tolerated and less toxic; however, certain patients may have side effects that are bothersome enough to discourage regular adherence. Regardless, patients who experience adverse reactions to medications [5, 28, 40] or who perceive side effects of ART to be a significant problem [38] are less likely to be adherent. In qualitative studies of patients with 100% adherence, the ability to integrate the taking of a regimen, regardless of the complexity, into a daily routine was found to be the most important factor to successful adherence rather the total pill burden [28, 31].

Clinician-specific barriers to adherence add a third layer of challenges. Current recommendations encourage clinicians to factor in patient readiness to take daily medication while determining when to initiate HIV treatment; this acknowledges that inconsistent adherence by ambivalent or unready patients can compromise future regimens [3]. While this is an important and reasonable recommendation, there is the potential for prescriber bias when assessing patients for treatment readiness if the provider has misinformed perceptions of which patients are likely to be adherent. Support for this potential misjudgment can be found by data suggesting that physicians misjudge patient adherence to ART from 41 to 76% of the time [24, 41] and that they underestimate adherence from 39 to 51% of the time [24, 26]. Beyond provider's impressions of patient adherence there is also suggestion that the physician–patient relationship itself can influence adherence, as patients who have greater trust in their clinical provider have been found to be more adherent [23, 31]. In addition, the quality of communication between patient and provider is essential to better adherence [42]. Greater physician experience with treating HIV-positive patients may also be related to improved adherence [27].

Finally, barriers to adherence for HIV treatment should be considered in the larger societal context. The HIV epidemic in the USA is predominant in vulnerable populations from men who have sex with men (MSM), intravenous drug users (IVDU), homeless, and increasingly in low-income African American populations [1]. Issues of unstable housing [43, 44] and transitions from recent incarceration

[45, 46] can also impact individual's adherence and clinical outcome. In addition, recent evidence suggests that some of the most vulnerable populations (e.g., young, female, African American, those without private insurance) are also more likely to discontinue a newly started ART regimen within the first year [47].

ART Medication Adherence Assessment

Timing is critical to adherence assessment in ART. It is important to identify potential barriers to adherence before starting ART in addition to ongoing monitoring of adherence once therapy has begun. Routine assessment of medication adherence is recommended even for patients whose adherence has been demonstrated to be excellent [42]. It is recommended that, when possible, barriers to adherence such as those described above can be addressed or considered prior to initiating therapy [3]. Rather than waiting for virologic failure to occur, monitoring adherence before viral rebound occurs creates an optimal time for intervention [10]. This approach is supported by the finding that adherence tends to be greatest at initiation of ART and wanes over time [4, 6]. If virologic failure can be avoided through improved adherence and prevention of resistance development, then patients can avoid heading down the "downward spiral" of increasingly complicated and burdensome regimens [10]. Because personal attributes are not consistently effective predictors of non-adherence [37], it is critical that HIV providers have other means of identifying which patients may need additional adherence support.

Measurement of adherence to ART in HIV-positive patients is performed using many of the same methods outlined in previous chapters – including indirect measures such as self-report [5, 6, 17, 19, 41], announced and unannounced pill counts [25, 26], pharmacy refill patterns [27, 48], and electronic medication caps (i.e., MEMs) [4, 22, 24, 33], as well as direct measures such as therapeutic drug monitoring. Given that most of these methods were reviewed in detail previously, here we will focus on HIV-specific adherence assessment techniques.

Two methods that are novel in HIV adherence are the CASE adherence index and pill recognition charts. Both of these methods were designed for use in the clinical setting, when time and practical limitations are driving forces. The CASE adherence index is a variation of self-report in which the clinician (or other designated individual) asks the patient a series of three questions (see Table 11.1) with set answers that correlate to a sum score. This index correlates strongly with three variables: a standard 3-day self-report tool, measures of HIV viral load, and CD4 count [49]. As with all self-report methods, there is some danger of patients becoming desensitized over time to the tool and the potential for social desirability bias [10, 50]; however, it is easily incorporated into clinical practice and gives a framework for adherence review at every visit [51]. Furthermore, self-reported medication adherence is consistently found to be a significant predictor of virologic outcome [6, 52].

Table 11.1 CASE adherence index questionnaire

---

1. How often do you feel that you have difficulty taking your HIV medication on time? By "on time" we mean no more than 2 h before or 2 h after the time your doctor told you to take it.
   a. 4 = Never
   b. 3 = Rarely
   c. 2 = Most of the time
   d. 1 = All of the time

2. On average, how many days per week would you say that you missed at least one dose of your HIV medications?
   a. 1 = Everyday
   b. 2 = 4–6 days/week
   c. 3 = 2–3 days/week
   d. 4 = Once a week
   e. 5 = Less than once a week
   f. 6 = Never

3. When was the last time you missed at least one dose of your HIV medications?
   a. 1 = Within the last week
   b. 2 = 1–2 weeks ago
   c. 3 = 3–4 weeks ago
   d. 4 = Between 1 and 3 months ago
   e. 5 = More than 3 months ago
   f. 6 = Never

Total >10 = good adherence; <10 = poor adherence

From [49]

Pill recognition charts are similarly practical for use in everyday practice, can be easily assembled, and are best made without names attached (see Fig. 11.2) [51]. Patients can be asked to identify their medications in a limited time interval, and successful rapid identification may be as accurate as other methods of self-report. Support for this type of adherence measurement comes from patient reports that they are not always able to recall the names of medications that they were taking, but that were better able to provide physical descriptions [28]. Visual identification has been used successfully in other measures of adherence [41].

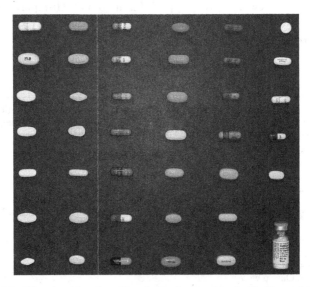

Fig. 11.2 Pill recognition chart. Permission for use given by Dr. Karam Mounzer

Therapeutic drug monitoring offers adherence assessment value that is similar in principle with ART treatment to other medications for chronic diseases. HIV drug monitoring is not currently recommended for routine use in clinical practice [3] due to limitations of access to the laboratory test, lack of standardization, and cost [50]. Drug monitoring has the advantage of being the only direct adherence monitoring method and can be useful for monitoring toxicity, especially in populations with altered pharmacokinetics such as pregnant women and patients with hepatic dysfunction [3, 50]. It has been used in research settings and may eventually be relevant to the practice setting, in particular in the management of patients with multidrug-resistant virus [53]. An upcoming Cochrane Collaboration review on this topic may lend additional insight into the appropriate role of this type of monitoring [54].

In addition to drug-level measurement, side effects of ART allow for alternative laboratory markers of adherence. For example, zidovudine and stavudine cause marked macrocytosis at therapeutic levels [55]. Similarly, the protease inhibitor atazanavir causes elevations of indirect bilirubin in a majority of patients at therapeutic doses [56]. Petersen et al. analyzed the bilirubin levels in 134 patients who were newly initiated on atazanavir and found that an absolute increase in bilirubin of 1.1 mg/dl predicted viral suppression, and presumably adherence, with a positive predictive value of 85% and a negative predictive value of 63% [57]. While this approach requires additional data to support its regular use, it is possible that alternative and potentially cheaper methods of laboratory monitoring to therapeutic drug levels may be available.

As with measurement of adherence in other settings, a common clinical challenge is finding a tool that is effective, economical, and feasible in a busy clinical setting. One consideration is choosing who should be performing the chosen assessment (i.e., clinician, non-clinical assistant, or self-administered) and whether or not it should coincide with the clinical visit at all. It remains clear that discussion of adherence that starts before initiation of ART and continues throughout treatment is essential for optimal clinical outcomes. Some would also suggest that no one measure of adherence is sufficient and that when possible, multiple methods should be used [50, 58]. Composite measures of adherence that combine various methods for adherence measurement have also been promoted, though primarily in the research setting [50].

Methods of ART Adherence Promotion

Multiple reviews have examined previous adherence interventions for ART in HIV-positive populations [29, 37, 59–62]. These reviews, especially those published in the early 2000s, have noted significant limitations of the available collection of adherence studies citing methodological weaknesses [60, 62], heterogeneous methods, small sizes [37], and generally underpowered designs [37]. While adherence interventions do appear to be effective, the effect sizes are generally small with respect to measured adherence [61], and there is minimal evidence to support an improvement in virologic control [59]. Despite these noted limitations, there are a few themes to the successful interventions.

One successful approach to adherence interventions is the targeting of practical medication management skills and providing supplemental resources [60]. The teaching of these basic skills is generally taught through various educational programs. Certain characteristics of these instructional programs seem to be important. For example, it appears that educational programs are more likely to be successful when conducted on an individual basis [35, 60] versus in a group setting [63–65]. One advantage of one-on-one programs is that they can be adapted to the needs of the individual [66]. Instructional methods for educational programs have included motivational interviewing [67, 68], knowledge acquisition [35, 69], self-efficacy training [35, 40, 69], and supplementary counseling [70]. Furthermore, not all instruction needs to be done in the clinic setting. Another promising tactic for management skills includes telephone behavioral support provided by registered nurses with opportunities for patients to ask questions about how to take their medications [71]. Finally, there is also evidence that interventions in general with longer durations (at least 12 weeks) are more likely to see a significant improvement in adherence rates than those of shorter duration [59, 60, 65, 69, 72].

In addition to the instructional component of medication management skills, there are tangible supports that can supplement this adherence promotion. One example is the use of reminder devices, which alert patients when they are supposed to take their medications. Such devices have shown promise and may be a simple, but effective solution for those patients who identify "forgetting" as a common reason for missing their medications. Numerous mechanisms exist for reminding patients to take their medications, including online pager systems [73] and programmable portable alarms [72, 74]. Reminder systems may be particularly helpful early on in the course of treatment [31] and for those with known memory impairment [74], though they may not be sufficient for long-term adherence promotion [72], especially for those with preexisting adherence problems [73]. However, despite the inherent appeal of such interventions, a recent systematic review of both published and unpublished studies of electronic reminder devices found that overall evidence was insufficient to support their widespread use in adherence of ART at this point [75].

Another ART adherence support tool is the use of pillbox organizers, something common to the treatment of multiple chronic diseases. They are cheap, easy to obtain, and can be used for treatments for multiple conditions simultaneously. Petersen et al. found support for the use of basic pillbox organizers in an urban, poor population and estimated an approximate $19,000 per QALY for the $5/month organizers [76]. A recent comparison of methods for prescription refills found that mail ordering and pharmacist-dispensed pill organizers were associated with improved adherence over pharmacy pick-up [48]. One significant limitation is that it requires someone to place the medication in the organizer (e.g., family, pharmacist, or clinician) or that the patient has a high level of cognitive function to use the organizer correctly on his or her own.

Beyond the way that adherence is promoted, there is evidence that certain groups can benefit most from such interventions. Amico et al. found that studies implemented in populations with known or anticipated problems with medication adherence had significantly larger intervention effect size [61]. While targeting those at risk for non-adherence may prove to be a successful strategy, it appears that targeting of marginalized populations is not a productive approach [60, 65].

An entirely different approach to the promotion of adherence to ART is through directly observed therapy (DOT) or modified DOT. While there has been extensive experience with DOT in the treatment of tuberculosis, its use in the treatment of HIV is still being explored. Clear differences between these diseases make the use of DOT non-parallel in these situations. For example, TB patient need to be chemically quarantined while HIV patient do not; and anti-TB medications make the patient noninfectious rapidly whereas HIV treatment is life-long [77]. However, there is some evidence of success in certain subpopulations. In particular, situations that include close proximity of patients to health-care workers [77] seem to have greater success and feasibility. Examples such as prisons [78, 79] and methadone clinics [80] in particular have had good outcomes as have those targeting specific populations, such as inner city drug users [81]. While DOT is not likely to be a reasonable option in most other settings, it is possible that either a modified version of DOT or a short duration of DOT might be successful [77]. Increasing numbers of accepted regimens that are once-daily may renew interest in this strategy, especially during the induction phase of antiretroviral therapy.

Despite these helpful findings, there are some unresolved questions about adherence interventions. Some have suggested that interventions targeted at maintenance of adherence should be different than efforts targeted at patients initiating ART or changing to a new regimen [61]. Furthermore, to be optimally successful, interventions would ideally simultaneously address multiple determinants of non-adherence [29]. There are a few groups that have attempted this multifaceted approach with some success [72, 82]. Another common question that remains unanswered is who should be performing the intervention and whether some individuals (pharmacists, clinical providers, or others) are best positioned for this task [60]. Finally, it is also worth noting that many of these studies used the cut-off of 95% adherence as the threshold for a successful intervention. If, as discussed previously, virologic control and successful clinical outcomes can be achieved through slightly lesser degrees of adherence, then perhaps the data supporting these adherence interventions would be more convincing.

Different adherence interventions can vary in intensity from demanding for both provider and patient (such as DOT) to passive for all involved (reminder devices). The lack of a universal "gold standard" for adherence promotion could be addressed by the development of a spectrum of interventions suitable to individual level needs over time, in research settings and in resource-poor settings, respectively [58, 61]. An understanding of case-specific barriers to adherence can allow for appropriate matching of suitable interventions to particular patients [10]. By using the information one knows about the barriers to adherence for a particular patient or patient population, one can make some choices about which adherence-promoting intervention may be most useful. One suggested way of matching of an adherence method to specific barriers to adherence is shown in Table 11.2.

Table 11.2 Suggested pairings for adherence barriers and support interventions

| | Adherence support interventions | | | | | | | |
| | | Tangible supports | | | | | | |
Barrier to adherence	Skills instruction	Reminder devices	Pillbox organizers	Change of regimen	Directly observed therapy	Intensive case management	Motivational interviewing	Counseling/therapy[a]
Simply forgetting	+	+						
Complexity of regimen (i.e., incl. # of pills, relation to meals)			+	+				
Side effects of medication	+			+				
Physician relationship							+	
Social issues (i.e., homeless, lack of social support)	+		+		+	+		
Substance abuse					+	+		+

Adapted with permission from [51]
[a]Can include support groups

Future Directions and New Technological Advances

While many existing adherence interventions are effective, there is always room for improvement, especially in the development of accessible and inexpensive methods that are readily applicable to the clinic setting. One possibility is the use of mobile phones as a medium for adherence reminders and support. Given their ubiquity across race and social class, they could overcome fears of being exposed by the bulkier and more obtrusive reminder devices and could allow for more sophisticated messages in different languages [75]. There is distinct appeal to this approach, though the reality of intermittent connectivity of personal mobile phones of some patients due to financial limitations may pose challenges to this approach. Another possibility is the use of the internet as a mechanism for promoting adherence. Early use of online paging systems has shown promise [83] and could likely be combined with mobile phones rather than pagers. Alternatively, the use of audio-computer-assisted self-interviewing (audio-CASI) has been successful in improving self-reported risk behaviors [84] and measuring adherence [41], and the use of online or computer-based adherence promotion programs might be an option to reach additional patients without time constraints or office-based limitations.

In addition to improving adherence interventions, work is also underway to develop newer treatment options that are more forgiving due to higher genetic barriers. This sort of compensation would complement behavioral interventions, especially for those with adherence in the particularly dangerous range for resistance development. Some have also suggested that alternative methods of medication delivery, for example, implantable/depot formulations [9], would be helpful to overcome patient adherence problems stemming from the forgetting of intermittent dosages. However, these sorts of medication delivery modes require a degree of chemical stability and a safe way to deal with toxicity if it occurs that do not currently exist.

Clinical and Policy Implications

The importance of adherence in the treatment of HIV cannot be overstated. The development of resistance on the individual level can be personally devastating with consequences ranging from increasingly complex and burdensome regimens to limited or absent treatment options. Fortunately, with the recent development of new generations of existing classes (darunavir, etravirine) to new classes of ART altogether (integrase inhibitors, CCR5 inhibitors), it is currently rare for a patient to be without treatment options that could lead to virologic suppression [53]. However, the impact of non-adherence is felt not just on the individual level.

Virologic resistance that does not compromise viral fitness (e.g., K103N associated with NNRTIs or Q148H/KR + G140S associated with raltegravir) is transmissible from person to person [11] and therefore can become a population-level threat if increasing numbers of patients are developing resistance due to non-adherence. Not only does non-adherence put patients at risk for development of virologic resistance, but non-adherence is also coexistent with higher viral loads [5]. Higher viral loads are the most important risk factor for increased transmission of the HIV virus [85] and so patients who are nonadherent are potentially jeopardizing the population at-large. Evidence suggests that increasing proportions of new infections in the USA are with drug-resistant virus [12]. Recent data from a cohort in New York City suggest that prevalence of transmitted resistance has increased by 10% from 1995 to 2004 [13]. Given this increased prevalence of resistant virus in newly infected patients, current guidelines recommend a baseline resistance test upon entry into care [3]. Focusing on adherence strategies and the prevention of resistance development may decrease opportunities for development and spread of multidrug-resistant virus.

Cost-effectiveness analyses are still in development for adherence interventions in HIV-positive populations. Logically, one could suppose that effective interventions could allow patients to remain on earlier, more effective and less expensive regimens for longer and defer use of costly and cumbersome regimens [86]. Goldie et al. created a simulation model which showed that an adherence interventions decreasing virologic failure by 10–20% would likely be cost-effective at the standard marker of $50,000 per QALY and that even expensive interventions in populations with advanced disease and those with lower baseline levels of adherence would be cost-effective [87]. One recent study found a cost of $14,100 per QALY gained with a home nursing intervention which led to improved self-reported adherence and overall improved survival [86]. These findings support the idea that effective adherence interventions could be cost-effective.

Issues of cost are especially important in resource-poor areas that are affected by the HIV epidemic. This is particularly true in developing countries, but is also a challenge domestically. As noted previously, issues of income, homelessness, and access to insurance are common themes in the US HIV epidemic [1, 47], with suggestions that hospital costs are higher in certain vulnerable populations [88]. The cost of care provision for HIV-positive patients has become an important theme [89] and varies significantly [88]. Wait lists in certain states for publicly funded ART have posed significant challenges to access to standard of care for many patients without private health insurance [90, 91]. Efforts to improve adherence could have considerable impact on national funding needs for individual clinical care through avoidance of more complicated regimens and, on the population level, by preventing the development and spreading of multidrug-resistant virus.

Other Infectious Diseases

Tuberculosis

While the annual incidence of tuberculosis has started to decline since a peak in 1992, it is still a disease that plagues public health officials in the USA with a case rate of 4.4 per 100,000 in 2007 [92]. Official recommendations for the treatment of TB include the administration of multiple medications requiring dosing multiple times per day for at least 6 months [93], thus presenting potential challenges to adequate adherence. Adherence to treatment for tuberculosis (TB) carries some similarities to HIV in importance and challenges. Both are infectious diseases that require treatment with combination therapy and both have the potential to develop resistance to standard medications in the setting of poor adherence which can then be transmitted to others [77] and are ultimately costly to society [94]. One significant difference is that the fast replication rate of HIV (around 10 billions copies per day), combined with the high error prone rate of the reverse transcriptase, generates a multitude of quasi-species of viral particles that are a fertile ground for selecting resistance under the selective pressure of a single antiretroviral agent. In contrast, infectious agents like *Mycobacterium tuberculosis* have a longer generation time, a lower mutational rate, thus are slower to develop resistance [77]. Nevertheless, with a high transmission rate, resistant strains of *Mycobacterium tuberculosis* tend to have serious epidemiologic consequences.

Adherence to TB treatment is suboptimal, especially across high-risk groups [95], and non-adherence to anti-TB therapy correlates with poor clinical outcome [96]. Identification of barriers to adherence is also a recommended part of the patient-centered approach to TB treatment [97]. However, particular risk factors for poor adherence to TB therapy are inconsistent [95] though substandard housing and substance abuse have been reported [96, 98].

As with HIV, adherence to anti-TB therapy has used multiple mechanisms of patient support. Pozsik et al. [99] reported successful methods of promoting adherence to anti-tuberculosis therapy as used in South Carolina and New York in the late 1980s and early 1990s. They report a spectrum of support ranging from incentives (i.e., tangible items like food and clothing), enablers (i.e., free transportation), free medication, coordinated alcohol and drug-treatment programs, directly observed therapy (DOT), as well as involuntary commitment to inpatient treatment for those patients with histories of repeated non-adherence. South Carolina noted an increase in overall completion of anti-tuberculosis therapy from 93.9 to 96.5% and a decrease in new cases per year from 593 to 410 using these strategies. Cost of these interventions ranged from $0.95 to $20 for incentives/enablers, to $653 per patient for DOT, and up to $66,000 per patient for commitment to inpatient management [99]. Incentives and enablers have also been recommended in national guidelines [97], including supplementation with special efforts to reach isolated populations [94]. A recent systematic review of trials largely in developing countries found use of late patient tracers (mechanisms for finding patients who do not complete treatment) and various reminder systems also to be useful [100].

DOT has become the cornerstone in optimizing adherence to anti-tuberculosis treatment, especially for those patients who are thought to be at highest risk for non-adherence and greatest risk for infection transmission [101]. While national guidelines advocate using the least restrictive method of adherence promotion needed to achieve successful eradication of disease, the use of DOT should be considered in every patient and is the preferred method of adherence assurance initially [97]. One aspect of anti-TB therapy that makes it amenable to DOT is that there is some flexibility in dosing allowing for larger doses given less frequently than daily [9]. Often, the term DOT refers not only to the actual supervised consuming of anti-tuberculosis medications, but a comprehensive strategy to support adherence that includes such activities when needed [102]. Free DOT provided on the local health department level has been shown to be feasible as well as effective in decreasing rates of TB resistance and treatment failure [103]. A study of 372 cases of culture-positive tuberculosis treated in San Francisco between 1998 and 2000 found that patients treated with DOT were significantly more likely to achieve cure and less likely to die of tuberculosis than those treated by self-administered therapy (SAT) [101]. Despite widespread enthusiasm and recommendations for this approach to treatment of TB, some have questioned whether or not there is sufficient randomized controlled trial data to justify this level of support [102].

More extreme measures of TB control have been used in the past, but thankfully today involuntary hospitalization has been used rarely to ensure adherence to treatment and is only used when less restrictive measures have failed [97].

Bacterial Infections

Compared with treatment of HIV and TB, limited data exist about patient adherence to antimicrobial regimens. Some fundamental differences exist with treatment for bacterial infections. The majority of bacterial infections tend to be more forgiving than HIV infection, primarily because the host immune system plays a critical role in containing the infection and because antimicrobial therapy enhances its eradication from the host. In addition, most infections and consequently the corresponding antibiotic course are short-lived, simple to administer with predictable drug-associated adverse events. Certain infections are less forgiving than others (e.g., infectious bacterial endocarditis and meningitis) in which case it is critical to maintain a bactericidal antibiotic level at the site of infection. In these settings adherence is paramount and usually achieved with intravenous therapy, often in the hospital setting.

While many might suspect that symptoms from acute infections would ensure that patients comply with clinician instructions for antimicrobial treatment, this is not always the case. What data do exist, supports the idea that patient adherence to antimicrobial regimens is generally suboptimal and tends toward underdosing [9]. Some specific examples can be seen in the treatment of sexually transmitted infections (STI) and other common infections.

In general, evidence from common outpatient infections such as upper respiratory tract infections, Gonorrhea, Chlamydia, and urinary tract infections suggests adherence is a significant problem. Recorded adherence rates for STI treatment have been noted to range from 25 to 63% [104, 105] and for other acute outpatient infections from 55 to 60% [106]. Some suggest that adherence to antibiotics for respiratory tract infections is greater than it is for other infections and can approach 100% [107]. Patients often over-report adherence to antibiotics. One study that compared self-report of adherence to MEMs caps data found a drastic difference with 91% of patients reporting taking all of their medication for Chlamydia as directed as opposed to 16% recorded to have been fully adherent by electronic data [108]. Unlike in chronic diseases, characteristics of non-adherence behavior in short courses of antibiotic treatment include the omission of single doses, premature discontinuation, and alternate dosing frequency [106, 107]. Fewer measurements of improper dosing schedule are available for antibiotics, but it is noted that erratic dosing schedules can also cause treatment failure, even if all prescribed doses are taken [108]. In fact, non-adherence was found to be the most important risk factor of repeated infection in women with recurrent lower urinary tract infection receiving chemoprophylaxis [109].

Common reasons for antibiotic non-adherence seem to be side effects (especially gastrointestinal symptoms), dosing frequency, length of treatment, and differing outcome expectations for acute infections [106, 107]. Little conclusive evidence exists about how to improve adherence to antibiotics. The use of pre-packaged blister cards was found to improve adherence to treatment for sexually transmitted infections and was acceptable to patients in one South African study [110]. Other interventions, such as the use of follow-up telephone calls from a community pharmacist to improve antibiotic adherence, have been interesting but not particularly successful [111]. Finally, other suggested strategies include sharing simple instructions about antimicrobial therapy which include information about adverse reactions [106, 107]. Given the rise in resistant and serious community bacterial infections, such as methicillin-resistant *Staphylococcus aureus* [112], it is clear that adherence to short-course antibiotic therapy is an important area of discussion and deserves further exploration.

Summary

Adherence is particularly important in the treatment of HIV infection. Not only does it correlate with clinical outcome in the short term, but it can determine available therapeutic options and clinical outcomes in the long term as poor adherence can lead to virologic resistance and limited treatment options. Non-adherence to ART can be caused by barriers on multiple levels from patient-specific (i.e., forgetfulness or daily routine) to regimen-specific (genetic barrier of a given ART) to provider-specific (quality of communication) or societal-specific (such as inadequate housing). Furthermore, barriers to adherence for an individual can change over time. Consequently, assessment of adherence is important both at the initiation of ART and throughout the duration of treatment, which, for most patients, is indefinite.

Assessment of adherence can be made through multiple mechanisms, many of which are similar to those used with other chronic diseases. The most common of these are measures of self-report, pharmacy refill patterns, and MEMs. After adherence has been assessed, particular methods for promoting adherence can be identified and matched to the case-specific needs. An example of how to match interventions for the particular needs of a patient was illustrated in Table 11.2. Successful interventions for HIV adherence focus on patient education of practical management skills, supportive tools, and those that are conducted in the individual setting. Better adherence results are also seen in those with known poor adherence at baseline. Providers should factor in the needs of their patient population and resources at hand to choose the best and most cost-effective options available.

Adherence to medication is also important for other infectious diseases. Anti-tuberculosis treatment poses similar challenges to adherence as HIV. However, TB has a slower replication rate causing slower accumulation of mutations and anti-TB treatment is notable for being time limited (usually 6–12 months). Poor adherence is common and resistance to anti-TB treatment is widely recognized as a public health threat. The mainstay of treatment for TB has been directly observed therapy with adjuvant use of various enablers, incentives, and treatment for coexisting diseases. There is significantly less information available about the prevalence of adherence to antimicrobial therapy for bacterial infections and how to improve adherence to this type of treatment. What data do exist from sexually transmitted infections and upper respiratory infections suggests that adherence is poor and generally overestimated. The recent increase in serious infections from resistant bacterial strains, such as MRSA, implies a need for further exploration in this area.

Acknowledgments I would like to acknowledge the helpful input and guidance of Dr. Karam Mounzer in the development of this chapter, as well as Jeremy Goldstein for assistance with images and layout.

References

1. CDC. HIV and AIDS in the United States: A picture of today's epidemic. 2008. Available at: http://www.cdc.gov/hiv/topics/surveillance/resources/reports/2007report/default.htm. Accessed January 9, 2009.
2. Gifford AL, Groessl EJ. Chronic disease self-management and adherence to HIV medications. *J Acquir Immune Defic Syndr*. 2002;31:S163–S166.
3. Panel on antiretroviral guidelines for adults and adolescents. Guidelines for the use of antiretroviral agents in HIV-1-infected adults and adolescents. Department of Health and Human Services. 2008;1–139. Available at: http://www.aidsinfo.nih.gov/ContentFiles/AdultandAdolescentGL.pdf
4. Gross R, Bilker W, Friedman H, et al. Effect of adherence to newly initiated antiretroviral therapy on plasma viral load. *AIDS*. 2001;15:2109–2117.
5. Ickovics J, Cameron A, Zackin R, et al. Consequences and determinants of adherence to antiretroviral medication: results from Adult AIDS Clinical Trials Group protocol 370. *Antiviral Ther*. 2002;7:185–193.
6. Mannheimer S, Friedland G, Matts J, et al. The consistency of adherence to antiretroviral therapy predicts biologic outcomes for human immunodeficiency virus-infected persons in clinical trials. *Clin Infect Dis*. 2002;34:1115–1121.
7. Press N, Tyndall M, Wood E, et al. Virologic and immunologic response, clinical progression, and highly active antiretroviral therapy adherence. *J Acquir Immune Defic Syndr*. 2002;31:S112–S117.
8. Perno CR, Ceccherini-Silberstein F, De Luca A, et al. Virologic correlates of adherence to antiretroviral medications and therapeutic failure. *J Acquir Immune Defic Syndr*. 2002;31:S118–S122.
9. Vrijens B, Urquhart J. Patient adherence to prescribed antimicrovial drug dosing regimens. *J Antimicrob Chemother*. 2005;55:616–627.

10. Bangsberg DR. Preventing HIV antiretroviral resistance through better monitoring of treatment adherence. *J Infect Dis.* 2008;197:S272–S278.

11. Hecht FM, Grant RM, Petropoulos CJ, et al. Sexual transmission of an HIV-1 variant resistant to multiple reverse-transcriptase and protease inhibitors. *N Engl J Med.* 1998;339:307–311.

12. Little SJ, Holte S, Routy JP, et al. Antiretroviral-drug resistance among patients recently infected with HIV. *N Engl J Med.* 2002;347:385–394.

13. Shet A, Berry L, Mohri H, et al. Tracking the prevalence of transmitted antiretroviral drug-resistant HIV-1: a decade of experience. *J Acquir Immune Defic Syndr.* 2006;41:439–446.

14. Hogg RS, Heath K, Bangsberg D, et al. Intermittent use of triple-combination therapy is predictive of mortality at baseline and after 1 year of follow-up. *AIDS.* 2002;16:1051–1058.

15. El-Sadr WM, Lundgren JD, Neaton JD, et al. CD4+ count-guided interruption of antiretroviral treatment. *N Engl J Med.* 2006;355:2283–2296.

16. DART Trial Team. Fixed duration interruptions are inferior to continuous treatment in African adults starting therapy with CD4 cell counts < 200 cells/microl. *AIDS.* 2008;22:237–247.

17. Parienti JJ, Massari V, Descamps D, et al. Predictors of virologic failure and resistance in HIV-infected patients treated with nevirapine- or efavirenz-based antiretroviral therapy. *Clin Infect Dis.* 2004;38:1311–1316.

18. Haubrich RH, Little SJ, Currier JS, et al. The value of patient-reported adherence to antiretroviral therapy in predicting virologic and immunologic response. *AIDS.* 1999;13:1099–1107.

19. Nieuwkerk PT, Sprangers MAG, Burger DM, et al. Limited patient adherence to highly active antiretroviral therapy for HIV-1 infection in an observational cohort study. *Arch Intern Med.* 2001;161:1962–1968.

20. Tam LWY, Chui CKS, Brumme CJ, et al. The relationship between resistance and adherence in drug-naive individuals initiating HAART is specific to individual drug classes. *J Acquir Immune Defic Syndr.* 2008;49:266–271.

21. Bangsberg DR. Less than 95% adherence to nonnucleoside reverse-transcriptase inhibitor therapy can lead to viral suppression. *Clin Infect Dis.* 2006;43:939–941.

22. Golin C, Liu H, Hays R, et al. A prospective study of predictors of adherence to combination antiretroviral medication. *J Gen Intern Med.* 2002;17:756–765.

23. Bangsberg DR, Charlebois ED, Grant RM, et al. High levels of adherence do not prevent accumulation of HIV drug resistance mutations. *AIDS* 2003;17:1925–1932.

24. Paterson DL, Swindells S, Mohr J, et al. Adherence to protease inhibitor therapy and outcomes in patients with HIV infection. *Ann Intern Med.* 2000;133:21–30.

25. Kalichman SC, Amaral CM, Stearns H, et al. Adherence to antiretroviral therapy assessed by unannounced pill counts conducted by telephone. *J Gen Intern Med.* 2007;22:1003–1006.

26. Miller LG, Liu H, Hays RD, et al. How well do clinicians estimate patients' adherence to combination antiretroviral therapy? *J Gen Intern Med.* 2002;17:1–11.

27. Gross R, Yip B, Lo Re V, et al. A simple, dynamic measure of antiretroviral therapy adherence predicts failure to maintain HIV-1 suppression. *J Infect Dis.* 2006;194:1108–1114.

28. Catz SL, Kelly JA, Bogart LM, et al. Patterns, correlates, and barriers to medication adherence among persons prescribed new treatments for HIV disease. *Health Psychol.* 2000;19:124–133.

29. Ickovics J, Meade C. Adherence to antiretroviral therapy among patients with HIV: a critical link between behavioral and biomedical sciences. *J Acquir Immune Defic Syndr.* 2002;31:S98–S102.

30. Ammassari A, Trotta MP, Murri R, et al. Correlates and predictors of adherence to highly active antiretroviral therapy: overview of published literature. *J Acquir Immune Defic Syndr.* 2002;31:S123–S127.

31. Sidat M, Fairley C, Grierson J. Experiences and perceptions of patients with 100% adherence to highly active antiretroviral therapy: a qualitative study. *AIDS Patient Care and STDs.* 2007;21:509–520.

32. Arnsten JH, Li X, Mizuno Y, et al. Factors associated with antiretroviral therapy adherence and medication errors among HIV-infected injection drug users. *J Acquir Immune Defic Syndr.* 2007;46:S64–S71.

33. Arnsten JH, Demas PA, Grant RW, et al. Impact of active drug use on antiretroviral therapy adherence and viral suppression in HIV-infected drug users. *J Gen Intern Med.* 2002;17:377–381.

34. Ingersoll K. The impact of psychiatric symptoms, drug use, and medication regimen on non-adherence to HIV treatment. *AIDS Care.* 2004;16:199–211.

35. Goujard C, Bernard N, Sohier N, et al. Impact of a patient education program on adherence to HIV medication: a randomized clinical trial. *J Acquir Immune Defic Syndr.* 2003;34:191–194.

36. Falagas ME, Zarkadoulia EA, Pliatsika PA, Panos G. Socioeconomic status (SES) as a determinant of adherence to treatment in HIV infected patients: a systematic review of the literature. *Retrovirology.* 2008;5:13.

37. Fogarty L, Roter D, Larson S, Burke J, Gillespie J, Levy R. Patient adherence to HIV medication regimens: a review of published and abstract reports. *Patient Educ Couns.* 2002;46:93–108.

38. Trotta MP, Ammassari A, Melzi S, et al. Treatment-related factors and highly active antiretroviral therapy adherence. *J Acquir Immune Defic Syndr.* 2002;31:S128–S131.

39. Viciana P, Rubio R, Ribera E, et al. Longitudinal study on adherence, treatment satisfaction, and effectiveness of once-daily versus twice-daily antiretroviral therapy in a Spanish cohort of HIV-infected patients (CUVA study). *Enferm Infecc Microbiol Clin.* 2008;26:127–134.

40. Smith SR, Rublein JC, Marcus C, et al. A medication self-management program to improve adherence to HIV therapy regimens. *Patient Educ Couns.* 2003;50:187–199.

41. Bangsberg DR, Bronstone A, Hofman R. A computer-based assessment detects regimen misunderstandings and nonadherence for patients on HIV antiretroviral therapy. *AIDS Care*. 2002;14:3–15.
42. Murri R, Ammassari A, Nappa S, et al. Physician estimates of adherence and the patient-physician relationship as a setting to improve adherence to antiretroviral therapy. *J Acquir Immune Defic Syndr*. 2002;31:S158–S162.
43. Kidder DP, Wolitski RJ, Campsmith ML, et al. Health status, health care use, medication use, and medication adherence among homeless and housed people living with ENDS. *Am J Public Health*. 2007;97:2238–2245.
44. Leaver CA, Bargh G, Dunn JR, et al. The effects of housing status on health-related outcomes in people living with HIV: a systematic review of the literature. *AIDS Behav*. 2007;11:S85–S100.
45. Spaulding A, Stephenson B, Macalino G, Ruby W, Clarke JG, Flanigan TP. Human immunodeficiency virus in correctional facilities: a review. *Clin Infect Dis*. 2002;35:305–312.
46. Binswanger IA, Stern MF, Deyo RA, et al. Release from prison – A high risk of death for former inmates. *N Engl J Med*. 2007;356:157–165.
47. Robison LS, Westfall AO, Mugavero MJ, et al. Short-term discontinuation of HAART regimens more common in vulnerable patient populations. *AIDS Res Hum Retroviruses*. 2008;24:1347–1355.
48. Gross R, Zhang Y, Grossberg R. Medication refill logistics and refill adherence in HIV. *Pharmacoepidemiol Drug Safety*. 2005;14:789–793.
49. Mannheimer SB, Mukherjee R, Hirschhorn LR, et al. The CASE adherence index: a novel method for measuring adherence to antiretroviral therapy. *AIDS Care*. 2006;18:853–861.
50. Berg KM, Arnsten JH. Practical and conceptual challenges in measuring antiretroviral adherence. *J Acquir Immune Defic Syndr*. 2006;43:S79–S87.
51. Mounzer, K. Choosing an optimal second-line regimen for a patient with intermittent adherence [Clinical care options web site]. 2008. Available at: http://www.clinicaloptions.com/HIV.aspx. Accessed January 9, 2009.
52. Glass TR, De Geest S, Hirschel B, et al. Self-reported non-adherence to antiretroviral therapy repeatedly assessed by two questions predicts treatment failure in virologically suppressed patients. *Antiviral Ther*. 2008;13:77–85.
53. Kaplan S, Mounzer K. Antiretroviral therapy in HIV-infected patients with multidrug-resistant virus: applying the guidelines to practice. *AIDS Patient Care STDs*. 2008;22:931–940.
54. Kredo T, Van der Walt J, Siegfried N, et al. Therapeutic drug monitoring of antiretrovirals for people with HIV. Cochrane Database Syst Rev. 2008; (Issue 3). Art. No.: CD007268. DOI:10.1002/14651858.CD007268.
55. Dolin R, Masur H, Saag M. *AIDS therapy*. Philadelphia, PA: Churchill Livingstone; 1999.
56. Barrios A, Rendon AL, Gallego O, et al. Predictors of virological response to atazanavir in protease inhibitor-experienced patients. *HIV Clin Trials*. 2004;5:201–205.

57. Petersen K, Riddle MS, Jones LE, et al. Use of bilirubin as a marker of adherence to atazanavir-based antiretroviral therapy. *AIDS*. 2005;19:1700–1702.
58. Chesney MA. The elusive gold standard. Future perspectives for HIV adherence assessment and intervention. *J Acquir Immune Defic Syndr*. 2006;43:S149–S155.
59. Simoni JM, Pearson C, Pantalone D, et al. Efficacy of interventions in improving highly active antiretroviral therapy adherence and HIV-1 RNA viral load: a meta-analytic Review of Randomized Controlled Trials. *J Acquir Immune Defic Syndr*. 2006;43:S23–S35.
60. Rueda S, Park-Wyllie L, Bayoumi A, et al. Patient support and education for promoting adherence to highly active antiretroviral therapy for HIV/AIDS. Cochrane Database Syst Rev. 2006; (Issue 3). Art. No.: CD001442.DOI:10.1002/14651858.CD001442.pub2.
61. Amico KR, Harman J, Johnson B. Efficacy of antiretroviral therapy adherence interventions: a research synthesis of trials, 1996–2004. *J Acquir Immune Defic Syndr*. 2006;41:285–297.
62. Simoni J, Frick P, Pantalone D, et al. Antiretroviral adherence interventions: a review of current literature and ongoing studies. *Topics HIV Med*. 2003;11:185–198.
63. Jones DL, McPherson-Baker S, Lydston D, et al. Efficacy of a group medication adherence intervention among HIV positive women: The SMART/EST women's project. *AIDS Behav*. 2007;11:79–86.
64. Jones DL, Ishii M, LaPerriere A, et al. Influencing medication adherence among women with AIDS. *AIDS Care*. 2003;15:463–474.
65. Rawlings MK, Thompson M, Farthing C, et al. Impact of an educational program on efficacy and adherence with a twice-daily Lamivudine/Zidovudine/Abacavir regimen in underrepresented HIV-infected patients. *J Acquir Immune Defic Syndr*. 2003;34:174–183.
66. Wagner G, Kanouse D, Golinelli D, et al. Cognitive-behavioral intervention to enhance adherence to antiretroviral therapy: a randomized controlled trial (CCTG 578). *AIDS*. 2006;20:1295–1302.
67. Golin C, Earp J, Tien H-C, et al. A 2-Arm, randomized, controlled trial of a motivational interviewing-based intervention to improve adherence to antiretroviral therapy (ART) among patients failing or initiating ART. *J Acquir Immune Defic Syndr*. 2006;42:42–51.
68. DiIorio C, McCarty F, Resnicow K, et al. Using motivational interviewing to promote adherence to antiretroviral medications: a randomized controlled study. *Aids Care*. 2008;20:273–283.
69. Tuldra A, Fumaz C, Ferrer MJ, et al. Prospective randomized two-arm controlled study to determine the efficacy of a specific intervention to improve long-term adherence to highly active antiretroviral therapy. *J Acquir Immune Defic Syndr*. 2000;25:221–228.
70. Pradier C, Bentz L, Spire B, et al. Efficacy of an educational and counseling intervention on adherence to highly active antiretroviral therapy: French prospective controlled study. *HIV Clin Trials*. 2003;4:121–131.

71. Reynolds N, Testa M, Su M, et al. Telephone support to improve antiretroviral medication adherence: a multisite, randomized controlled trial. *J Acquir Immune Defic Syndr*. 2008;47:62–68.

72. Mannheimer S, Morse E, Matts J, et al. Sustained benefit from a long-term antiretroviral adherence intervention: results of a large randomized clinical trial. *J Acquir Immune Defic Syndr*. 2006;43:S41–S47.

73. Safren SA, Hendriksen ES, Desousa N, et al. Use of an on-line pager system to increase adherence to antiretroviral medications. *AIDS Care*. 2003;15:787–793.

74. Andrade A, McGruder H, Wu A, et al. A programmable prompting device improves adherence to highly active antiretroviral therapy in HIV-infected subjects with memory impairment. *Clin Infect Dis*. 2005;41:875–882.

75. Wise J, Operario D. Use of electronic reminder devices to improve adherence to antiretroviral therapy: a systematic review. *AIDS Patient Care STDs*. 2008;22:495–504.

76. Petersen M, Wang Y, van der Laan M, et al. Pillbox organizers are associated with improved adherence to HIV antiretroviral therapy and viral suppression: a marginal structural model analysis. *Clin Infect Dis*. 2007;45:908–915.

77. Lucas G, Flexner C, Moore R. Directly administered antiretroviral therapy in the treatment of HIV infection: benefit or burden? *AIDS Patient Care STDs*. 2002;16:527–535.

78. Kirkland LR, Fischl MA, Tashima KT, et al. Response to lamivudine-zidovudine plus abacavir twice daily in antiretroviral-naive, incarcerated patients with HIV infection taking directly observed treatment. *Clin Infect Dis*. 2002;34:511–518.

79. Babudieri S, Aceti A, D'Offizi GP, Carbonara S, Starnini G. Directly observed therapy to treat HIV infection in prisoners. *JAMA*. 2000;284:179–180.

80. Lucas G, Mullen A, Weidle P, Hader S, McCaul M, Moore R. Directly administered antiretroviral therapy in methadone clinics is associated with improved HIV treatment outcomes, compared with outcomes among concurrent comparison groups. *Clin Infect Dis*. 2006;42:1628–1635.

81. Altice FL, Maru D, Bruce RD, Springer S, Friedland G. Superiority of directly administered antiretroviral therapy over self-administered therapy among HIV-infected drug users: a prospective, randomized, controlled trial. *Clin Infect Dis*. 2007;45:770–778.

82. Levy RW, Rayner CR, Fairley CK, et al. Multidisciplinary HIV adherence intervention: a randomized study. *Aids Patient Care and Stds* 2004;18:728–735.

83. Safren SA, Boswell S, Johnson W, Salomon L, Mayer K. Initial outcome of an on-line paging system (Medimom) to increase adherence to antiretroviral medications. In: Conference on Retroviruses and Opportunistic Infections. Chicago, IL; 2001:Abstract No. 480.

84. Des Jarlais DC, Paone D, Milliken J, et al. Audio-computer interviewing to measure risk behaviour for HIV among injecting drug users: a quasi-randomised trial. *Lancet*. 1999;353:1657–1661.

85. Quinn TC, Wawer MJ, Sewankambo N, et al. Viral load and heterosexual transmission of human immunodeficiency virus type 1. Rakai Project Study Group. *N Engl J Med*. 2000;342:921–929.

86. Freedberg KA, Hirschhorn LR, Schackman BR, et al. Cost-effectiveness of an intervention to improve adherence to antiretroviral therapy in HIV-infected patients. *J Acquir Immune Defic Syndr*. 2006;43:S113–S118.

87. Goldie SJ, Paltiel AD, Weinstein MC, et al. Projecting the cost-effectiveness of adherence interventions in persons with human immunodeficiency virus infection. *Am J Med*. 2003;115:632–641.

88. Bozzette SA, Joyce G, McCaffrey DF, et al. Expenditures for the care of HIV-infected patients in the era of highly active antiretroviral therapy. *N Engl J Med*. 2001;344:817–823.

89. Freedberg KA, Losina E, Weinstein MC, et al. The cost effectiveness of combination antiretroviral therapy for HIV disease. *N Engl J Med*. 2001;344:824–831.

90. ADAP programs fight for survival with less money and more clients. North Carolina's list tops 700 by midyear. *AIDS Alert*. 2004;19:85, 7–9.

91. More patients seek drugs through ADAPs, creating $50 million deficit. *AIDS Alert*. 2001;16:53–56.

92. CDC. reported tuberculosis in the United States, 2007. 2008. Available at: http://www.cdc.gov/tb/statistics/reports/2008/default.htm. Accessed on January 9, 2009.

93. Horsburgh CR, Feldman S, Ridzon R. Practice guidelines for the treatment of tuberculosis. *Clin Infect Dis*. 2000;31:633–639.

94. Chaulk CP, Kazandjian VA. Directly observed therapy for treatment completion of pulmonary tuberculosis – consensus statement of the public health tuberculosis guidelines panel. *J Am Med Assoc*. 1998;279:943–948.

95. Hirsch-Moverman Y, Daftary A, Franks J, et al. Adherence to treatment for latent tuberculosis infection: systematic review of studies in the US and Canada. *Int J Tubercular Lung Dis*. 2008;12:1235–1254.

96. Burman WJ, Cohn DL, Rietmeijer CA, et al. Noncompliance with directly observed therapy for tuberculosis. Epidemiology and effect on the outcome of treatment. *Chest*. 1997;111:1168–1673.

97. Blumberg HM, Burman WJ, Chaisson RE, et al. American thoracic society/centers for disease control and prevention/infectious diseases society of America: treatment of tuberculosis. *Am J Respir Crit Care Med*. 2003;167:603–662.

98. Franke MF, Appleton SC, Bayona J, et al. Risk factors and mortality associated with default from multidrug-resistant tuberculosis treatment. *Clin Infect Dis* 2008;46:1844–1851.

99. Pozsik C, Kinney J, Breeden D, et al. Approaches to Improving Adherence to Antituberculosis Therapy – South Carolina and New York, 1986–1991. *Morb Mortal Wkly* Rev. 1993;42:74–75, 81.

100. Liu Q, Abba K, Alejandria M, et al. Reminder systems and late patient tracers in the diagnosis and management of tuberculosis. Cochrane Database Syst Rev. 2008:Art. No.:CD006594. DOI: 10.1002/14651858.CD006594.pub2.

101. Jasmer R, Seaman C, Gonzalez L, et al. Tuberculosis treatment outcomes: directly observed therapy compared with self-administered therapy. *Am J Respir Crit Care Med.* 2004;170:561–566.

102. Volmink J, Garner P. Directly observed therapy for treating tuberculosis. *Cochrane Database of Syst Rev.* 2007:Art. No.: CD003343. DOI: 10.1002/14651858.CD003343.pub3.

103. Weis SE, Slocum PC, Blais FX, et al. The effect of directly observed therapy on the rates of drug-resistance and relapse in tuberculosis. *N Engl J Med.* 994;330:1179–1184.

104. Augenbraun M, Bachmann L, Wallace T, et al. Compliance with doxycycline therapy in sexually transmitted diseases clinics. *Sex Transm Dis.* 1998;25:1–4.

105. Katz BP, Zwickl BW, Caine VA, et al. Compliance with antibiotic therapy for Chlamydia trachomatis and Neisseria gonorrhoeae. *Sex Transm Dis.* 1992;19:351–354.

106. Reyes H, Guiscafre H, Munoz O, et al. Antibiotic noncompliance and waste in upper respiratory infections and acute diarrhea. *J Clin Epidemiol.* 1997;50:1297–1304.

107. Kardas P. Patient compliance with antibiotic treatment for respiratory tract infections. *J Antimicrob Chemother.* 2002;49:897–903.

108. Bachmann LH, Stephens J, Richey CM, et al. Measured versus self-reported compliance with doxycycline therapy for Chlamydia-associated syndromes: high therapeutic success rates despite poor compliance. *Sex Transm Dis.* 1999;26:272–278.

109. Alexiou Z, Mouktaroudi M, Koratzanis G, et al. The significance of compliance for the success of antimicrobial prophylaxis in recurrent lower urinary tract infections: the Greek experience. *Int J Antimicrob Agen.* 2007;30:40–43.

110. Wright J, Htun Y, Leong G, et al. Evaluation of the use of calendar blister packaging on patient compliance with STD Syndromic Treatment Regimens. *Sex Transm Dis.* 1999;26:556–563.

111. Beaucage K, Lachance-Demers H, Ngo TT, et al. Telephone follow-up of patients receiving antibiotic prescriptions from community pharmacies. *Am J Health Sys Pharm.* 2006;63:557–563.

112. Moran GJ, Krishnadasan A, Gorwitz RJ, et al. Methicillin-resistant S. aureus infections among patients in the emergency department. *N Engl J Med.* 2006;355:666–674.

Chapter 12
Adherence and Substance Use

A. Meade Eggleston, Jennifer L. Strauss, Vito S. Guerra, and Patrick S. Calhoun

As reported in other chapters of this volume, the misuse of alcohol and other substances can contribute to treatment non-adherence across a range of medical and mental health service settings. In this chapter, our focus is specific to non-adherence in the context of treatment programs that directly target substance misuse and substance use disorders. In such treatment settings, problems with adherence are prevalent and, as elaborated below, significantly impact treatment outcomes.

There are notable interrelationships between alcohol and other drug use disorders, which support reviewing them together [1]. Alcohol and illicit drug dependence are treated in similar contexts and with similar protocols, and treatment outcomes overlap considerably [2, 3]. While nicotine dependence shares many features of other substance dependence, treatment of nicotine dependence is far more likely to be time limited and to occur in primary care contexts, with treatment attrition rates significantly lower than those found in alcohol and other drug dependence treatment. Thus, nicotine dependence is not addressed in this chapter [2, 4]. Readers are encouraged to seek guidance from Chapter 5.

A.M. Eggleston (✉)
Veterans Affairs Mid-Atlantic Mental Illness, Research, and Clinical Center, Durham Veterans Affairs Medical Center, Durham, NC, USA
e-mail: a.meade.eggleston@gmail.com

H. Bosworth (ed.), *Improving Patient Treatment Adherence*,   289
DOI 10.1007/978-1-4419-5866-2_12,
© Springer Science+Business Media, LLC 2010

Problem Overview

Substance misuse and substance use disorders, which include substance abuse and dependence, are prevalent and damaging problems in the USA. Substance abuse is characterized by recurrent substance use resulting in failure to fulfill major role obligations at work, school, or home; persistent or recurrent substance-related interpersonal, social, or legal problems; and/or recurrent substance use in hazardous situations. Substance dependence is characterized by impaired control over substance use, compulsive substance use, preoccupation with substance use, withdrawal symptoms, and/or tolerance to the substance.

Fifty-two percent of Americans consume alcohol [5]. Of these, 22% exceed recommended limits (no more than one drink per day for women; two drinks daily for men) [6] and are considered high-risk drinkers because their alcohol consumption significantly increases their risk of negative social and medical consequences. Risky drinking (i.e., drinking above recommended limits) is a significant public health problem and accounts for as much disability and mortality as tobacco use and hypertension [7]. According to the annual National Survey on Drug Use and Health, approximately 30.5 million people 12 years or older drove under the influence of alcohol at least once in the previous year [8]. Alcohol consumption above recommended limits significantly and negatively impacts risk for adverse medical outcomes, including diabetes, hypertension, chronic pain, and various cancers [9–12].

While risky drinking is more prevalent than alcohol use disorders [13], as many as 9% of American adults who drink alcohol meet criteria for alcohol use disorders. Five percent of those who drink both exceed the recommended limits and experience some consequences, but do not experience withdrawal or tolerance (formally diagnosed as alcohol abuse). The other 4% drink heavily and nearly daily and have a variety of symptoms including physiological dependence. These rates of moderate and severe misuse correspond to past year alcohol abuse and dependence rates, as per criteria set forth in the *Diagnostic and Statistical Manual of Mental Disorders, 4th edition* [14]. These percentages translate into approximately 17.6 million adults in the USA meeting criteria for an alcohol use disorder [15, 16].

Illicit substance use, including use of cannabis, cocaine, heroin, and other drugs, is prevalent and problematic as well. Approximately 4.2 million Americans (2%) meet criteria for some other substance use disorder [15, 16]. Over 6% of individuals aged 18 years and older report use of an illicit substance in the past month [17]. The 1988 National Household Survey on Drug Abuse found that nearly 28 million Americans aged 12 years or older, approximately one out of seven Americans, used illicit substances at least once in the past year [18]. While data suggest that marijuana is the illicit drug most commonly used, more than one million people reported "past year" crack cocaine use and nearly 600,000 people reported past year heroin use. Of note, there have also been increases in nonmedical use of prescription drugs among young adults (18–25 years old), the reported rates of use rising from 5.4 to 6.4% between 2002 and 2006 [8].

Like many mental and medical illnesses, prevalence of alcohol and other substance use disorders varies according to gender, socioeconomic status, and race, among other factors. Rates of alcohol and other substance use tend to be higher among men than women [19]. Among both men and women, more individuals aged 25–34 years meet criteria for alcohol and other substance abuse and dependence than any other age group. Rates of abuse steadily decline after 35 years of age [19]. Lower socioeconomic status is associated with increased alcohol and other substance misuse and abuse/dependence across populations [19].

Drinking habits and use of illicit drugs also vary according to race. In 2000, reported use of illicit drugs in the past month was highest among American Indian/Alaskan Native populations (13%) and individuals who self-identified as multi-racial (15%). Rates of illicit drug use were similar among Caucasians (6%), Hispanics (5%), and African-Americans (6%). Regarding alcohol use, an estimated 51% of Whites, 42% of persons reporting more than one race, and 40% of Hispanics reported drinking alcohol in the past month. Asians reported both the lowest drinking rate (28%) and the lowest binge drinking rate (12%) and American Indians/Alaskan Natives reported the highest binge drinking rate (26%; note that 35% endorsed drinking in the past month) [19].

Treatment Adherence

Researchers and clinicians have broadly defined adherence as the "extent to which a person's behavior coincides with medical or health advice" [20, 21]. Adherence to pharmacological treatment, for example, is often defined in terms of whether or not a person takes a prescribed medication at the correct dose on the correct schedule; use of the medication can be gauged in a variety of ways, including pill counts, monitoring devices on medication bottles, self-reports, and plasma levels [22]. Adherence to psychosocial treatments (e.g., individual, group, or family therapy), which comprise the bulk of substance use treatment programs, can be more difficult to define and assess reliably. Adherence to psychosocial substance use treatment can be described vis-à-vis both (1) retention-related factors (i.e., whether an individual remains in treatment) and (2) treatment-specific factors (i.e., whether or not the patient performs the tasks required by the treatment) [20]. Retention-related indicators include the number of prescribed sessions attended, the frequency of rescheduling, the number of sessions attended when intoxicated, and the premature discontinuation of treatment ("dropping out"). Examples of treatment-specific indicators of non-adherence include failure to complete between-session homework assignments, failure to attend recommended Alcoholics Anonymous (AA)/Narcotics Anonymous (NA) meetings, failure or refusal to bring spouse or family for family therapy, and failure to provide requested breath/urine/blood samples.

While there is consensus that the most important indicator of adherence in substance use treatment is treatment attendance, high attendance does not imply that patients have been fully adherent with treatment. Indeed, multiple measures of both retention-related and treatment-specific factors are needed to assess adherence in a treatment trial. Unfortunately, the majority of substance use treatment research has focused only on treatment retention, as defined above, with specific attention to dropout rates. Other aspects of adherence, such as homework compliance, are rarely monitored or reported [20].

Prevalence of Non-adherence

There is a wide range of estimates of treatment retention in substance use treatment. Substance use treatment researchers operationalize treatment retention in different ways, making it difficult to directly compare retention rates reported across studies [2, 23]. For example, some researchers consider leaving a program against medical advice equivalent to expulsion from a program, whereas others distinguish between these two types of discharges. Investigators sometimes collapse total visits/sessions into "levels" of attendance (e.g., 1–5, 6–8) when reporting retention rates. Others elect to report retention rates without collapsing these data. Alternatively, investigators may elect to operationalize retention in terms of the period of time (e.g., number of months) during which a patient remains in contact with the program.

Against this backdrop of methodological variability, reported rates of attrition in substance use treatment range from 25 to 90% [23, 24]. The Substance Abuse and Mental Health Services Administration determined that over half of patients admitted to addiction treatment do not complete their intended treatment because they leave against staff advice, are administratively discharged for various infractions such as drug distribution within the program, or are transferred to other treatments [25]. Given that substance abuse is strongly related to poor adherence, many psychotherapy trials for disorders other than substance abuse actively exclude those with a substance use diagnosis [20]. As reported in this volume, substance abuse is a correlate of poor adherence in medical populations as well.

Consequences of Non-adherence

No matter how effective a treatment is, high rates of dropout will mitigate against its success. In the substance abuse field, available treatments are often considered effective to the degree to which they retain participants [20]. As common sense might suggest, treatment adherence has positive effects on treatment outcome [26–28]. For example, reductions in drug use among methadone-maintained patients increase as treatment duration increases [2]. For individuals in outpatient and long-term residential inpatient treatment programs, overall and primary drug use appears to improve incrementally with treatment duration until about one year [29]. More generally, reductions in drug use have a direct association with time in treatment across a number of substance use treatment modalities [29].

Conversely, terminating treatment early has a clear negative outcome in substance-abusing patients. Clinicians and researchers have long acknowledged that high attrition significantly limits substance abuse treatment effectiveness. Indeed, a review by Baekeland and Lundwall, over 30 years ago, found that individuals who terminated outpatient or inpatient alcoholism treatment early had worse outcomes than individuals who completed treatment [23]. Substance-dependent individuals who complete detoxification or comprehensive treatment programs are more likely to remain abstinent from alcohol and other drugs, have lower relapse rates, and report better psychosocial outcomes, such as lower unemployment and arrest rates, than treatment dropouts [2]. A notable exception to these findings is found in the literature on methadone maintenance treatment; the relationship between treatment completion and positive outcomes among those on methadone maintenance becomes insignificant when length of stay is controlled statistically [2].

Similar to findings examining treatment retention, the length of stay or contact with a treatment program appears positively associated with treatment outcomes. A large number of studies of both inpatient and outpatient treatment programs document a positive relationship between long-term outcomes and length of stay [23]. Moreover, individuals who leave treatment before at least six months of abstinence or appreciable improvement are unlikely to maintain improvements after treatment. On the other hand, 80% of outpatients with one year of abstinence or appreciable improvements maintain these gains after treatment [23].

Predictors of Good and Poor Adherence

In a review of the literature examining factors related to non-adherence in substance abuse treatment, Carroll notes that investigators have persistently focused on identifying patient characteristics associated with poor adherence including age, gender, socioeconomic status, race, substance use factors, social functioning, and motivation. A brief review of the findings in this area is presented below.

Age: The findings examining the relationship between age and adherence in substance abuse treatment are mixed. The bulk of the evidence, however, suggests that there is either no relationship or an inverse relationship between age and attrition, i.e., as age increases, rates of attrition are lower [2, 23]. Reviews of the relationship between age and adherence in this area suggest that any apparent relationship between age and adherence is likely better explained by other age-related factors such as substance use history, treatment history, and social context [2, 23].

Gender: Findings are mixed regarding whether men or women are more likely to stay in substance abuse treatment. Baekland and Lundwall determined that gender was related to discontinuing alcoholism treatment in nearly half (45%) of the studies they reviewed [23]. In a more recent comprehensive review of both alcohol and other substance abuse treatment, findings related to whether gender was associated with attrition were also equivocal [2].

There is some evidence, however, that gender may moderate the relationship between social and personality factors and attrition [2]. Research is consistent in the presence of differences in this regard, although which factors and treatment modalities best or most reliably predict retention and attrition among men and women is not straightforward. Like the measurement of adherence itself, each researcher examines unique aspects of substance use, social functioning, personality, and other constructs such as years of drug use, treatment episodes, treatment tenure, perceived pressure to attend treatment, current use, history of incarceration, family history, and health beliefs. Individual findings are thus difficult to compare and synthesize. In a review of this work, Stark concluded that specific substance use factors, personality, and social characteristics are generally stronger predictors of treatment retention for men than for women [2].

Education and socioeconomic status: Generally, socioeconomic status factors that provide resources to support treatment seeking and attendance, such as adequate insurance and income, predict treatment retention. Conversely, socioeconomic factors that are either unrelated to treatment or may interfere with treatment seeking and attendance, such as work-related scheduling conflicts, produce a negligible or negative effect on treatment seeking and attendance [2]. Findings that educational attainment has a negligible association with treatment retention suggest that education is only helpful as it relates to having necessary treatment resources. As a result of such findings, many have argued for the need to make treatment more accessible and less expensive in order to improve treatment retention.

Race: Several studies have documented that African-American patients are more likely than Caucasian patients to discontinue treatment prematurely [30–33]. The pattern of results examining race and treatment initiation and retention in substance use interventions is consistent with decreased access and use of health-care services overall for African-Americans compared to Caucasians [34].

Substance use habits, prior treatment history, and comorbidity: Current substance use severity has been consistently related to attrition rates whereas alcohol and drug use histories have not. Current substance use severity indicators associated with higher dropout include intoxication at admission, combined alcohol and other drug use, and greater number of dependence symptoms [2].

Social functioning: Social isolation and levels of affiliation influence treatment retention [2]. Social isolation can be measured by assessing the patient's ties to family, friends, and a wider social community such as church, although most researchers examine marital status alone. Evidence to suggest that marital status and satisfaction are related to treatment retention is mixed [2]. The depth and breadth of connections – to children, other family, and supportive people – are more consistently related to attrition.

Patient motivation: Almost by definition, negative or ambivalent attitudes toward treatment and globally poor treatment motivation do not bode well for starting or staying in substance use treatment. Institutionally referred patients, typically compelled into treatment by legal charges, child custody concerns, and employers, are more likely to drop out than those who are self-referred [23]. Perceptions of needing help, believing return visits are important, and expecting improvements based on adherence with treatment are associated with greater treatment retention for alcoholism [2].

As noted earlier, evidence of demographic findings related to adherence in substance abuse interventions is extremely mixed. Results often are not replicated across settings and treatment approaches [20]. One finding that has emerged consistently, however, is that the majority of those who drop out of treatment do so within the first month [20]. Carroll and others have noted, in many settings, that patient heterogeneity is met with treatment homogeneity. In other words, regardless of a patient's background or preferences, the severity of their substance use problems, or other personal circumstances, many treatment programs offer only a single type of treatment. As a result, many researchers have argued that early attrition may reflect a process of self-selection, where patients find themselves in a treatment setting that may not meet their needs or preferences [20].

Interventions to Improve Adherence

Identifying Non-adherence

A major obstacle to understanding, and thus addressing, adherence problems in substance use treatment is the diverse and numerous adherence indicators used in research studies. Carroll notes that "different indicators of compliance may not converge.... Thus multiple indicators of compliance may be needed to fully assess compliance and its effects on process and outcome" (p. 10) [20]. As noted earlier, although the majority of studies in this area have utilized treatment retention as the primary outcome, a more comprehensive view of the behaviors related to adherence and treatment outcome is warranted. Adapted from Carroll [20], Table 12.1 lists variables associated with adherence to substance use interventions. Many of these indicators can be derived from routinely collected treatment data and patient self-report. A direction for future research is to determine whether and how each of these measures are associated with treatment outcome.

Improving Adherence

Empirical evaluation of substance dependence treatment has led to the recognition that (1) substance abuse treatment is effective and (2) no single approach is useful for all people [35]. Reviews by the Institute of Medicine have noted that there is significant heterogeneity in substance use treatment across sites. This heterogeneity has led many to advocate matching patients to specific aspects of treatment including setting (e.g., inpatient versus outpatient), modality (individual versus group), and orientation (e.g., cognitive-behavioral versus psychodynamic) to enhance treatment effects [35]. Others have suggested that matching patients with clinicians on the basis of gender or race might improve outcomes through increased self-disclosure and development of a stronger therapeutic alliance.

Table 12.1 Indicators of adherence and non-adherence in addiction treatment

Adherence-related indicators in psychosocial treatments
- Number of prescribed sessions attended
- Number of sessions missed
- Lateness to sessions
- Repeated rescheduling of sessions
- Failure to call to cancel sessions
- Attending sessions while intoxicated
- Use of other psychoactive substances
- Leaving treatment against medical advice

Adherence-related indicators in pharmacological treatments
- Failure or refusal to take medication
- Taking medication at the wrong times
- Discontinuing medication because feeling better
- Discontinuing medication because feeling worse
- Failure or refusal to refill medication
- Medication plasma levels
- Pill counts
- Record of bottle opening via Medication Event Monitoring System cap
- Use of contraindicated substances or medications

Treatment-specific indicators in psychosocial treatments
- Failure to complete practice assignments
- Incomplete practice assignments
- Failure to attend Narcotics Anonymous/Alcoholic Anonymous meetings
- Failure or refusal to bring spouse or family for family therapy
- Overt resistance (e.g., silence, hostility)
- Failure to provide breath/urine/blood samples

However, these hypotheses have not borne out the empirical investigations of matching procedures in substance abuse treatments [35, 36].

On the other hand, research that has examined contingency management interventions, specifically the use of voucher-based incentive programs for the treatment of substance dependence, has received relatively strong support (for a review, see [37]). Voucher-based incentives, typically exchangeable for retail items, are "earned" by patients when they meet some well-defined therapeutic goal. Most often this goal is biochemically verified abstinence from substance use. As patients must remain in treatment in order to receive vouchers, this approach often is associated with an increase in treatment retention [37].

Table 12.2 lists other practical strategies that address the correlates of non-adherence and point to interventions that have been found successful in clinical practice and research [23]. As summarized in Table 12.2, important first-line strategies include early identification of alcohol and other drug use, providing brief advice and recommendations immediately, and directing the individual to specialized treatment or mental health triage as appropriate.

Table 12.2 Strategies to improve adherence

- Identify alcohol and other drug dependence early and direct the individual to specialized treatment or mental health triage
- Eliminate waiting lists/offer immediate admission
- Orient the patient to treatment: explain justification for and goals of treatment, clarify role expectations for provider and patient, describe treatment course and expected outcomes
- Explore motivation, especially as it related to past treatment dropout (or completion), and current treatment
- Maintain contact with significant individual(s) in the patient's life and elicit participation from them
- Focus on rapid symptom relief. Do not withhold medication that might help

Alcohol screening and brief intervention is recommended by the U.S. Preventive Services Task Force, although this organization currently finds insufficient evidence to recommend screening for illicit substance use [38, 39]. Nevertheless, while assessing alcohol and other substance use is a standard part of clinical work in addiction-oriented treatment, many primary care and other providers do not reliably screen for these behaviors [40–42]. In a nationally representative sample of adult primary care patients, only 28% reported that their general medical provider screened for substance use or mental health problems during the past year [43, 44]. Primary care and other providers may choose not to follow screening recommendation because of competing demands during a typically brief medical visit, because behavioral health screening is not generally reimbursable or because they do not know how to proceed following a positive screen [44, 45].

Screening and referral, however, do not need to be time consuming or complicated. Simply engaging in screening and brief interventions may improve adherence to other medical treatments and is an efficacious intervention for mild-to-moderate alcohol use and possibly drug use [39, 46]. Self-reported hazardous alcohol use can be assessed with the Alcohol Use Disorder Identification Test – Consumption (AUDIT-C; see Appendix), which is comprised of the first three consumption items of the World Health Organization's 10-item Alcohol Use Disorders Identification Test [47, 48]. The AUDIT-C has demonstrated reliability and validity in numerous studies that have compared results to interview-based diagnostic assessment of hazardous drinking and alcohol abuse and dependence in both the Veterans Affairs (VA) medical centers, where annual alcohol use screening is mandated, and the general U.S. population [48–51]. According to studies in the VA and general populations, hazardous drinking has been defined as AUDIT-C scores ≥ 4 for men and ≥ 3 for women [48, 51–53]. Cutting scores that maximized sensitivity and specificity in previous studies conducted in the general and VA populations are AUDIT-C scores ≥ 4 for women and ≥ 6 for men [48, 51, 53]. Furthermore, the National Institute on Alcohol Abuse and Alcoholism (NIAAA) provides excellent guidelines for clinicians exploring alcohol use, which can organize information gathering for both addiction specialist and other care providers: http://pubs.niaaa.nih.gov/publications/Practitioner/pocketguide/pocket_guide.htm. These NIAAA guidelines are a rubric for providing brief, immediate interventions and specialty referrals. The wording of these questions can be altered to investigate other substance use as well. Any use of illicit substances warrants consideration for a referral to a mental health or addiction specialist.

The American Medical Association approved two codes, based on time required for service provision, that address alcohol and other drug screening and intervention: 99408 and 99409. Providers can bill for health behavioral assessment and interventions, as they relate to treatment or management of patients diagnosed with physical health problems.

Second, eliminate waiting lists/offer immediate admission. Clear evidence suggests that scheduling patients with an immediate appointment or an appointment in the first week after treatment initiation or screening increases session attendance [54]. For example, one study found that when patients calling to enroll in a cocaine treatment center were given a same day appointment, as many as 59% attended their scheduled intake appointment versus 33% of those in an alternative group who received a later appointment [55]. Similar studies have demonstrated that those scheduled within 48 hours are more likely to attend than those given later appointments even when those with later appointments received reminder calls [56]. Other studies have demonstrated that patients given an appointment in the week after screening are more likely to attend treatment than those scheduled beyond 1 week from screening [57].

Third, orient the patient to treatment: Many patients have no experience with formal mental health or substance use treatment. It is good practice and important for clinicians to explain the goals of treatment, clarify role expectations for the patient and the therapist, and describe the expected treatment course and outcomes. It is also important to assess what patients expect and to elicit any feelings they have toward treatment. Eliciting feelings or concerns about treatment has shown to effectively reduce the likelihood of premature withdrawal [58]. Patients are more likely to drop out of treatment if there are misunderstandings between the patient and the therapist regarding the course and nature of treatment [59].

Fourth, explore motivation, especially as it relates to current treatment and past treatment dropout (or completion). As noted above, motivation for treatment is associated with treatment retention and outcomes. Increasing evidence suggests that specific cognitive-behavioral techniques which target ambivalence about treatment may lead to positive behavior change. Specifically, motivational interviewing (MI) is a directive, patient-centered approach for eliciting behavior change by assisting patients in exploring and resolving ambivalence [60]. MI has shown promise in a variety of treatment contexts [61].

A therapist working from an MI perspective will focus on expressing empathy, developing a discrepancy between current behavior and broader goals, avoiding arguments and use of labels, supporting self-efficacy, and using resistance as a problem-solving exercise [62]. A helpful resource for information on training related to motivational interviewing, as well as a bibliography and review of studies that have examined MI is hosted by the University of New Mexico and found at the following web address: http://www.motivationalinterview.org/.

A significant aspect of motivational enhancement is identifying and reducing obstacles to achieving target behavior (e.g., attending treatment). Individuals with addictions identify very real and salient obstacles to treatment attendance which can be acknowledged and, hopefully, addressed by providers. Potential barriers to treatment that clinicians should consider include [63] the following:

- *Traveling distance to treatment facility.* If patients must travel lengthy distances to treatment, they are more likely to terminate treatment prematurely.

- *Reliability of transportation.* Similarly, patients are more likely to terminate treatment or attend intermittently if they cannot get to treatment facilities reliably. Identifying patient transportation needs early in the treatment process, providing transportation assistance (i.e., bus vouchers, program van), and generating a concrete plan in cooperation with the patient are often overlooked aspects of treatment planning.
- *Legal difficulties.* Patients with substance use disorders frequently face legal difficulties. Ask the patient about any pending or current legal charges, speak directly with probation or other court officers to confirm and elaborate on legal issues, and develop a clearly delineated plan which includes program, provider, and patient expectations.
- *Childcare arrangements.* Childcare can be a significant barrier to treatment participation. Helping patients find or arrange appropriate resources for childcare can improve treatment retention. Provision of childcare during the appointment by the treatment facility has been shown to increase attendance of pregnant women with substance use disorders [64].
- *Psychiatric or medical problems.* Other psychiatric and medical problems can be barriers for completing substance abuse treatment. Coordinating care with other treatment providers is good clinical practice and may lead to improved adherence.

Fifth, maintain contact with significant individual(s) in the patient's life and elicit their participation. As Carroll [20] summarizes, significant others can provide information and encouragement and help the patient identify needed resources, develop realistic goals, identify and express feelings, find meaning, and develop a sense of belonging. There is evidence that patients are more likely to remain in treatment if their significant others are involved in treatment sessions. Further, involving significant others in treatment allows them to express concerns, ask questions, and participate in treatment planning which may prevent them from directly or inadvertently sabotaging treatment [20].

Sixth, focus on rapid symptom relief. Do not withhold medication that might help. There are a number of pharmacological treatments for substance abuse which are supported by at least two randomized, placebo-controlled clinical trials including disulfiram, naltrexone, and acamprosate for the treatment of alcohol use disorders; naltrexone, methadone, and buprenorphine for opiate dependence; disulfiram and topiramate for cocaine addiction; and rimonabant for marijuana abuse.

Summary and Conclusions

Poor treatment retention and adherence is a clear problem in substance use treatment settings. From a policy perspective, continued screening and expansion of existing services are essential to improving access to care. Reimbursement for alcohol and other drug screening and brief intervention is cost-effective. Untreated alcohol and substance-dependent people incur health care and other costs at nearly twice the rate of their age- and gender-matched peers; however, this trend begins reversing at treatment initiation [65, 66]. Data suggest, however, that our current delivery system is inadequate as only 9% of all people who need alcohol or other substance use treatment receive care [67]. As noted earlier, common barriers to initiation and retention in existing treatments include distance, transportation, and time to next available appointments. Overcoming such barriers to enhance access to care may increase treatment adherence and ultimately reductions in morbidity and mortality associated with continued substance use.

Clinicians need to continue to develop flexible treatment approaches that are responsive to the specific needs of their patients and to view treatment adherence and retention as a partnership between themselves and the patient. This is reflected, for example, in taking time to discuss patient expectations about treatment and providing education about the treatment process. Flexibly meeting the needs of the patient may also include modifying service policies to eliminate/reduce wait lists, allowing same day or same week first appointments, providing telephone reminders, providing access to transportation (e.g., bus passes or use of a treatment van), and offering flexible clinic hours to more easily allow patients who work and/or have limited child care, as well as their partners, be involved in treatment. The use of contingency management strategies such as vouchers and cognitive-behavioral interventions aimed at improving motivation for behavior change is well supported for use with those with substance abuse or dependence. Providers are encouraged to implement these approaches into practice after receiving appropriate training.

Appendix. Alcohol Use Disorders Identification Test – Consumption (AUDIT-C)

Patient name_____

Date of visit_____

1. How often do you have a drink containing alcohol?

- o Never (0)
- o Monthly or less (1)
- o 2–4 times per month (2)
- o 2–3 times per week (3)
- o 4 or more times a week (4)

2. How many standard drinks containing alcohol do you have on a typical day?

- o 1 or 2 (0)
- o 3 or 4 (1)
- o 5 or 6 (2)
- o 7 to 9 (3)
- o 10 or more (4)

3. How often do you have six or more drinks on one occasion?

- o Never (0)
- o Monthly or less (1)
- o 2–4 times per month (2)
- o 2–3 times per week (3)
- o 4 or more times a week (4)

Did you use any of these in the **past month**? Check all that apply.		Did you use any of these in the **past year**? Check all that apply.	
alcohol		alcohol	
marijuana		marijuana	
heroin		heroin	
cocaine		cocaine	
hallucinogens (like mushrooms, acid)		hallucinogens (like mushrooms, acid)	
stimulants (like crystal meth., speed)		stimulants (like crystal meth., speed)	
prescription pain killers		prescription pain killers	
nicotine (like cigarettes, dip)		nicotine (like cigarettes, dip)	
something else		something else	

If you did not feel comfortable answering this honestly, check here:

References

1. Battjes RJ. Smoking as an issue in alcohol and drug abuse treatment. *Addict Behav.* 1988;13(3):225–230.

2. Stark MJ. Dropping out of substance-abuse treatment – a clinically oriented review. *Clin Psychol Rev.* 1992;12(1):93–116.

3. National Institute on Drug Abuse. *Main findings for drug abuse treatment units: September 1982. Data from the National Drug and Alcoholism Treatment Utilization Survey (NDATUS).* Washington, DC: Govt Printing Office; 1983. Series F, No. 10, DHHS Publication No. ADM 83-1284.

4. Bastian LA, Molner SL, Fish LL, McBride CM. Smoking cessation and adherence. In: Bosworth HB, Oddone EZ, Weinberger M, eds. *Patient treatment adherence concepts, interventions and measurement.* Mahwah, NJ: Lawrence Erlbaum Associates; 2006:125–146.

5. Grant BF. Alcohol consumption, alcohol abuse and alcohol dependence. The United States as an example. *Addiction.* 1994;89:1357–1365.

6. Willenbring M. Alcoholism isn't what it used to be: new research on the nature and diagnosis of alcohol use disorders. NIAAA Videoconference Series https://webmeeting.nih.gov/p27471408/. Accessed May 7, 2009.

7. Room R, Babor T, Rehm J. Alcohol and public health. *Lancet.* 2005;365(9458):519–530.

8. National Institute on Drug Abuse. 2008 *NIDA InfoFacts: Nationwide trends.* http://www.drugabuse.gov/infofacts/nationtrends.html. Accessed May 7, 2009.

9. Howard AA, Arnsten JH, Gourevitch MN. Effect of alcohol consumption on diabetes mellitus. *Ann Intern Med.* 2004;140(3):211–219.

10. McFadden CB, Brensinger CM, Berlin JA, Townshend RR. Systematic review of the effect of daily alcohol intake on blood pressure. *Am J Hypertens.* 2005;18:276–286.

11. Martell BA, O'Connor PG, Kerns RD, et al. Systematic review: opioid treatment for chronic back pain: prevalence, efficacy, and association with addiction. *Ann Intern Med.* 2007;146(2):116–127.

12. Terry MB, Zhang FF, Kabat G, et al. Lifetime alcohol intake and breast cancer risk. *Ann Epidemiol.* 2006;16(3):230–240.

13. Grant BF, Dawson DA, Stinson FS, Chou SP, Dufour MC, Pickering RP. The 12-month prevalence and trends in DSM-IV alcohol abuse and dependence: United States, 1991–1992 and 2001–2002. *Drug Alcohol Depend.* 2004;74(3):223–234.

14. American Psychiatric Association. *Diagnostic and statistical manual of mental disorders. 4th Ed.* Washington, DC: American Psychiatric Association; 1994.

15. Compton WM, Thomas Y, Stinson F, Grant BF. Prevalence, correlates, disability, and comorbidity of DSM-IV drug abuse and dependence in the United States: results from the National Epidemiologic Survey on Alcohol and Related Conditions. *Arch Gen Psychiatry.* 2007;64(5):566–576.

A.M. Eggleston et al.

16. Hasin D, Stinson F, Ogburn E, Grant BF. Prevalence, correlates, disability, and comorbidity of DSM-IV alcohol abuse and dependence in the United States: results from the National Epidemiologic Survey on Alcohol and Related Conditions. *Arch Gen Psychiatry.* 2007;64(7):830–842.

17. Hughes AL. The prevalence of illicit drug use in six metropolitan areas in the United States: results from the 1991 National Household Survey on Drug Abuse. *Br J Addict.* 1992;87(10):1481–1485.

18. National Institute on Drug Abuse. National household survey on drug abuse: main findings 1985. *U.S. Department of health and human services PHS, alcohol, drug abuse, and mental health administration.* Rockville, MD: Department of Health and Human Services; 1990.

19. Substance Abuse and Mental Health Services Administration. *Summary of findings from the 2000 national household survey on drug abuse.* Rockville, MD: Department of Health and Human Services, Office of Applied Studies; 2001. DHHS Publication No. SMA 01–3549.

20. Carroll K, ed. Improving compliance with alcoholism. Rockville, MD: NIAAA; 1977. Project MATCH Monograph Series; No. 6, DHHS Publication No. 97–4143.

21. Haynes RB. Strategies to improve compliance with referrals, appointments, and prescribed medical regimens. In: Haynes RB, Taylor DW, Sackett DL, eds. *Compliance in health care.* Baltimore, MD: Johns Hopkins University Press; 1979:2–3.

22. Bosworth HB. *Medical treatment adherence in patient treatment adherence: Concepts, interventions and measurements.* Mahwah, NJ: Lawrence Erlbaum Associates; 2006.

23. Baekeland F, Lundwall L. Dropping out of treatment: a critical review. *Psychol Bull.* 1975;82(5):738–783.

24. Wickizer T, Maynard C, Atherly A, Frederick M. Completion rates of clients discharged from drug and alcohol treatment programs in Washington State. *Am J Public Health.* 1994;84(2):215–221.

25. Substance Abuse and Mental Health Services Administration. *National survey of substance abuse treatment (NSSAT): Data for 2000 and 2001.* Washington, DC: Department of Health and Human Services; 2002. DHHS Publication No. SMA 98–3176.

26. Hubbard RL, Arsden ME, Rachal JV, Harwood HJ, Cavanaugh ER, Ginzburg H. *Drug abuse treatment: A national study of effectiveness.* Chapel Hill, NC: University of North Carolina Press; 1989.

27. McKay JR, McLellan AT, Alterman AI, Cacciola JS, Rutherford MJ, O'Brien CP. Predictors of participation in aftercare sessions and self-help groups following completion of intensive outpatient treatment for substance abuse. *J Stud Alcohol.* 1998;59(2):152–162.

28. Hoffman JA, Caudill BD, Koman JJ, Luckey JW. Psychosocial treatments for cocaine abuse: 12-month treatment outcomes. *J Subst Abuse Treat.* 1996;13(1):3–11.

29. Zhang Z, Friedmann PD, Gerstein DR. Does retention matter? Treatment duration and improvement in drug use. *Addiction.* 2003;98(5):673–684.

30. McCaul ME, Svikis DS, Moore RD. Predictors of outpatient treatment retention: patient versus substance use characteristics. *Drug Alcohol Depend.* 2001;62(1):9–17.

31. Kleinman P, Kang S, Lipton D, Woody GE, Kemp J, Millman RB. Retention of cocaine abusers in outpatient psychotherapy. *Am J Drug Alcohol Abus.* 1992;18:29–43.

32. Agosti V, Nunes E, Ocepeck-Welikson K. Patient factors related to early attrition from an outpatient cocaine research clinic. *Am J Drug Alcohol Abus.* 1996;22:29–39.

33. Saxon JJ, Wells EA, Fleming C, Jackson TR, Calsyn DA. Pre-treatment characteristics, program philosophy and level of ancillary services as predictors of methadone maintenance treatment outcome. *Addiction.* 1996;91: 1197–1209.

34. Himmelstein DU, Woodhandler S. Care denied: U.S. residents who are unable to obtain needed medical services. *Am J Public Health.* 1995;85:341–344.

35. Sterling RC, Gottheil E, Weinstein SP, Serota R. The effect of therapist/patient race-and-sex matching in individual treatment. *Addiction.* 2001;96: 1015–1022.

36. Project Match Research Group. Matching alcoholism treatments to client heterogeneity: project MATCH posttreatment drinking outcomes. *J Stud Alcohol.* 1997;58(1):7–29.

37. Higgins ST, Alessi SM, Dantona RL. Voucher-based incentives: a substance abuse treatment innovation. *Addict Behav.* 2002;27:887–910.

38. U.S. Preventive Services Task Force. *Screening for illicit drug use: U.S. preventive services task force recommendation statement.* Rockville, MD: Agency for Healthcare Research and Quality; 2008. AHRQ Publication No. 08-05108-EF-3.

39. U.S. Preventive Services Task Force. *Screening and behavioral counseling interventions in primary care to reduce alcohol misuse.* Rockville, MD: Agency for Healthcare Research and Quality; 2004. AHRQ Publication No. 04-0533A.

40. Cleary P, Miller M, Bush BT, Warburg MM, Delbanco TL, Aronson MD. Prevalence and recognition of alcohol abuse in a primary care population. *Am J Med.* 1988;85:466–471.

41. Buchsbaum D, Buchanan R, Poses RM, Schnoll SH, Lawton MJ. Physician detection of drinking problems in patients attending a general medicine practice. *J Gen Intern Med.* 1992;7:517–521.

42. Friedmann PD, McCullough D, Saitz R. Screening and intervention for illicit drug abuse: a national survey of primary care physicians and psychiatrists. *J Gen Intern Med.* 2001;161:248–251.

43. Edlund MJ, Unützer J, Wells KB. Clinician screening and treatment of alcohol, drug, and mental problems in primary care: results from healthcare for communities. *Med Care.* 2004;42(12):1158–1166.

44. Yarnall KSH, Pollak KI, Østbye T, Krause KM, Michener JL. Primary care: is there enough time for prevention? *Am J Public Health.* 2003;93(4): 635–641.

45. Spandorfer JM, Israel Y, Turner BJ. Primary care physicians' views on screening and management of alcohol abuse: inconsistencies with national guidelines. *J Fam Pract.* 1999;48(11):899–902.

46. U.S. Preventive Services Task Force. *Counseling to prevent tobacco use and tobacco-caused disease.* Rockville, MD: Agency for Healthcare Research and Quality; 2003. AHRQ Publication No. 04-0526.

47. Barbor TF, Higgins-Biddle JC, Saunders JB, Monteiro M. *AUDIT: The alcohol use disorders identification test: Guidelines for use in primary health care.* Geneva: World Health Organization; 2001.

48. Bush K, Kivlahan DR, McDonell MB, Fihn SD, Bradley KA. The AUDIT alcohol consumption questions (AUDIT-C): an effective brief screening test for problem drinking. *Arch Intern Med.* 1998;158(16):1789–1795.

49. Reinert DF, Allen JP. The Alcohol Use Disorders Identification Test (AUDIT): a review of recent research. *Alcohol Clin Exp Res.* 2002;26(2):272–279.

50. Reinert DF, Allen JP. The alcohol use disorders identification test: an update of research findings. *Alcohol Clin Exp Res.* 2007;31(2):185–199.

51. Bradley KA, Bush KR, Epler AJ, et al. Two brief alcohol-screening tests from the Alcohol Use Disorders Identification Test (AUDIT): validation in a female Veterans Affairs patient population. *Arch Intern Med.* 2003;163(7):821–829.

52. Bradley KA, Williams EC, Achtmeyer CE, Volpp B, Collins BJ, Kivlahan DR. Implementation of evidence-based alcohol screening in the Veterans Health Administration. *Am J Manag Care.* 2006;12(10):597–606.

53. Dawson DA, Grant BF, Stinson FS. The AUDIT-C: screening for alcohol use disorders and risk drinking in the presence of other psychiatric disorders. *Compr Psychiatry.* 2005;46(6):405–416.

54. Lefforge NL, Donohue B, Strada MJ. Improving session attendance in mental health and substance abuse settings: a review of controlled studies. *Behav Therap.* 2007;38(1):1–22.

55. Festinger DS, Lamb RJ, Kirby KC, Marlowe DB. The accelerated intake: a method for increasing initial attendance to outpatient cocaine treatment. *J Appl Behav Analy.* 1996;29:387–389.

56. Stasiewicz PR, Stalker R. A comparison of three "interventions" on pretreatment dropout rates in an outpatient substance abuse clinic. *Addict Behav.* 1999;24:579–582.

57. Gariti P, Alterman AI, Holub-Beyer E, Volpicelli JR, Prentice N, O'Brien CP. Effects of an appointment reminder call on patient show rates. *J Substan Abuse Treat.* 1995;12:207–212.

58. Zweben A, Bonner M, Chaim G, Stanton P. Facilitative strategies for retaining the alcohol-dependent client in outpatient treatment. *Alcohol Treat Q.* 1988;5:3–23.

59. Zweben A, Li S. The efficacy of role induction in preventing early dropout from outpatient treatment of drug dependency. *Am J Drug Alcohol Abuse.* 1981;8:171–183.

60. Miller D. Addictions and trauma recovery: an integrated approach. *Psychiatric Quarter.* 2002;73(2):157–170.

61. Burke BL, Arkowitz H, Menchola M. The efficacy of motivational interviewing: a meta-analysis of controlled clinical trials. *J Consult Clin Psychol.* 2003;71(5):843–861.
62. Miller WR, Rollnick S. *Motivational interviewing: Preparing people to change addictive behavior.* New York, NY: The Guilford Press; 1991.
63. Kabela E, Kadden RM. Practical strategies for improving client compliance with treatment. In: Carroll KM, ed. *Improving compliance with alcoholism treatment.* Vol NIH publication No. 97-4143. Bethesda, MD: National Institute of Health, National Institute of Alcohol Abuse and Alcoholism (NIAAA); 1997:15–50.
64. Comfort M, Loverro J, Kaltenback K. A search for strategies to engage women in substance abuse treatment. *Soc Work in Health Care.* 2000;31:59–70.
65. Holder HD. Cost benefits of substance abuse treatment: an overview of results from alcohol and drug abuse. *J Ment Health Policy Econ.* 1998;1(1):23–29.
66. French MT. Economic evaluation of drug abuse treatment programs: methodology and findings. *Am J Drug Alcohol Abuse.* 1995;21(1):111–1135.
67. Substance Abuse and Mental Health Services Administration. *Results from the 2004 National Survey of Drug Use and Health: National findings.* Rockville, MD: Office of Applied Studies; 2005. DHHS Publication No. SMA 05-4062.

Chapter 13
Special Considerations of Medication Adherence in Childhood and Adolescence

Alex R. Kemper, Elizabeth Landolfo, and Emmanuel B. Walter

Introduction

Nearly all children and adolescents will at some point require medication therapy for an acute illness, usually a prescribed antibiotic or an over-the-counter medication such as acetaminophen or ibuprofen for symptomatic relief. Many children also require medications for chronic illnesses such as asthma or allergic rhinitis. The number of children with chronic health conditions which could benefit from medication therapy has also been rising [1], due to a wide range of factors such as improved survival of premature infants and the increasing prevalence of childhood obesity.

Identifying strategies to improve medication adherence in children and adolescents must take into account their changing development, the role of parents, autonomy, and the health consequences of nonadherence. In this chapter, we illustrate these considerations through four clinical scenarios: over-the-counter medication use for symptomatic relief of an acute illness; prescription medication use for two prevalent chronic conditions, asthma and attention deficit hyperactivity

A.R. Kemper (✉)
Division of Children's Primary Care, Department of Pediatrics, Duke University Medical Center, Durham, NC, USA
e-mail: kempe006@mc.duke.edu

H. Bosworth (ed.), *Improving Patient Treatment Adherence*,
DOI 10.1007/978-1-4419-5866-2_13,
© Springer Science+Business Media, LLC 2010

disorder (ADHD); and a rare chronic condition, type 1 diabetes mellitus (T1DM). We then conclude by summarizing the key lessons that clinicians can use to foster improved adherence.

Over-the-Counter Medications

Bobby is 18 months old and has had many ear infections. He wakes up at 4 am crying and with a fever. His mom, who is exhausted, reaches into their medicine cabinet and gives ¾ teaspoon of acetaminophen elixir (160 mg per 5 ml). Bobby is still fussy an hour later. His dad, unaware that Bobby has already been given acetaminophen, reaches into the medicine cabinet. He finds that they are running out of elixir, so he gives ¾ teaspoon of acetaminophen concentrated drops (80 mg per 0.8 ml). At 7 am, Bobby's grandmother comes to watch him for the day. Bobby's mother tells the grandmother that Bobby is due to receive another dose of acetaminophen. She takes Bobby to the drug store, where she buys junior strength meltaways (160 mg) and gives one to him in the car on the way to the pediatrician. The pediatrician says that Bobby does not have an ear infection and he likely has a virus. The pediatrician recommends acetaminophen or ibuprofen for symptomatic relief, but does not review dosing instructions.

Over-the-counter medications are usually perceived as safe. However, overdose of drugs like acetaminophen can lead to serious morbidity and rarely even mortality. Acetaminophen is one of the most commonly used of all drugs and a common cause of poisoning. Importantly, up to 26% of acetaminophen overdoses are accidental [2].

Implementing strategies for proper adherence to over-the-counter medications is challenging. There are numerous preparations of even single-ingredient drugs such as acetaminophen or ibuprofen, making specific recommendations about dosing amount difficult. Young children usually take these medications in liquid formulation and such liquids are often difficult to measure appropriately. Errors of dosing frequency and amount can occur as tired parents try to help control fever of their young children over night. Perhaps more concerning is the difference between drug product label dosing for consumers and professional recommendations [3]. The drug product label often recommends doses lower than would be recommended by health-care providers. Such differences may confuse parents and lead to inappropriate dosing.

There are two strategies that have been found in clinical trials to approve adherence with treatment recommendations with over-the-counter medications for young children. A standardized pictogram illustrating dosing improved adherence by overcoming language problems, which is especially important for caregivers with low literacy [4]. A separate study found that color-coded syringes are effective in assuring proper dosage for children [5]. We are not aware of any study that has evaluated strategies to improve adherence with over-the-counter medications specifically in adolescents. This is an important gap because adolescents often self-medicate with these seemingly safe over-the-counter medications.

In our practice, we give parents "dosing cards" during routine preventive visits. These cards describe which formulations of acetaminophen and ibuprofen that we recommend parents keep in their medication cabinet and how the drugs should be administered.

Asthma

Carlos is an 8-year-old with a history of asthma. Every winter since he was 3 years old, Carlos has required at least three visits to the emergency department for asthma flares. Although he has never been hospitalized for asthma, he seems to regularly be treated with oral steroids for his asthma. Carlos has been prescribed two medications for his asthma: albuterol and fluticasone, both as metered dose inhalers. The fact that Carlos' mother has asthma is a great help to the pediatric office and decreases the amount of education that the office needs to provide about signs of asthma flares and acute management. Carlos does not have an asthma action plan. Carlos' mother also understands how to use inhalers. Like she does, Carlos holds the inhaler directly to his mouth and inhales deeply when the inhaler is pressed. Although a spacer device has been prescribed for Carlos, no one has reviewed its use after it was initially recommended when Carlos was 5 years old. No medical staff person has ever observed Carlos using his inhalers.

Asthma is the most common chronic disease of childhood, affecting about five million American children in the United States [6].

Appropriate treatment of asthma often requires daily use of a controller medication and acute uses of a rescue medication during exacerbations of the illness. Because children feel well in between acute exacerbations, adherence to the controller medication is particularly challenging [7]. Overall, fewer than half [7] of children and one-third [8] of adolescents adhere to recommended asthma inhalation medication regimens.

Written asthma action plans that describe steps for both prevention and treatment of asthma have been shown in numerous studies to improve outcomes through better adherence and self-management [9]. Unfortunately, many health-care providers do not provide these. Barriers for providers include lack of knowledge, lack of self-efficacy, and time constraints within the typical short office visit [10]. One of the major challenges that we have found is finding the appropriate time to develop asthma action plans with families. Parents are too distracted to discuss chronic management during an acute exacerbation of asthma. Unfortunately, many families do not follow-up for asthma-related office visits when their children are well, which would be the ideal time to discuss the asthma action plan.

Other important barriers to adherence include the inability to properly use an inhaler [11–15]. Proper technique education is essential for adherence to asthma regimens [16, 17]. One small retrospective study suggests that treatment with an oral controller medication (montelukast) may lead to better adherence than an inhaled controller medication (fluticasone) [18]. However, overall adherence was low, and we would not suggest treatment with montelukast solely for issues of adherence. Training kits are available for use in the office setting to teach children and their caregivers about the proper use of inhalers and spacer devices. In addition, the American Academy of Pediatrics provides educational material for health-care providers and families on the Internet (http://www.aap.org/healthtopics/asthma.cfm).

Adolescents report a wide range of reasons for why they are not adherent with medication, none of which are surprising. These include forgetfulness, denial, and the difficulty and inconvenience of using inhalers [19]. However, these barriers can be reduced. Educational programs for self-management of asthma are effective for both children and adolescents [20]. In our experience, clinicians need to closely partner with parents and their children to develop an individualized plan to transition to independence over time and need to continually emphasize proper asthma care at both acute care and health maintenance visits.

Attention Deficit Hyperactivity Disorder (ADHD)

Mary is in the fourth grade and her teacher has noted that Mary's behavior and academic performance are inconsistent. At times she is inattentive and disruptive in class. Mary's former teachers are surprised to hear that she is having so many problems. The teachers remembered that Mary has ADHD and that she was taking methylphenidate in the morning before coming to school and again at lunch time. The teachers also remembered that sometimes the medication ran out at the beginning of each month, during which time Mary had some problems. After a few days, however, the medication was back and Mary was a fine student. The fourth grade teachers had a conversation with Mary's mother about the behavior problems during which time they learned that Mary's parents have recently divorced and have a joint custody arrangement. Although Mary's mother gives the methylphenidate in the morning, Mary's father is opposed to such medication and does not give it to Mary when she stays with him.

Estimates of the prevalence of ADHD range from 4 to 12% during childhood [21]. Stimulant medication therapy is an important component of care for many children [22]. Unfortunately, the rate of non-adherence with stimulant medication can be high [23]. Carefully assessing adherence among those with ADHD is particularly important to avoid inappropriate dose escalation.

In our experience, there are numerous factors that may contribute to poor adherence to stimulant medications. First, by the nature of the condition, remembering to take the medication can be challenging. For example, those with co-morbid oppositional defiant disorder are much more likely to discontinue therapy [24]. Stimulant medications are controlled substances requiring new prescriptions monthly, causing barriers to timely and convenient prescription refills. Some families are concerned about the risks of stimulant therapy and therefore discontinue its use [25], sometimes surreptitiously. There may also be disagreement between parents about the use of stimulant medications for ADHD. Children of divorced or separated parents with joint custody arrangements face additional logistical challenges to medication adherence. When children transition from one parent's house to another, medications can often be forgotten or left behind. Lastly, some parents and children complain about stimulant medication side effects such as loss of appetite, weight loss, or they don't like the way the medication makes them feel.

Some evidence suggests that extended-release stimulant medication which requires only once-daily treatment improves adherence [23]. Unfortunately, these long-acting medications are more expensive than short acting ones and may not be covered by health insurance. It is a major challenge for clinicians to keep track of which, if any, extended-release stimulant medications are included on the formulary of the major health plans that cover their patients.

We have found that the best strategy for improving adherence is to work carefully with families to help them develop systems for assuring adherence. Often this also involves the school system for those children that require a midday stimulant dose. It is also critical to have a system within the medical office to facilitate timely new prescriptions for families. Furthermore, families must understand how the system works, including when and how the families should contact the office. Also it is important to acknowledge parental disagreements about stimulant medication use, educate parents and children about known medication side effects, weigh the potential risks and benefits of medication therapy, and teach strategies to ameliorate potential side effects.

Type 1 Diabetes Mellitus (T1DM)

Hannah is a 17-year-old girl with T1DM. Until this year, her T1DM has always been under excellent control and outside of when she was first diagnosed at age 11, Hannah has never been hospitalized. Her parents feel that they should get a lot of credit for her excellent diabetes management because they directly oversee most of the care. Hannah silently disagrees and feels that she should get more credit for making wise decisions about diet and exercise. Her parents realize that Hannah will soon be leaving home for college, which will be at least 300 miles away. Hannah's parents want to help her foster independence but are worried about her having worsening control. This has been a source of many arguments at home. Over the year, Hannah has taken more charge of her diabetes care. Hannah sometimes forgets to check her blood sugar levels, especially during the weekend when she spends more time with her friends. Furthermore, she is embarrassed to give herself insulin. Hannah wonders if she could get an insulin pump, which she thinks might be less obtrusive.

About 1 or 2 children per 1,000 have T1DM [26]. The management of T1DM is complex and in addition to the central role of insulin therapy requires regular monitoring of blood glucose levels and close attention to diet, exercise, overall health, and growth. Adherence to all components of diabetes care is often considered to be poor. However, there is great opportunity to help affected individuals and their families with the complexity of care imposed by T1DM.

Family and child education plays a central role in the management of T1DM [27]. Education has to be continuous and adjusted to the development of the child. Although school-aged children can assume some management tasks, parent support is important throughout adolescence [27]. As with asthma care, transition to independence needs to be personalized and planned for well in advance. Some children and adolescents as well as their families benefit from psychological support services to help with diabetes management and transition to independence.

In addition to educational and psychological support, new technology such as the insulin pump can facilitate adherence to T1DM treatment [28]. However, these devices require protection and are not fully automated, requiring adjustment to the amount of insulin that is provided. Studies have shown that insulin pumps can be safely used in young children with parental involvement [29] and that insulin pumps may be particularly important in allowing for transition to independence among adolescents [30].

Summary

Regardless of the medication indication, developmentally appropriate, family-centered education is critical to improving adherence. We believe that these issues of adherence need to be considered at all patient encounters, and issues related to family dynamics are of critical importance. Clearly, some strategies for improving adherence are outside of what can be modified by clinicians. These include improving drug product labels and dosing formulations. However, there are several important opportunities to improve adherence through office-based activities.

First, we recommend that all health-care providers actively reconcile all medications that their patients receive and where possible, simplify the regimen. This includes minimizing dose frequency where possible. During this reconciliation process, health-care providers should ask families about barriers to and facilitators of adherence.

We recommend that practices routinely counsel families and separately adolescents about the role of over-the-counter medications and provide easy-to-read documents about appropriate dosing. These forms should include a review of the indications and risks for these medications. We strongly advocate providing the contact information for the local poison control center on these documents and discussing the role of such centers.

Family education about how to use medications, especially those that are not just swallowed is critical. Practices should have demonstration kits available and patients taking such medications should routinely be asked to demonstrate their ability to appropriately use them. Health-care providers should also be aware of community resources for education of chronic medical conditions.

Practices should not be a barrier to medication refills for chronic medical conditions. Careful systems need to be put in place to facilitate refills while at the same time not allow families to miss necessary follow-up appointments by simply always getting refills.

Transition to self-management is an important component of assuring adherence for chronic conditions which persist into adulthood. The strategy of such transitions will depend on many considerations, including the developmental status of the adolescent, family support, the condition, and the complexity of care. We believe that planning for the transition begins much earlier than when it will occur and that families are involved in the planning process.

References

1. van Dyck PC, Kogan MD, McPherson MG, Weissman GR, Newacheck PW. Prevalence and characteristics of children with special health care needs. *Arch Pediatr Adolesc Med.* 2004;158:884–890.
2. Nourjah P, Ahmad SR, Karwoski C, Willy M. Estimates of acetaminophen (paracetamol)-associated overdoses in the United States. *Pharmacoepidemiol Drug Saf.* 2006;15:398–405.

3. Orr KK, Matson KL, Cowles BJ. Nonprescription medication use by infants and children: product labeling versus evidence-based medicine. *J Pharm Pract*. 2006;19:286–294.
4. Yin HS, Dreyer BP, vanSchaick L, Foltin GL, Dinglas C, Mendelsohn AL. Randomized controlled trial of a pictogram-based intervention to reduce liquid medication dosing errors and improve adherence among caregivers of young children. *Arch Pediatr Adolesc Med*. 2008;162:814–822.
5. Frush KS, Luo X, Hutchinson P, Higgins JN. Evaluation of a method to reduce over-the-counter medication dosing error. *Arch Pediatr Adolesc Med*. 2004;158:620–624.
6. Redd SC. Asthma in the United States: burden and current theories. *Environ Health Perspect*. 2002;110:557–560.
7. Bender BG. Overcoming barriers to nonadherence in asthma treatment. *J Allergy Clin Immunol*. 2002;109:S554–S559.
8. Burkhart PV, Sabate E. Adherence to long-term therapies: evidence for action. *J Nurs Scholarsh*. 2003;35:207.
9. Gibson PG, Powell H. Written action plans for asthma: an evidence-based review of the key components. *Thorax*. 2004;59:94–99.
10. Cabana MD, Rand CS, Becher OJ, Rubin HR. Reasons for pediatrician nonadherence to asthma guidelines. *Arch Pediatr Adolesc Med*. 2001;155: 1057–1062.
11. Buck M. Improving compliance with medication regimens. *Pediatr Pharmacother*. 1997;3:1–3.
12. Rand CS, Wise RA. Measuring adherence to asthma medication regimens. *Am J Respir Crit Care Med*. 1994;149:S69–S76.
13. Kelloway JS, Wyatt RA, Adlis SA. Comparison of patients' compliance with prescribed oral and inhaled asthma medications. *Arch Intern Med*. 1994;154:1349–1352.
14. Weinstein AG. Clinical management strategies to maintain drug compliance in asthmatic children. *Ann Allergy Asthma Immunol*. 1995;74:304–310.
15. Farber HJ, Capra AM, Finkelstein JA, et al. Misunderstanding of asthma controller medications: association with nonadherence. *J Asthma*. 2003;40:17–25.
16. Fish L, Lung CL. Adherence to asthma therapy. *Ann Allergy Asthma Immunol*. 2001;86:24–30.
17. Celano M, Geller RJ, Phillips KM, Ziman R. Treatment adherence among low-income children with asthma. *J Pediatr Psychol*. 1998;23:345–349.
18. Sherman J, Patel P, Hutson A, Chesrown S, Hendeles L. Adherence to oral montelukast and inhaled fluticasone in children with persistent asthma. *Pharmacotherapy*. 2001;21:1464–1467.
19. Buston KM, Wood SF. Non-compliance amongst adolescents with asthma: listening to what they tell us about self-management. *Fam Prac*. 2000;17: 134–138.
20. Guevara JP, Wolf FM, Grum CM, Clark NM. Effects of educational interventions for self management of asthma in children and adolescents: systematic review and meta-analysis. *BMJ*. 2003;326:1308–1309.

21. Brown RT, Freeman WS, Perrin JM, et al. Prevalence and assessment of attention-deficit/hyperactivity disorder in primary care settings. *Pediatrics.* 2001;107:e43.

22. Jensen PS, Hinshaw SP, Swanson JM, et al. Findings from the NIMH Multimodal Treatment Study of ADHD (MTA): implications and applications for primary care providrs. *J Dev Behav Pediatr.* 2001;22:60–73.

23. Swanson J. Compliance with stimulants for attention-deficit/hyperactivity disorder: issues and approaches for improvement. *CNS Drugs.* 2003;17:117–131.

24. Thiruchelvam D, Charach A, Schachar RJ. Moderators and mediators of long-term adherence to stimulant treatment in children with ADHD. *J Am Acad Child Adolesc Psychiatry.* 2001;40:922–928.

25. Berger I, Dor T, Nevo Y, Goldzweig G. Attitudes toward attention-deficit hyperactivity disorder (ADHD) treatment: parents' and children's perspectives. *J Child Neurol.* 23:1036–1042.

26. Kemper AR, Dombkowski KJ, Menon RK, Davis MM. Trends in diabetes mellitus among privately insured children, 1998–2002. *Ambul Pediatr.* 2006;6:178–181.

27. Silverstein J, Klingensmith G, Copeland K, et al. Care of children and adolescents with type 1 diabetes. *Diabetes Care.* 2005;28:186–212.

28. Scheiner G, Sobel RJ, Smith DE, et al. Insulin pump therapy: guidelines for successful outcomes. *Diabetes Educ.* 2009;35:29S–41S.

29. Plotnick LP, Clark LM, Brancati FL, Erlinger T. Safety and effectiveness of insulin pump therapy in children and adolescents with type 1 diabetes. *Diabetes Care.* 2003;26:1142–1146.

30. Low KG, Massa L, Lehman D, Olshan JS. Insulin pump use in young adolescents with type 1 diabetes: a descriptive study. *Pediatric Diabetes.* 2005;6:22–31.

Chapter 14
Special Considerations of Adherence in Older Adults

S. Nicole Hastings, Janine C. Kosmoski, and Jason M. Moss

Optimizing medication adherence is a significant challenge for clinicians caring for older adults, particularly those with multiple chronic health conditions. Nearly half of all adults aged 65 or older take five or more medications regularly; however, adherence to chronic pharmacological therapies is often poor [1]. Overall, 40% of older Medicare beneficiaries reported one or more forms of medication non-adherence in the previous year [1]. Older patients are often more susceptible to the outcomes of poor adherence including worsening symptoms of disease and disease severity, increased hospital admissions, costs, and mortality [2, 3]. Older adults face many of the barriers to adherence discussed in previous chapters; however, age-related physical or cognitive impairments, multiple chronic health conditions, and/or complex treatment regimens frequently create distinct challenges related to adherence in this population. The aims of this chapter are to discuss special considerations related to medication adherence in older adults and to offer practical advice for improving medication adherence in this population.

S.N. Hastings (✉)
Geriatrics, Duke University Medical Center, Durham, NC, USA
e-mail: hasti003@mc.duke.edu

H. Bosworth (ed.), *Improving Patient Treatment Adherence*,
DOI 10.1007/978-1-4419-5866-2_14,
© Springer Science+Business Media, LLC 2010

Barriers and Challenges

Physiological Barriers to Adherence

Older adults often develop physical limitations such as decreased vision and hearing, reduced manual dexterity, and impaired cognition that can have a negative impact on adherence. Visual, hearing, and cognitive deficits create communication barriers between patient and provider, so that patients may not fully understand what treatment is being recommended, the rationale for the treatment, and/or instructions for how to carry it out. Visual and manual dexterity problems can also lead to problems taking medications as prescribed (e.g., reading labels and opening pill bottles). Patients with cognitive impairments may have difficulty not only obtaining information but also retaining it (e.g., remembering to schedule appointments or take scheduled medications).

Visual impairment. One-third of older adults have a chronic disease that can lead to vision problems such as macular degeneration, diabetes, glaucoma, or cataracts [4]. Among all adults aged 65 and older the prevalence of visual impairment is approximately 17% [5]. Among nursing home residents, it is even higher at 26% [6]. Visual deficits can result in improper medication use because of inability to recognize medications by color or shape and difficulty reading labels on pill bottles. Additionally, misinterpretation of clinicians' written instructions or other educational materials can occur.

Hearing impairment. Hearing impairment is a common problem and its prevalence increases with age. Approximately 28% of community-dwelling seniors aged 65–79 and 37% of those aged 80 or older have hearing loss [5]. Difficulty with speech comprehension is one of the early consequences of age-related decline in hearing [7]; thus, patient/provider communication can be compromised, which in turn can have a negative impact on treatment adherence.

Reduced manual dexterity. About 1 in 15 seniors report difficulty with grasping objects or writing [8]. Motor impairment may be even more common in patients who suffer from cognitive decline or dementia [9]. Many seniors suffer from chronic diseases such as osteo- and rheumatoid arthritis, neuropathies from chronic diseases, or general joint stiffness that contribute to these motor deficits [10]. Reduced manual dexterity can affect adherence by making it difficult for patients to manipulate medication packaging such as vial caps or blister packs or pill organizers.

Impaired cognition. Cognitive impairments in older adults span a broad clinical spectrum, ranging from subtle deficits to disabling dementia. Although mild cognitive impairment can be difficult to detect, it often has a serious effect on patients' ability to understand and follow through with treatment recommendations. Impairment in executive function, defined as higher order cognitive abilities involved with the planning and monitoring of goal-directed activities and problem solving, has been shown to predict miscomprehension of medical information [11]. Impaired memory is also correlated with reduced adherence [12]. Patients with memory deficits can have difficulty remembering to take medications or inadvertently overuse medications. Patients with more severe dementia may have caregivers to observe or supervise medication administration, but these individuals can still experience adherence problems because of inadequate education and preparation of caregivers or patient resistance to taking medications.

Complexity of Regimen

Older adults who have several chronic conditions (i.e., multimorbidity) often have complex treatment regimens that include multiple prescription medications, a myriad of lifestyle interventions, and frequent testing and follow-up appointments [13]. Older adults with multimorbidity have worse adherence when compared to well elders [1], likely related to polypharmacy, medication side effects, multiple providers, and frequent health-care transitions.

Polypharmacy. Nearly 75% of complex, chronically ill seniors take five or more prescription medications [1]. Because elderly patients often require many medications to treat multiple disease states, it is problematic to define polypharmacy based on a predetermined number of medications [14]. Defined as the "prescription, administration, and/or use of more medications than clinically indicated" [14–16], polypharmacy is very common among older adults. Studies from a variety of clinical settings have shown that 40–60% of older adults received at least one unnecessary prescription medication [17] and that one of the main consequences of polypharmacy is non-adherence [14].

Medication side effects. Older adults frequently report that adverse experiences with medications lead to non-adherence [1]. Overall, 25% of older adults reported skipping doses or stopping a medication because it was making them feel worse or because they did not feel it was helping [1]. Older patients are particularly susceptible to adverse effects from renally cleared medications because chronic kidney disease is prevalent, and often unrecognized, in this population [18]. Polypharmacy is also a well-established risk factor for drug interactions and adverse drug effects [19]. Patients with dementia may have reduced ability to report early adverse effects from medications, which could increase their risk for developing more severe problems [20].

Multiple providers/transitions. More than half of older adults have received prescriptions from more than one provider, and many also receive medications from more than one pharmacy [1].Because of multimorbidity, older patients are commonly treated by several clinicians, but having multiple prescribers has been associated with greater risk of unnecessary medication use and adverse drug effects. Health-care transitions, such as discharge from the hospital, have also been associated with adverse drug events, which in turn contribute to poor adherence [21].

Low Health Literacy

Low health literacy, defined as the inability to obtain, process, and understand the basic health information needed to make appropriate health decisions [22], is prevalent in many populations, but it is especially problematic in older adults. Approximately one-third of Medicare enrollees aged 65 years or older were found to have inadequate or marginal health literacy [23]. General reading ability is also lower among older adults. In certain patient populations, such as in urban public hospitals, the prevalence of inadequate or marginal functional health literacy has been reported as high as 82% [24]. Reduced literacy and health literacy contributes to non-adherence by making it difficult for patients to read prescription bottle labels, appointment slips, and written instructions from providers. Low health literacy has also been shown to dissuade patients from playing an active role in the decision-making process and to make them feel that they lacked the knowledge to make a contribution to health-care decisions [25].

High Costs

Cost remains a barrier to treatment adherence for many older patients, despite the implementation of Medicare Part D. In the biggest change to the Medicare system since its establishment in 1965, Medicare Part D, a prescription drug benefit, was launched in January 2006 in an effort to help seniors afford medications [26]. Although there is some evidence that cost-related medication non-adherence decreased after the start of Medicare Part D (14% in 2005, 11.5% in 2006), cost still leads to non-adherence in one out of every nine seniors [27]. Among Medicare beneficiaries with poor to fair baseline health, cost-related medication non-adherence was 22%, and this number did not change after the launch of Medicare Part D [27].

Interventions

Review of Screening Methods

The most common method of screening for non-adherence is information garnered in clinical practice from patient or caregiver interview. This is understandable because there is no gold standard for measuring medication adherence in seniors [28], but there are limitations to this approach. Patient self-report may not be a useful assessment tool if close-ended questions are used, such as "Do you take all your medications as prescribed?" Faced with this type of question, most patients will answer "yes" and, thus, true adherence cannot be assessed [28, 29].

Other methods of assessing adherence include pill count, prescription claims processing reports, and electronic monitoring. All of these methods have the advantage of brevity, but there are caveats to their use. Pill counts can give an overall estimate of adherence, but do not provide information about the timing of doses. This method has also been shown to lead to "pill dumping" before pill count visits which overestimates adherence [30]. Pill counts can also underestimate adherence if patients get prescriptions filled early [31]. Refill records confirm that a patient is getting their medications refilled, but do not give information about correct administration or missed doses.

In addition, refill records prove most helpful when a patient fills all of their medications at a single pharmacy, which is not always the case. Electronic monitoring is a novel method to track medication adherence and may be the most reliable since it records the time and date a medication vial was opened; however, an opened vial does not necessarily correspond to adherence with that dose. Furthermore electronic or microchip medication vials are not useful for patients who use pillboxes and may not be easily accessible due to cost [29].

Screening for medication-taking ability. A slightly different approach is to screen older adults for their *ability* to be adherent to a medication regimen. It can be hard to disentangle intentional non-adherence from patient error; therefore, a number of tools have been developed aimed at evaluating patients' medication-management skills [32]. One of these tools is the Drug Regimen Unassisted Grading Scale (DRUGS) [33]. The performance-based DRUGS tool evaluates a patient's ability to identify their own medications, open the container, remove the appropriate dosage, and demonstrate the appropriate timing of administration with each of their prescription and over-the-counter medications. The DRUGS tool has demonstrated reliability and has been correlated with cognition [33, 34], but its usefulness in clinical practice has yet to be established.

Review of General Medication Adherence Improvement Strategies

Many different types of programs have been developed to enhance adherence among older adults, with somewhat mixed results. One challenge in interpreting these data is that relatively few studies have tested *single* strategies for improving adherence among older patients. Adherence improvement programs tend to be complex and multi-faceted; therefore, it can be difficult to disentangle the most effective components of an intervention. Much of the data from smaller trials on adherence improvement strategies have been synthesized in systematic review articles which shed light on the most important strategies for improving adherence among elderly patients [35–37].

Education. Patient education has been described as a necessary, but not sufficient step in improving patient adherence. In one study performed in ambulatory, chronically ill older patients, receiving copies of physician office visit notes made no difference in their adherence to medication regimens [38]. On the other hand, some form of medication education has been included in the majority of interventions that have been shown to improve medication taking in elderly patients [35]. A variety of forms of education have been studied, including face-to-face verbal, telephone- and computer-mediated, and written, without clear consensus on the preferred method. Few studies have described explicit involvement of families and caregivers in education strategies to improve medication adherence [35].

Simplification of regimen. Simplification of the drug and/or dosage regimen is widely regarded as a prudent strategy for improving medication adherence, although this has been most commonly studied as part of multicomponent interventions. One literature review noted that relatively few studies had employed dose reduction or simplification, but that those that did frequently reported significant improvements in medication adherence [35]. The dose modification interventions most commonly reported were changing dosing from three to two times daily or from twice daily to once daily.

Adherence aids. Adherence aids are frequently used in clinical practice, yet there is little data to suggest which patients may derive the most benefit from them. The most commonly used adherence aids are drug reminder systems (pill organizers, etc.) that rely on filling by patients or caregivers, although in some cases, pharmacy or nursing staff may provide this service. Other adherence aids include special packaging such as multi-medication blister packs. Blister packs organize medications in a disposable punch card according to daily dosing times. These serve the same purpose as traditional pill organizers except that patients do not have to work with multiple medication bottles. Blister packaging has been used as part of successful comprehensive programs to improve adherence, but it is not known how important this part of the intervention was [39]. There is little data to compare the effectiveness of pill organizer to blister packs. One study involving vitamin supplements found that pill organizers did not improve adherence, but blister packs did, particularly among those with lower baseline adherence [40]. Pill organizers are widely available at low cost to patients and families; however, they require that someone knowledgeable fill these containers. Blister packs may not be ideal when frequent dosage adjustments are required, and their cost-effectiveness is not known.

Pharmacy-led interventions. Many pharmacy-led interventions have shown improvements in medication adherence among older adults. In one study from the UK, a single telephone call from a pharmacist reduced self-reported non-adherence in patients 75 and older who were prescribed new medication for a chronic condition [41, 42]. Two reviews have also concluded that pharmacist-led medication review has a positive effect on adherence and on reducing unnecessary drug use [36, 37]. In these studies, medication review often included counseling patients on medications, giving advice on adherence, checking for drug efficacy and adverse events, and optimizing the medication regimen [36]. One of the largest and most rigorous trials of pharmacy-led interventions demonstrated that a comprehensive pharmacy care program could increase medication adherence by 35% among older patients taking at least four chronic medications [39]. The pharmacy care program in this study consisted of 6 months of standardized medication education, regular follow-up by pharmacists, and medications delivered in time-specific blister packs.

New Technologies and Advances in Health-Care Delivery

A number of technological advances have been developed to augment medication adherence. For example, automated and/or electronic medication reminder systems have been developed [29]. Devices are available that attach to standard pharmacy vial caps, metered dose inhalers, or pill boxes to emit reminder tones when it is time for the patient to take their medication. Pager-like devices and digital watches with reminder systems are also available. None of these devices are currently in widespread use and cost remains a barrier to wider dissemination.

Recent changes in the health-care delivery system have also aimed to improve adherence among older adults. The Medicare Modernization Act (MMA) of 2003 established that all Medicare Part D sponsors must develop and maintain Medication Therapy Management (MTM) programs. Beneficiaries targeted for MTM services include those who have multiple chronic diseases, are taking multiple Medicare Part D drugs, and are likely to spend a predetermined amount of money for all covered Medicare Part D drugs (the annual cost threshold was set at $4000 in 2006). Individual plans have the flexibility to select eligible disease states and methods of intervention. In 2008, over 98% of all MTM plans were utilizing pharmacists to conduct interventions that ranged from polypharmacy screenings to educational newsletters [43]. Adherence is one important outcome that MTM programs are designed to improve, but most programs have not yet reported on clinical outcomes.

Clinical Implications

Screening for Adherence

The recommended method for discussing adherence with patients and caregivers is using open-ended phrases such as "Tell me how you take your medications." This type of statement is non-judgmental, and will give the provider insight into the patient's true knowledge and understanding of their medication regimen [44]. Similarly, when a lifestyle intervention has been recommended, this is a useful way to begin the discussion (e.g., "Tell me about your walking program"). Although there is insufficient evidence to suggest a screening tool for medication-taking ability like the DRUGS for all patients, asking the patient to demonstrate how they take their medicines can be useful for identifying physiological barriers to adherence such as impaired manual dexterity. In this case, the opening phrase can be adapted to "Show me how you take your medications".

A crucial element of effective screening for adherence is the timing. For all new medications, the follow-up visit should include questioning about adherence, including specific queries about side effects and an assessment of whether the drug is effective. An often overlooked, but important concept is the patient's perception of whether the medication is working. If the medication is treating an asymptomatic condition such as hypertension, the clinician should give feedback about how they are monitoring the drug's effect, and whether there is any indication that the medication has been effective (e.g., "Since starting this medicine, your blood pressure has come down, so that tells me it's working"). For patients who take medications chronically, but have not started new ones or changed the dose, adherence screening should be performed routinely, usually once or twice per year. Screening for medication adherence is a task that can be performed well by many different types of health professionals including physicians, physician assistants, nurse practitioners, nurses, or pharmacists. For providers in integrated health systems with access to electronic medication information, refill records can also provide information about patients that may need more in-depth questioning about their medications.

Addressing Barriers and Challenges

Early recognition is the key for managing age-related physiological barriers to adherence.

Vision and hearing impairment. Routine eye examinations have been associated with reduced decline in visual and functional ability [45]. For patients with vision problems, interventions such as increased font size and use of only black and white ink colors on printed educational material can be helpful. Encouraging patients to use magnification devices as needed to read labels and fill pill organizers may also help improve adherence. Similarly, hearing examinations and hearing aids, when appropriate, can improve office communication about recommended interventions. Clinicians may also consider keeping equipment in the office, such as portable amplifiers, to facilitate communication. Various models of portable amplifiers, sometimes referred to as "pocket talkers," are available but common elements include a microphone and earphone or headphones.

Reduced manual dexterity. Evaluating and treating pain associated with conditions such as arthritis that contributes to reduce manual dexterity may be sufficient to restore the patient's ability to manipulate medication containers. For patients with chronic musculoskeletal or neurologic conditions that impair hand coordination, patients can request "easy off" caps from their pharmacy to make opening medication bottles easier, although this requires extra vigilance to keep medications out of the reach of young children. An alternative strategy is to engage a caregiver or family member to take over responsibility of filling a pill organizer (provided this is easier for the patient to manipulate).

Cognitive impairment. The Mini Mental State Examination (MMSE) is a well-known and useful tool for screening for cognitive impairment in a clinic setting. All patients who are known to have cognitive impairment or dementia should have a regular assessment of how they are taking their medications, and whether they are receiving any assistance with this task. Cognitively impaired patients without a caregiver assisting with medication management should be provided with an adherence aid such as a pill organizer or multi-dose medication blister packs.

The majority of cognitively impaired older adults do receive some level of assistance with medication management from caregivers [46], and this should be encouraged. Patients with memory disorders who rely on a caregiver have been shown to have higher adherence compared to those who do not [47]. Some medications such as bis-phosphonates require specific instructions for safe administration (e.g., take with water, remain sitting upright after ingestion). Inability to fol-low these instructions and potential delay in reporting adverse effects can introduce safety concerns as well as adherence problems [48].

Engaging caregivers. Caregivers often handle medications for seniors due to physical frailty, cognitive impairments, personal prefer-ence, or a combination of these factors. Thus, it is crucial to understand who has medication responsibility and to engage directly with a care-giver who has been given this charge. Make a specific plan with the caregiver about how they will assist the patient (will they cue patients, fill pill organizers, supervise medication administration, etc.). Educate caregivers about potential adverse effects of medications, so that they can monitor for signs of distress. If patients with dementia are resistant to taking medications, discuss the pros and cons of alternative deliv-ery strategies such as skin patches, if it is a medication that the patient needs to continue to take. Finally, recognize that managing the health of an older person can be a tremendous burden for caregivers; mon-itor for caregiver stress and recommend local support groups. Local chapters of the Alzheimer's Association often host support groups that can be a very helpful resource for caregivers who have a difficult time getting their loved ones to take needed medications.

Limited health literacy. Low health literacy is so prevalent among older adults that a "universal precautions" approach is preferable to implementing specific screening measures [49]. A "universal precau-tions" approach means that clinicians make it routine practice to use language and written communication materials that are appropriate for individuals with limited health literacy, without trying to determine the literacy level of each individual [49]. Physicians often use words that patients do not understand [50]. Clinicians should reflect on their communication and interview styles and ensure that they are using lay language as much as possible and avoiding or explaining terminology that may be unfamiliar to patients and families. Keep in mind that caregivers may also have limited health literacy. Communication methods such as the "teach back," asking patients or surrogates to repeat key information in their own words, are useful strategies for ensuring that patients and families have heard and processed the information appropriately [51, 52].

Reducing Complexity of Regimen

Prescriber interventions. All patients on chronic medications should have regular medication reviews. Medication review can be facilitated by encouraging patients to bring their medications with them to their appointment. Medication management in older adults is a dynamic ongoing process. It begins with careful attention to prescribing, but must be followed by frequent reevaluation of indications and outcomes of prescribing. The key step in medication review is eliminating unnecessary medications. Unnecessary medications may end up on an older adults' regimen for many reasons. For example, a sleeping medication used in the hospital may not be required once the patient has returned to his or her home environment. Patients may lose weight and require less medication to control chronic diseases such as diabetes or hypertension. Goals of care may also change, such that patients receiving palliative or end-of-life care may wish to forgo medications for primary prevention of disease such as cholesterol-lowering agents. Medication review should also include monitoring for duplicative therapy (two or medications of the same drug class) and drug interactions and to ensure that the lowest effective dose is being used. The plan for monitoring medications also needs review, that is, the plan for watching for the occurrence of adverse consequences and for evaluating the drugs' effectiveness [53].

Interdisciplinary team care. Nurses and pharmacists are invaluable members of interdisciplinary teams who can play an important role in optimizing medication adherence. In order to take full advantage of pharmacy providers, encourage patients to get their medications at one pharmacy. This minimizes the risk of missed therapeutic duplications or drug interactions and increases the likelihood that patients will build a relationship with a pharmacist. In settings with access to a clinical pharmacist for medication review or adherence counseling, utilize this resource. Nurses can perform a variety of tasks related to adherence, from screening to education. In some clinics, nurses fill pill organizers for patients who have particular difficulty performing this task.

Continuity and coordination of care. Older patients frequently transition between health-care settings. Providers should perform medication reconciliation after each health-care transition to minimize unnecessary drug use which leads to low adherence. It is well known that older patients receive medications from multiple providers; acknowledging and monitoring chronic medications that are started by other providers is a crucial piece of high-quality medication management for vulnerable elders [54]. Patients should also be encouraged to maintain a list of their active medications and to share this with all providers they encounter in all settings. Although review of individual medication containers may be ideal, reviewing a medication list is a reasonable alternative when providers do not have time to perform a "brown-bag" medication review.

Managing Costs

The most important intervention in managing costs is to talk openly about it with patients. Patients may feel embarrassed admitting difficulty affording their prescriptions and may find ways to save money by altering administration instructions to "stretch out their supply." Simply asking patients if they are able to afford medications and offering help, if needed, can be the first step toward increased adherence.

Cost-efficient prescribing. Forecasting problems for patients at the pharmacy counter may not always be possible, but there are concrete steps that providers can take to reduce the risk of this occurring. Encourage patients to bring their prescription insurance's formulary with them to office visits to facilitate cost-efficient prescribing. Formularies provide information about medication co-payment tiers, limitations, and restrictions including prior authorization, quantity limits, and step therapy. Knowing where to locate formulary information can be invaluable. Most Part D plans post their formularies online at the plan's Web site or can be found at Medicare's Web site www.medicare.gov. If formulary information is not available while writing a prescription, prescribing a generic medication can help to control costs for a patient. When a generic is not available, simply informing a patient that the prescribed medication may not be covered and establishing a plan of what the patient should do in this circumstance will lead to less frustration at the pharmacy.

Medicare Part D. Although a full review of the Medicare Part D benefit is beyond the scope of this chapter, it is important for providers to understand the basics of what this program does and does not offer seniors and where to go for more information. Some Medicare health plans (such as Medicare Advantage or Program of All-Inclusive Care for the Elderly) include prescription drug coverage. However, most beneficiaries do not participate in one of these plans, and thus must enroll in a free-standing prescription drug plan (PDP), which are offered by insurance companies that are approved by Medicare.

Patients should be encouraged to evaluate their Medicare Part D Plan every year during open enrollment from November 15 to December 31 to ensure that their current plan continues to be their most cost-effective option. Plans change every year which may cause patients' costs to go up even if they stay in the same plan and stay on the same medications. Individuals who are eligible for both Medicaid and Medicare, known as dual eligibles, are automatically enrolled in Medicare Part D and assigned a plan without consideration of their current medication regimen. It is especially important for a dual eligible to review their plan's formulary and consider switching plans if necessary. Dually eligible individuals have the ability to change plans once a month and are not restricted to the November 15 to December 31 open enrollment period.

While Medicare Part D was created to help seniors pay for prescriptions drugs, it does not come without its drawbacks. For example, when a patient's medication costs have reached an initial coverage limit termed the coverage gap or "donut hole" they must pay the full cost of their prescriptions without the aid of their drug plan. Patients with high medication costs should consider enrolling in a plan that offers some help during the coverage gap. Reviewing a patient's medication list and switching from a brand name to a generic alternative in the same or alternative class can also prove helpful. Many Medicare Part D plans offer Mail-Order Pharmacy Services that could save patients a considerable amount of money. However, this method of cost savings may come at a cost of lost monthly interaction with their community pharmacist. Patients who have hit the coverage gap may benefit from a referral to an available resource such as a social worker, State Health Insurance Program (SHIP), Medicare, or a community outreach program [55].When medically necessary medications are not covered under a patient's plan, Medicare Part D offers an appeals process. Additional information on Medicare Part D can be found at the Medicare Web site at www.medicare.gov or by calling the Medicare Hotline at 1-800-Medicare.

Payment assistance programs. Many state assistance programs and other community support resources, often at the county level, are available to help patients pay for prescription medications. State Pharmaceutical Assistance Programs (SPAP), established under the MMA, utilize state funds to pay for the cost of medications for specific groups of people who meet eligibility criteria. SPAPs provide secondary drug coverage to help pay monthly premiums, co-insurance or co-payments, annual deductibles, and coverage gap costs. State discount cards are also available to help patients pay for medication.

The US Social Security Administration also offers help for medication costs for certain Medicare beneficiaries who have limited income and resources through low-income subsidies (LIS). In order to be eligible, patients must be enrolled in a Medicare Part D PDP and must meet certain annual income and resource limits. Details about eligibility and application forms (*Application for Help with Medicare Prescription Drug Plan Costs* (SSA-1020)) are available at the Social Security Web site: http://www.ssa.gov/, by calling Social Security at: 1-800-772-1213 or in local Social Security Offices.

Lastly, patient assistance programs (PAPs) are programs set up by drug companies to offer free or low-cost medications to those who cannot afford them. These programs are limited to brand name drugs only. All major drug companies have PAPs, and eligibility and application requirements differ between plans. Generally, individuals must have incomes less than 200% of the federal poverty level, cannot have prescription coverage from any private/public source, and must be a US resident (some require that individuals do not have health insurance). Those with Part D benefits may or may not be eligible. Most people receiving LIS are not eligible; a letter from Social Security stating an individual is not eligible to receive LIS benefits is often required. Detailed information including applications can be found online at the Patient Assistance Program Center Web site: www.rxassist.org.

Summary and Recommendations for Clinicians

- Be alert to special barriers and challenges to medication adherence among older adults, especially vision, hearing, and cognitive impairments, limited health literacy, and costs.
- Use open-ended questions when asking patients and families about adherence. Consider asking patients to demonstrate medication management tasks (e.g., opening pill bottles, filling pill box).
- When providing information about medications or therapies, involve family members whenever possible. Use strategies such as the "teach back," to assess patient and family understanding of the new information.
- After starting any new medication, schedule a follow-up visit to ask about adverse effects and elicit the patient's perspective of whether the medication is working.
- Review medication lists regularly with the goal of reducing unnecessary medication use, using the lowest effective dose and making the regimen as simple and inexpensive as possible.
- Refer patients with low medication adherence to a comprehensive medication management program if available or engage other members of the interdisciplinary health team such as nurses or pharmacists to develop adherence support mechanisms.
- Use generic formulations and formulary choices from Medicare Part D (or other) drug plans to minimize financial barriers to adherence. Maintain a list of state and local resources to assist older patients and families with Medicare D and cost issues.

References

1. Safran DG et al. Prescription drug coverage and seniors: findings from a 2003 national survey. *Health Aff (Millwood)*. 2005;Suppl Web Exclusives: W5-152–W5-166.
2. Col N, Fanale JE, Kronhold P. The role of medication noncompliance and adverse drug reactions in hospitalization of the elderly. *Arch Intern Med.* 1990;150:841–845.

3. Sokol MC, McGuigan KA, Verbrugge RR, Epstein RS. Impact of medication adherence on hospitalization risk and healthcare cost. *MedCare* 2005;43: 521–530.

4. Ganley JP, Roberts J, eds. *Eye conditions and related need for medical care among persons 1–74 years of age, United States, 1971–72.* Hyattsville, MD: US Department of Health and Human Services, Public Health Service, National Center for Health Statistics;1983:DHHS Publication No. 83-1678.

5. Caban AL et al. Prevalence of concurrent hearing and visual impairment in US adults: the national health interview survey, 1997–2002. *Am J Public Health.* 2005;95(11):1940–1942.

6. Dey A. Characteristics of older nursing home residents: data from the 1995 National Nursing Home Survey. Advance Data from Vital and Health Statistics No. 289. Hyattsville, MD: National Center for Health Statistics, 1997.

7. Howarth A et al. Ageing and the auditory system. *Postgrad Med J.* 2006;82:166–171.

8. Iezzoni LI, Davis RB, Soukup J, O'Day B. Satisfaction with quality and access to health care among people with disabling conditions. *Int J Qual Health Care.* 2002;14(5):369–381.

9. Klugar A, Gianutsos JG, Golomb J, Ferris SH, George AE et al. Patterns of motor impairment in normal aging, mild cognitive decline, and early Alzheimer's disease. *JG:PS.* 1997;52B:28–39.

10. Dunlop DD, Manheim LM, Song J, Chang RW. Arthritis prevalence and activity limitations in older adults. *Arthritis Rheum.* 2001;44(1):212–221.

11. Royall DR, Cordes J, Polk M. Executive control and the comprehension of medical information by elderly retirees. *Exp Aging Res.* 1997;23(4): 301–313.

12. Isaac LM, Tamblyn RM. Compliance and cognitive function: a methodological approach to measuring unintentional errors in medication compliance in the elderly. McGill-Calgary Drug Research Team. *Gerontologist.* 1993;33(6):772–781.

13. Boyd CM, Darer J, Boult C, et al. Clinical practice guidelines and quality of care for older patients with multiple comorbid diseases: implications for pay for performance. *JAMA.* 2005;294:716–724.

14. Rollason V, Vogt N. Reduction of polypharmacy in the elderly: a systematic review of the role of the pharmacist. *Drugs Aging.* 2003;20(11):817–832.

15. Montamat SC, Cusack B. Overcoming problems with polypharmacy and drug misuse. *Clin Geriatr Med* 1992;8:143–158.

16. Hanlon JT, Schmader KE, Ruby CM, Weinberger M. Suboptimal prescribing in older inpatients and outpatients. *J Am Geriatr Soc.* 2001 49:200–209.

17. Haajar ER, Cafiero AC, Hanlon JT. Polypharmacy in elderly patients. *Am J Geriatr Pharmacother.* 2007;5(4):345–551.

18. Stevens LA, Fares G, Fleming J, Martin D, Murthy K, Qiu J, Stark PC, Uhlig K, Van Lente F, Levey AS. Low rates of testing and diagnostic codes usage in a commercial clinical laboratory: evidence for lack of physician awareness of chronic kidney disease. *J Am Soc Nephrol.* 2005;16(8):2439–2448.

19. Hanlon JT, Pieper CF, Hajjar ER, Sloane RJ, Lindblad CI, Ruby CM, Schmader KE. Incidence and predictors of all and preventable adverse drug reactions in frail elderly persons after hospital stay. *J Gerontol A Biol Sci Med Sci.* 2006;61(5):511–515.

20. Brauner DJ, Muir JC, Sachs GA. Treating nondementia illnesses in patients with dementia. *JAMA.* 2000;283:3230–3235.

21. Forster AJ, Murff HJ, Peterson JF, Gandhi TK, Bates DW. The incidence and severity of adverse events affecting patients after discharge from the hospital. *Ann Intern Med.* 2003;138(3):161–167.

22. Institute of Medicine. *Health literacy: a prescription to end confusion.* Washington, DC: National Academy; 2004.

23. Gazmararian JA et al. Health literacy among Medicare enrollees in a managed care organization. *JAMA.* 1999;281(6):545–551.

24. Williams MV et al. Inadequate functional health literacy among patients at two public hospitals. *JAMA.* 1995;274(21):1677–1682.

25. Belcher VN et al. Views of older adults on patient participation in medication-related decision making. *J Gen Intern Med.* 2006;21(4):298–303.

26. Stemple C, Cammisa CR, Evans S, Fenter TC, Gonzalez J, Lee H, Lewis SJ, Noga M. Current issues and trends in medicare Part D. JMCP. 2008;14(6 Suppl):1–28.

27. Madden JM, Graves AJ, Zhang F, Adams AS, Briesacher BA, Ross-Degnan D, Gurwitz JH, Pierre-Jacques M, Safran DG, Adler GS, Soumerai SB. Cost-related medication nonadherence and spending on basic needs following implementation of Medicare Part D. *JAMA.* 2008;299(16):1922–1928.

28. Vik SA, Maxwell CJ, Hogan DB. Measurement, correlates, and health outcomes of medication adherence among seniors. *Ann Pharmacother.* 2004;38(2):303–312.

29. MacLaughlin EJ, Raehl CL, Treadway AK, Sterling TL, Zoller DP, Bond CA. Assessing medication adherence in the elderly: which tools to use in clinical practice? *Drugs Aging.* 2005;22(3):231–255.

30. Rudd P, Byyny RL, Zachary V, et al. The natural history of medication compliance in a drug trial: limitations of pill counts. *Clin Pharmacol Ther.* 1989;46:169–176.

31. Grymonpre RE, Didur CD, Montgomery PR, Sitar DS. Pill count, self report, and pharmacy claims data to measure medication adherence in the elderly. *Ann Pharmacother* 1998;32(7–8):749–754.

32. Farris KB, Phillips BB. Instruments assessing capacity to manage medications. *Ann Pharmacother.* 2008:242:1026–1036.

33. Edelberg HK, Shallenberger E, Wei JY. Medication management capacity in highly functioning community-living older adults: detection of early deficits. *J Am Geriatr Soc.* 1999;47(5):592–596.

34. Hutchison LC, Jones SK, West DS, Wei JY. Assessment of medication management by community-living elderly persons with two standardized assessment tools: a cross-sectional study. *Am J Geriatr Pharmacother.* 2006;4(2):144–153.

35. Ruppar TM, Conn VS, Russell CL. *Res Theor Nurs Pract.* 2008;114–147.

36. Holland R, Desborough J, Goodyer L, Hall S, Wright D, Loke Y K Does pharmacist-led medication review reduce hospital admissions and deaths in older people? A systematic review and meta-analysis. *Br J Clin Pharmacol.* 2008;65(3):303–316.
37. Hanlon JT, Lindblad CI, Gray SL. Can clinical pharmacy services have a Positive impact on drug-related problems and health outcomes in community-based older adults? *Am J Geriatr Pharmacother.* 2004;2:3–13.
38. Bronson DL, Costanza MC, Tufo HM. Using medical records for older patient education in ambulatory practice. *Med Care.* 1986;24(4):332–339.
39. Lee JK, Grace KA, Taylor AJ. Effect of a pharmacy care program on medication adherence and persistence, blood pressure, and low-density lipoprotein cholesterol: a randomized controlled trial. *JAMA.* 2006;296(21): 2563–2571.
40. Huang H, Maguire MG, Miller ER, Appel LJ. Impact of pill organizers and blister packs on adherence to pill taking in two vitamin supplementation trials. *Am J Epi.* 2000;152:780–787.
41. Elliott RA, Barber N, Clifford S, Horne R, Hartley E. The cost effectiveness of a telephone-based pharmacy advisory service to improve adherence to newly prescribed medicines. *Pharm World Sci.* 2008;30(1):17–23.
42. Clifford S, Barber N, Elliott R, Hartley E, Horne R. Patient-centered advice is effective in improving adherence to medicines. *Pharm World Sci.* 2006;28(3):165–170.
43. Medicare Part D Medication Therapy Management Programs Fact Sheet. http://www.cms.hhs.gov/PrescriptionDrugCovContra/Downloads/MTMFact Sheet.pdf. Accessed June 26; 2009.
44. Raehl CL, Bond CA, Woods T, Patry RA, Sleeper RB. Individualized drug use assessment in the elderly. *Pharmacotherapy.* 2002;22(10):1239–1248.
45. Sloan FA et al. Longitudinal analysis of the relationship between regular eye examinations and changes in visual and functional status. *JAGS.* 2005;53:1867–1874.
46. Cotrell V, Wild K, Bader, T. Medication management and adherence among cognitively impaired older adults. *J Gerontol Soc Work.* 2006;47(3–4):31–46.
47. Ownby RL, Hertzog C, Crocco E, Duara R. Factors related to medication adherence in memory disorder clinic patients. *Aging Ment Health.* 2006;10(4):378–385.
48. Brauner DJ, Muir JC, Sachs GA. Treating nondementia illnesses in patients with dementia. *JAMA.* 2000;283:3230–3235.
49. Chugh A, Williams MV, Grigsby J, Coleman EA. Better transitions: improving comprehension of discharge instructions. *Front Health Serv Manage.* 2009;25(3):11–32.
50. Vieder JN, Krafchick MA, Kovach AC, Galluzzi KE. Physician-patient interaction: what do elders want? *J Am Osteopath Assoc.* 2002;102(2):73–78.
51. http://www.qualityforum.org/pdf/reports/safe_practices/txspexecsummary public.pdf. Accessed December 9; 2008.
52. Denham C, Dingman J, Foley M, et al. Are you listening…are you really listening? *J Patient Safety.* 2008;4(3):148–161.

53. Aspinall S, Sevick MA, Donohue J, Maher R, Hanlon JT. Medication errors in older adults: a review of recent publications. *Am J Geriatr Pharmacother.* 2007;5(1):75–84.
54. Wenger NS, Young RT. Quality indicators for continuity and coordination of care in vulnerable elders. *J Am Geriatr Soc.* 2007;55:S285–S292.
55. Federman AD, Alexander GC, Shrank WH. A practical physicians' guide to the Medicare drug benefit plan. *Mayo Clin Proc.* 2006;81(9):1217–1221.

Index

Note: The letters 'f' and 't' following the locators refer to figures and tables respectively.

H. Bosworth (ed.), *Improving Patient Treatment Adherence*,
DOI 10.1007/978-1-4419-5866-2,
© Springer Science+Business Media, LLC 2010